...LIC HEALTH AND HEALTH PROMOTION PRACTICE

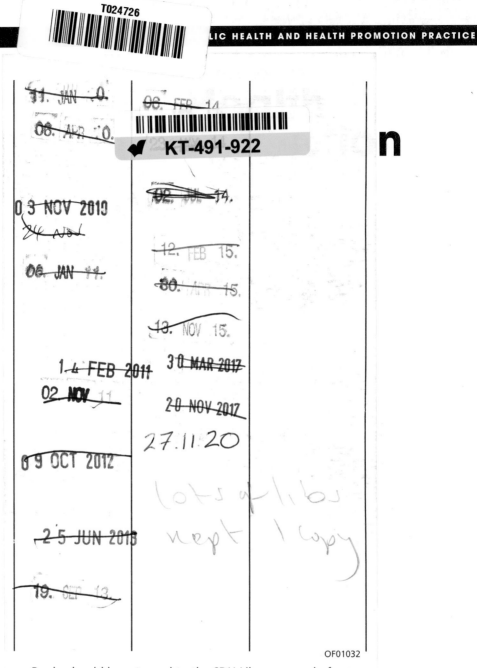

Books should be returned to the SDH Library on or before
the date stamped above unless a renewal has been arranged

Salisbury District Hospital Library

Telephone: Salisbury (01722) 336262 extn. 4434 / 33
Out of hours answer machine in operation

For Elsevier

Commissioning Editor: *Mairi McCubbin*
Development Editor: *Fiona Conn*
Project Manager: *Anne Dickie and Nayagi Athmanathan*
Designer/Design Direction: *Charles Gray*
Illustration Manager: *Gillian Richards*
Illustrator: *HL Studios*

PUBLIC HEALTH AND HEALTH PROMOTION PRACTICE

Foundations for
Health
Promotion

THIRD EDITION

Jennie Naidoo BSc MSc PGDip PGCE
Principal Lecturer, Health Promotion and Public Health,
University of the West of England, Bristol, UK

Jane Wills BA MA MSc PGCE
Professor of Health Promotion, London South Bank University, London, UK

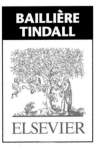

BAILLIÈRE
TINDALL

ELSEVIER

Edinburgh   London   New York   Oxford   Philadelphia   St Louis   Sydney   Toronto   2009

BAILLIÈRE
TINDALL
ELSEVIER

© Elsevier Limited 2000
© Elsevier Limited 2009. All rights reserved.

Second edition 2000
Third edition 2009

ISBN 978-0-7020-2965-3

British Library Cataloguing in Publication Data
A catalogue record for this book is available from the British Library

Library of Congress Cataloging in Publication Data
A catalog record for this book is available from the Library of Congress

Notice
Neither the Publisher nor the Authors assume any responsibility for any loss or
injury and/or damage to persons or property arising out of or related to any use of the
material contained in this book. It is the responsibility of the treating practitioner,
relying on independent expertise and knowledge of the patient, to determine the best
treatment and method of application for the patient.

The Publisher

Printed in China

Contents

PART 1: The theory of health promotion

Contents

Preface

Health promotion is a core aspect of the work of a wide range of health care workers and those engaged in education and social welfare. It is an emerging area of practice and study, still defining its boundaries and building its own theoretical base and principles. This book aims to provide a theoretical framework for health promotion which is vital to clarify practitioners' intentions and desired outcomes. It offers a foundation for practice which encourages practitioners to see the potential for health promotion in their work, to be aware of the implications of choosing from a range of strategies and to be able to evaluate their health promotion interventions in an appropriate and useful manner.

This third edition of *Health Promotion: Foundations for Practice* has been comprehensively updated and expanded to reflect recent research findings and major organizational and policy changes over the last decade. Our companion volume *Public Health and Health Promotion: Developing Practice* (Naidoo & Wills 2005) discusses in more detail some of the challenges and dilemmas raised in this book, e.g. partnership working, tackling inequalities and engaging the public.

The book is divided into four main parts. The first part provides a theoretical background, exploring the concepts of health, health education and health promotion. Part 1 concludes that health promotion is working towards positive health and well-being of individuals, groups and communities. Health promotion includes health education but also acknowledges the social, economic and environmental factors which determine health status. Ethical and political values inform practice and it is important for practitioners to reflect upon these values and their implications. The aim of the first part is to enable readers to understand and reflect upon these theoretical drivers of health promotion practice within the context of their own work.

The second part explores strategies to promote health and some of the dilemmas that they pose. Using the Ottawa Charter (World Health Organization 1986) framework to identify the range of strategies, the potential, benefits and challenges of adopting each strategy are discussed. Examples of interventions using the different strategies are presented.

The third part focuses on the provision of supportive environments for health, identified as a key strategy in the Ottawa Charter. Part 3 explores how a range of different settings in which health promotion interventions take place can be oriented towards positive health and well-being. The settings discussed in this part – schools, workplaces, neighbourhoods, health services and prisons – have all been targeted by national and international policies as key settings for health promotion. Reaching specific target groups such as young people, adults and older people within these settings is also covered in part 3.

Part 4 focuses on the implementation of health promotion interventions. Each chapter in this part discusses a different stage in the implementation process, from needs assessment through planning to the final stage of evaluation. This part is designed to help practitioners to reflect on their practice through examining what drives their choice of practical implementation strategies. A range of real-life examples helps to illustrate the options available and the criteria that inform the practitioner's choice of approach.

This book is suitable for a wide range of professional groups and this is reflected in the choice of examples and illustrative case studies. The text includes interactive exercises designed to encourage readers to reflect on their values, debate the issues and apply their knowledge and understanding to practice situations. Where appropriate, feedback has been given, but this is often not feasible because the issues are open-ended and contested. The aim is to encourage readers to consider these issues for themselves, and not have their views prescribed or limited.

The book is targeted at a range of students, including those in basic and post-basic training and qualified professionals. By combining an academic critique with a readable and accessible style, this book will inform, stimulate and encourage readers to engage in ongoing enquiry and reflection regarding their health promotion practice. The intention, as always, is to encourage readers to develop their health promotion practice through considering its foundation in theory, policy and clear principles.

Jennie Naidoo
Jane Wills
Bristol and London

References

Naidoo J, Wills J 2005 Public health and health promotion: developing practice, 2nd edn. Baillière Tindall, London.

World Health Organization 1986 Ottawa Charter for health promotion. WHO, Geneva.

Acknowledgements

It is 15 years since the publication of the first edition of this book, which was initially prompted by our teaching on the first postgraduate specialist courses in health promotion. Students and colleagues at the University of the West of England and London South Bank University have, as always, contributed to this edition through their ideas, debates and practice examples. We continue to be committed to the development of health promotion as a discipline.

We would like to thank Susie Sykes, who has been an invaluable critical reader offering comment, key links and examples and material on community development, and Nick de Viggiani, who contributed material for the new Chapter 17 on health promotion in prisons.

We dedicate this third edition to our children: Declan, Jessica, Kate and Alice.

How to use this book

The book is clearly structured and signposted for ease of reading and study. Each chapter starts with key points and an overview outlining the contents of the chapter. A summary and recommendations for further reading are included at the end of each chapter. There are also questions to encourage further discussion and debate either by the individual reader or by student groups.

A number of boxes appear throughout and these are identified by the following icons:

 Example, to illustrate the content or topic being discussed

 Activity, for the reader to undertake, linked to the text and with some feedback provided on possible responses

 Discussion point, for the reader to consider and debate – broader and more open-ended than the activities

The theory of health promotion	What are the key theoretical frameworks and principles for health promotion?	**Part 1**
Concepts of health	What informs my understanding of health and ill health? What informs the understanding of others (lay people and practitioners) regarding health and ill health?	Chapter 1
Influences on health	What social, cultural, economic and societal factors have an impact on the health of individuals and populations that I work with? How can I tackle inequalities in health in my role?	Chapter 2
Measuring health	Why do I need to be able to measure the health of people I work with? What methods of measuring, analysing and describing health can I use? How do these measurements relate to my concept of health? What other ways are there of measuring health and well-being?	Chapter 3
Defining health promotion	How can I define health promotion to others? What is unique about health promotion? What activities are entailed in promoting health? Is health promotion different from public health?	Chapter 4
Models and approaches to health promotion	What frameworks exist that seek to analyse health promotion approaches? What are the key differences between these different frameworks or models? What are the major different approaches towards health promotion?	Chapter 5
Ethical issues in health promotion	What are the major ethical schools and how do they differ from each other? What ethical issues are involved in promoting health? What are, and what should be, the ethical principles underpinning my professional practice? How can I resolve the dilemmas that arise from trying to use ethical principles when promoting health?	Chapter 6
The politics of health promotion	How do different political ideologies view health promotion? In what sense can health promotion be understood as a political activity? How can I interpret and assess the impact of policy at a local level?	Chapter 7
Strategies and methods	What are the key strategies used to promote and protect the health of the public? What knowledge, skills and competences are needed to use these strategies effectively?	**Part 2**
Reorienting health services	How can I ensure my practice is oriented towards prevention? How can I ensure my practice is holistic? Who are the relevant stakeholders that I need to engage with?	Chapter 8

Developing personal skills	What explains the decisions that people make in relation to their health? What personal skills do people need to take greater control over their health? How can I support and enable people to take greater control over their health? How can I address individual lifestyles and behaviours in a non-victim-blaming manner?	Chapter 9
Strengthening community action	How can I develop links with different local communities? How can I facilitate the involvement of different communities in assessing and articulating their own health and well-being needs? How can I enable communities and groups to address their needs and promote their health? How can I help communities to ensure that any developments they introduce are sustainable?	Chapter 10
Developing healthy public policy	How can I help to make healthy choices easier? What is my role in framing and implementing policy? How can I work with others to build healthy public policy?	Chapter 11
Using media in health promotion	How can I provide relevant and accessible information for my clients? What are the most effective means of communication? How can I use the mass media to promote health?	Chapter 12
Settings for health promotion	Opportunities for health promotion activity take place in many contexts, including schools, hospitals, the workplace, neighbourhoods and prisons. How can I embed a concern for positive health and well-being within settings that are designed for other purposes? How can I ensure that these settings promote the health of all those who use them?	**Part 3** Chapters 13–17
Implementing health promotion	What are the main stages in an integrated and systematic approach to health promotion project planning?	**Part 4**
Assessing health needs	What methods are there for conducting needs assessment? How can I ensure my practice is based on the needs of my clients?	Chapter 18
Planning health promotion interventions	How can I become organized and systematic in planning projects and interventions? What are the different stages in planning interventions? What aspects do I need to consider and address in planning?	Chapter 19
Evaluation in health promotion	Why is it important to evaluate my work? What aspects of my work should I evaluate? What criteria should I use to evaluate my work? What challenges are there in demonstrating the effectiveness of health promotion? How can I be evidence-informed in my practice?	Chapter 20

Part 1

The theory of health promotion

This part explores the concepts of health, health education and health promotion. Those who promote health need to be clear about their intentions and how they perceive the purpose of health promotion. Is it to encourage healthy lifestyles? Or is it to redress health inequalities and empower people to take control over their lives?

Chapter One

Concepts of health

OVERVIEW

Everyone engaged in the task of promoting health starts with a view of what health is. However, there is a wide variety of these views, or concepts, of health. It is important at the outset to be clear about the concepts of health which are personally adhered to, and to recognize where these differ from those of your colleagues and clients. Otherwise, you may find yourself drawn into conflicts about appropriate strategies and advice that are actually due to different ideas concerning the end goal of health. This chapter introduces different concepts of health and traces the origin of these views. The western scientific medical model of health is dominant but challenged by social and holistic models. Working your way through this chapter will enable you to clarify your own views on the definition of health and to locate these views in a conceptual framework.

Defining health, disease, illness and ill health

Health

Health is a broad concept which can embody a huge range of meanings, from the narrowly technical to the all-embracing moral or philosophical.

The word 'health' is derived from the Old English word for heal (*hael*) which means 'whole', signalling that health concerns the whole person and his or her integrity, soundness or well-being. There are 'common-sense' views of health which are passed through generations as part of a common cultural heritage. These are termed 'lay' concepts of health, and everyone acquires a knowledge of them through their socialization into society. Different societies or different groups within one society have different views on what constitutes their 'common sense' about health.

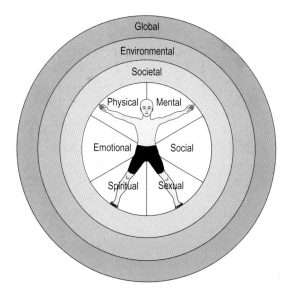

Figure 1.1 • Dimensions of health.

 Box 1.1

What are your answers to the following?
• I feel healthy when ...
• I am healthy because ...
• To stay healthy I need ...
• I become unhealthy when ...
• My health improves when ...
• (A person) affected my health by ...
• (An event) affected my health by ...
• (A situation) affected my health by ...
• ... is responsible for my health.

Health has two common meanings in everyday use, one negative and one positive. The negative definition of health is the absence of disease or illness. This is the meaning of health within the western scientific medical model, which is explored in greater detail later on in this chapter. The positive definition of health is a state of well-being, interpreted by the World Health Organization in its constitution as 'a state of complete physical, mental and social well-being, not merely the absence of disease or infirmity' (World Health Organization 1946).

Health is holistic and includes different dimensions, each of which needs to be considered. Holistic health means taking account of the separate influences and interaction of these dimensions. Figure 1.1 shows a diagrammatic representation of the dimensions of health.

The inner circle represents individual dimensions of health.
• Physical health concerns the body, e.g. fitness, not being ill.
• Mental health refers to a positive sense of purpose and an underlying belief in one's own worth, e.g. feeling good, feeling able to cope.
• Emotional health concerns the ability to feel, recognize and give a voice to feelings and to develop and sustain relationships, e.g. feeling loved.
• Social health concerns the sense of having support available from family and friends, e.g. having friends to talk to, being involved in activities with other people.
• Spiritual health is the recognition and ability to put into practice moral or religious principles or beliefs and the feeling of having a purpose in life.
• Sexual health is the acceptance and ability to achieve a satisfactory expression of one's sexuality.

The three outer circles are broader dimensions of health which affect the individual. Societal health refers to the link between health and the way a society is structured. This includes the basic infrastructure necessary for health (for example, shelter, peace, food, income), and the degree of integration or division within society. We shall see in Chapter 2 how the existence of patterned inequalities between groups of people harms health. Environmental health refers to the physical environment in which people live, and the importance of good-quality housing, transport, sanitation and pure water facilities and involves caring for the planet and ensuring its sustainability for the future.

Box 1.2

What are the implications of a holistic model of health for the professional practice of health workers?

Disease, illness and ill health

Disease, illness and ill health are often used interchangeably, although they have very different meanings. Disease derives from *desaise*, meaning uneasiness or discomfort. Nowadays, disease implies an objective state of ill health, which may be verified by accepted canons of proof. In our society, these accepted canons of proof are couched in the language of scientific medicine. For example, microscopic analysis may yield evidence of changes in cell structure, which may in turn lead to a diagnosis of cancer or disease. Disease is the existence of some pathology or abnormality of the body which is capable of detection. Disease can be due to exogenous (outside the body, e.g. viral infection) or endogenous (inside the body, e.g. inadequate thyroid function) factors. Health then is the normal functioning of the body as a biological entity.

Illness is the subjective experience of loss of health. This is couched in terms of symptoms, for example the reporting of aches or pains, or loss of function. One way that illness is given meaning is through the narratives we construct about how we fall sick. The process of making sense of illness is a task most sick people engage in to answer the question 'why me?' Illness and disease are not the same, although there is a large degree of coexistence. For example, someone may be diagnosed as having cancer through screening, even when there have been no reported symptoms. That is, a disease may be diagnosed in someone who has not reported any illness. When someone reports symptoms, and further investigations such as blood tests prove a disease process, the two concepts, disease and illness, coincide. In these instances, the term ill health is used. Ill health is therefore an umbrella term used to refer to the experience of disease plus illness. Health then is not being ill, the absence of symptoms.

Social scientists view health and disease as socially constructed entities. Health and disease are not states of objective reality waiting to be uncovered and investigated by scientific medicine. Rather, they are actively produced and negotiated by ordinary people. In Cornwell's (1984) study of London's Eastenders, they referred to three categories of health problems:

1. Normal illness, e.g. childhood infections

2. Real illness, e.g. cancer

3. Health problems, e.g. ageing, allergies.

Illness has often been conceptualized as deviance – as different from the norm and a source of stigma. Goffman (1968) identifies three sources of stigma:

1. Abominations of the body, e.g. psoriasis

2. Blemishes of character, e.g. human immunodeficiency virus (HIV)/acquired immunodeficiency syndrome (AIDS)

3. Tribal stigma of race, nation and religion.

The subjective experience of feeling ill is not always matched by an objective diagnosis of disease. When this happens, doctors and health workers may label such sufferers 'malingerers', denying the validity of subjective illness. This can have important consequences, for example a sick certificate may be withheld if a doctor is not convinced that someone's reported illness is genuine. The acceptance of a behaviour as an illness then becomes an issue of how to manage it. Several conditions, such as chronic fatigue syndrome and repetitive strain injury (RSI), have taken a long time to be recognized as illnesses.

Box 1.3

Homosexuals, formerly considered to be sinners, were labelled as ill – not bad but mad. Commitments to mental institutions, hormonal treatments, and castrations were used to deal with unwanted sexual behaviour.... treatments for homosexual men – such as aversion therapy – continued until, and beyond, 1973, when the American Psychiatric Association redesigned homosexuality as non-pathological (Hart & Wellings 2002).

Can you think of other examples of a condition or behaviour where its medicalization has led to its acceptance or otherwise?

It is also possible to experience no symptoms or signs of disease, but to be labelled sick as a result of examination or screening. Hypertension and precancerous changes to cell structures are two examples where screening may identify a disease even though the person concerned may feel perfectly healthy. Figure 1.2 gives a visual representation of these discrepancies. The central point is that subjective perceptions cannot be overruled, or invalidated, by scientific medicine.

The western scientific medical model of health

In modern western societies, and in many other societies as well, the dominant professional view of health adopted by most health care workers during their training and practice is labelled western scientific

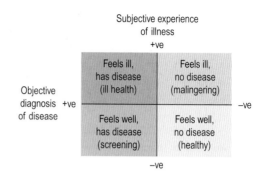

Figure 1.2 • The relationship between disease and illness.

medicine. Western scientific medicine operates within a medical model of explanation using a narrow view of health, which is often used to refer to no disease or no illness. In this sense, health is a negative term, defined more by what it is not than by what it is.

This view of health is extremely influential, as it underpins much of the training and ethos of a wide variety of health workers. These definitions become powerful because they are used in a variety of contexts, not just in professional circles. For example, the media often present this view of health, disease and illness in dramas set in hospitals or in documentaries about health issues. By these means, professional definitions become known and accepted in society at large.

The scientific medical model arose in western Europe at the time of the Enlightenment, with the rise of rationality and science as forms of knowledge. In earlier times, religion provided a way of knowing and understanding the world. The Enlightenment changed the old order, and substituted science for religion as the dominant means of knowledge and understanding. This was accompanied by a proliferation of equipment and techniques for studying the world. The invention of the microscope and telescope revealed whole worlds which had previously been invisible. Observation, calculation and classification became the means of increasing knowledge. Such knowledge was put to practical purposes, and applied science was one of the forces which accompanied the Industrial Revolution. In an atmosphere when everything was deemed knowable through the proper application of scientific method, the human body became a key object for the pursuit of scientific knowledge. What could be seen, and measured, and catalogued, was 'true' in an objective and universal sense.

This view of health is characterized as:

- *Biomedical* – health is assumed to be a property of biological beings.
- *Reductionist* – states of being such as health and disease may be reduced to smaller and smaller constitutive components of the biological body.
- *Mechanistic* – it conceptualizes the body as if it were a machine, in which all the parts are interconnected but capable of being separated and treated separately.
- *Allopathic* – it works by a system of opposites. If something is wrong with a body, treatment consists of applying an opposite force to correct the sickness, e.g. pharmacological drugs which combat the sickness.
- *Pathogenic* – it focuses on why people become ill.
- *Dualistic* – the mind and the body can be treated as separate entities.

Health is predominantly viewed as the absence of disease. This view sees health and disease as linked, as if on a continuum, so that the more disease a person has, the further away he or she is from health and 'normality'.

The pathogenic focus on finding the causes for ill health has led to an emphasis on risk factors. Antonovsky (1993) has called for a *salutogenic* approach which looks instead at why some people remain healthy. He identifies coping mechanisms which enable some people to remain healthy despite adverse circumstances, change and stress. An important factor for health, which Antonovsky labels a 'sense of coherence', involves the three aspects of understanding, managing and making sense of change. These are human abilities which are in turn nurtured or obstructed by the wider environment.

The medical model focuses on aetiology and the belief that disease originates from specific and identifiable causes. The causes of contemporary long-term chronic diseases in developed countries are often 'social'. Medicine and medical practice thus recognize that disease and the diseased body must be placed in a social context. Nevertheless the professional training of many health care workers provides an exaggerated view of the benefits of treatment and pays little attention to prevention. In part this is due to the dominant concern of the biomedical model with the organic appearance of disease and malfunction as the cause of ill-health.

Box 1.4

John is 19 and cannot go to the local college because he uses a wheelchair. He is given a place at a day centre because it is thought that this will suit his needs better.
- What view of disability is evident here?
- How does a medical model of health view disability?
- What factors of society may contribute to the individual and collective disadvantage of disabled people?

Table 1.1 contrasts the traditional views of a medical model with that of a social model of health.

A critique of the medical model

The role of medicine in determining health

The view that health is the absence of disease and illness, and that medical treatment can restore the body to good health, has been criticized. The distribution of health and ill health has been analysed from a historical and social science perspective. It has been argued that medicine is not as effective as is often claimed. The medical writer, Thomas McKeown, showed that most of the fatal diseases

Table 1.1 The medical and social model of health

Medical model	Social model
Health is the absence of disease	Health is a product of social, biological and environmental factors
Health services are geared towards treating the sick and disabled	Services emphasize all stages of prevention and treatment
High value is placed on specialist medical services	Less emphasis is placed on the role of specialists – there is more attention to self-help and community activity
Health workers diagnose and treat and sanction 'the sick role'	Health workers enable people to take greater control over their own health
The pathogenic focus emphasizes finding biological cause	A salutogenic focus emphasizes understanding why people are healthy

of the 19th century had disappeared before the arrival of antibiotics or immunization programmes. He concluded that social advances in general living conditions, such as improved sanitation and better nutrition made available by rising real wages, have been responsible for most of the reduction in mortality achieved during the last century. Although his thesis has been disputed, there is little disagreement that the contribution of medicine to reduced mortality has been minor, when compared with the major impact of improved environmental conditions.

Box 1.5

- What effects do medical advances in knowledge have on death rates?
- What other reasons could account for declining death rates?

The rise of the evidence-based practice movement (see Chapter 20) is attributed to Archie Cochrane (1972). His concern was that medical interventions were not trialled to demonstrate effectiveness prior to their widespread adoption. Rather, many procedures rest on habit, custom and tradition rather than rationality. Cochrane advocated greater use of the randomized controlled trial as a means to scientific knowledge and the key to progress.

The role of social factors in determining health

The modern UK is characterized by profound inequalities in income and wealth and these in turn are associated with persistent inequalities in health (Shaw et al 1999). The impact of scientific medicine on health is marginal when compared to major structural features such as the distribution of wealth, income, housing and employment. Tarlov (1996) has claimed that medical services contributed only 17% to the gain in life expectancy in the 20th century. As Chapter 2 will show, the distribution of health mirrors the distribution of material resources within society. In general, the more equal a society is in its distribution of resources, the more equal, and better, is the health status of its citizens (Wilkinson 1996).

Medicine as a means of social control

Social scientists argue that medicine is a social enterprise closely linked with the exercise of professional power (Stacey 1988). This derives from its role in legitimizing health and illness in society and the socially exclusive and autonomous nature of the profession. Medicine is a powerful means of social control, whereby the categories of disease, illness, madness and deviancy are used to maintain a status quo in society. Doctors who make the diagnosis are in a powerful position. The role of the patient during sickness as conceptualized by Parsons (1951) is illustrated in Table 1.2.

Table 1.2 The sick role

Rights	Responsibilities
Patient is relieved of normal responsibilities and tasks	Patient must want to recover as soon as possible and only then can he or she be seen as 'sick'
Patient is given sympathy and support	Patient must seek professional advice and comply with treatment
Patient has the right to a diagnosis, examination and treatment	

Increasingly, too, doctors are involved in decisions relating to the beginning and ending of life (terminations, assisted reproduction, neonatal care). The encroachment of medical decisions into these stages of life subverts human autonomy and gives to medicine an authority beyond its legitimate area of operation (Illich 1975).

The medical profession has long been regarded as an institution for securing occupational and social authority. Access to such power is controlled by professional associations that have their own vested interests to protect (Freidson 1986). The 1858 Medical Act established the General Medical Council which was authorized to regulate doctors, oversee medical education and keep a register of qualified practitioners. The Faculty of Public Health Medicine opened membership to non-medically qualified specialists in 2003, becoming the Faculty of Public Health.

Box 1.6

The following is a list of labels which are attached to people at certain stages of their life. Some are universal (everyone is born and dies); others only happen to some people at some stages of their lives. For each label identify:

- Who is responsible for attaching the label in a recognized or socially approved manner as part of his or her professional duties?
- Who is likely to receive the label?
- What are the likely consequences of being so labelled?
- Birth
- Death
- Illness requiring a prescription
- Illness requiring a sick certificate
- Long-term or chronic illness
- Being in need of continual care and attendance
- Being disabled
- Mental illness
- Mental illness requiring hospitalization
- Having a child on the at-risk register
- Having a learning difficulty
- Being convicted of a crime
- Terminal illness requiring hospice care.

Medicine as surveillance

Public health medicine has been concerned with the regulation and control of disease. Historically this may have included the containment of bodies, whether those infected with plague, tuberculosis or venereal disease. Mass screening programmes have given rise to what has been called medical surveillance. The wish to identify the 'abnormal' few with 'invisible' disease justifies monitoring the entire target population. Another critique of the pervasive power of medicine suggests the mapping of disease and identification of risk have subtly handed responsibility of health to individuals. This may invite new forms of control in the name of health, e.g. random drug testing or linking deservedness of surgery to lifestyle factors (Bunton et al 1995). The ability to identify risk also means there can be a moral discourse in which reducing one's risk factors are seen as a good thing, e.g. eating 'sensibly,' living 'well.'

Medicine as harm

According to Illich (1975), doctors and health workers contribute to ill health and create harm (iatrogenesis):

- Clinical iatrogenesis is ill health caused by medical intervention, for example side-effects caused by prescribed medicine, dependence on prescribed drugs and cross-infection in medical settings such as hospitals.
- Social iatrogenesis is the loss of coping and the right to self-care which have resulted from the medicalization of everyday life.
- Cultural iatrogenesis is the loss of the means whereby people cope with pain and suffering, which results from the unrealistic expectations generated by medicine.

Box 1.7

The Health Promotion Agency (HPA) for Northern Ireland launched a campaign to reduce antibiotic prescribing:
  'Against colds and flu, there's nothing antibiotics can do.'
  To what extent do you think society has become dependent on medicine? Is this true of developing countries?

Challenges to medicine

The dominance of medicine has been challenged in recent years by:

- Managerialism and challenges to clinical autonomy
- A rise in complementary therapies
- Consumerism and rise in the number of informed patients
- Social movements and advocacy
- Patient-centred care and shared decision-making.

These trends are related to wider forces that challenge the expertise of professionals. The response of most professions including medicine has been to introduce democratic decision-making, giving far more credence to lay knowledge. This has led to new concepts such as the 'expert patient'.

Box 1.8

What changes have you noticed in the practice of medicine and health care?

Lay concepts of health

For people concerned with the promotion of health, there is another problem with the dominance of scientific medicine. This is the focus within medicine on illness and disease, and the neglect of health as a positive concept in its own right. Many researchers have studied the general public's beliefs about health or lay concepts of health. The findings present an interesting picture, where there are continuities in definitions but also differences attributable to age, sex and class.

Blaxter (1990) identified five common concepts of health:

1. 'Health as not-ill' – health is the absence of symptoms or medical input widely used by all groups.
2. 'Health as physical fitness' – health as having energy and strength – mostly used by younger men.
3. 'Health as social relationships'– mostly used by women.
4. 'Health as function' – health is the ability to carry out tasks and activities – mostly used by older people of both sexes.
5. 'Health as psychosocial well-being' – less used by young men, most used by higher socioeconomic groups.

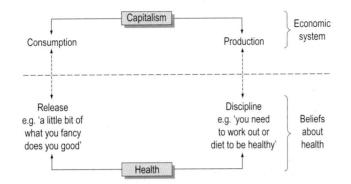

Figure 1.3 • Cultural views about health in capitalist society. Adapted from Crawford (1984).

The concepts of 'control' and 'release' are also commonly found in lay accounts – release is the taking of known risks (e.g. binge drinking) whereas control is the management of health. As illustrated in Figure 1.3 Crawford (2000) suggests that capitalism also requires individuals to be healthy consumers, having fun and seeking immediate gratification. Adherence to healthy lifestyles has to be offset by pleasure or release. In capitalist societies we are encouraged to be disciplined and controlled about pleasures such as alcohol. This is couched as being balanced and moderate.

Box 1.9

Is 'a little bit of what you fancy' healthy advice?

Researchers have found these issues of control and release in many accounts of health together with a moral view about taking risks. The following extract is from a study of lay men's views:

I eat healthy food generally and I cheat now and again. Alcohol is bad for you, but we all drink. Mostly everyone I know likes a drink 'cause its good for you, it actually cheers you up ... we've got like this throwaway society and I think

people's perceptions are changing, everybody wants everything yesterday ... and that's it, get fit one day, get drunk the next (Robertson 2006, p. 179).

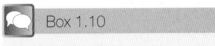

Box 1.10

Do men and women have different views on health?

There is often a difference between lay and professional concepts of health. The gap between the two has been identified by health workers as a problem, giving rise to concern. The concern centres around two issues: (1) the perceived lack of communication or poor communication between health worker and client; and (2) clients' lack of compliance with prescribed treatment regimes. However, there is also a cross-over between lay and professional beliefs about health. Health workers acquire their professional view of health during training. These beliefs overlie their original views of health adopted at an early age from family and society, so professionals are familiar with both. The general public is also aware of, and operates with, both sets of beliefs. In searching for meaning, lay patients frequently adopt professionals' explanations and interpretations about health and illness. So the two sets of beliefs, scientific medicine and lay public, are not discrete entities but overlap each other and exist in tandem.

Cornwell (1984) describes how people operate with both official and lay beliefs about health. Cornwell's study of London's Eastenders found that accounts of health were either public or private. Public accounts are couched in terms of scientific medicine and reflect these dominant beliefs. Health and illness are related to medical diagnosis and treatment, and medical terms and events are used to explain health status. These public accounts were offered first in Cornwell's interviews. What Cornwell terms private accounts reflect lay views of health, which typically use more holistic and social concepts to explain health and illness. For example, private accounts related health to general life experiences, such as employment, housing and perceived stress. Private accounts were offered in subsequent interviews, when a relationship had been established between Cornwell and the women she was interviewing. Cornwell suggests that people are therefore aware of both systems of beliefs and can use either when asked to talk about health. In encounters with strangers who are perceived as professionals, people use public accounts. However, in more informal settings, people use private accounts.

Box 1.11

People's explanations for their health and illness are complex. Why is it important for health promoters to understand the health beliefs of those with whom they work? How might they do this?

Box 1.12

How would your account of your health over the last month differ if you were talking to:
- Your doctor?
- Your friend?
- A member of your family?
- A researcher?

Cultural views of health

We are able to think about health using the language of scientific medicine because that is part of our cultural heritage. We do so as a matter of course, and think it is self-evident or common sense. However, other societies and cultures have their own common-sense ways of talking about health which are very different. Many cultures view disease as the outcome of malign human or supernatural agencies, and diagnosis is a matter of determining who has been offended. Treatment includes ceremonies to propitiate these spirits as an integral part of the process. Ways of thinking about health and disease reflect the basic preoccupations of society, and dominant views of society and the world. Anthropologists refer to this phenomenon as the cultural specificity of notions of health and disease.

Box 1.13

The Gnau of New Guinea refer to illness and other general misfortunes by the same word, *wala*. They also use the pidgin English *sik* to refer to bodily misfortunes. Sickness is a particular type of misfortune which is caused by evil beings or by magic and sorcery. People who are sick act in certain ways (shunning certain foods, eating alone) which oblige others to find out and treat the illness (Lewis 1986).

In any multicultural society such as the UK, a variety of cultural views coexist at any one time. For example, traditional Chinese medicine is based on the dichotomy of yin and yang, female and male, hot and cold, which is applied to symptoms, diet and treatments, such as acupuncture and Chinese herbal medicine. Complementary therapists offer therapies based on these cultural views of health and disease alongside (or increasingly within) the National Health Service, which is based on scientific medicine.

A unified view of health

Is there any unifying concept of health which can reconcile these different views and beliefs? Attempts at such a synthesis have come from philosophers such as Seedhouse (1986) and from organizations concerned with health, such as the World Health Organization.

> ## Box 1.14
>
> Figure 1.4 shows four theories of health:
> 1. Health as an ideal state
> 2. Health as mental and physical fitness
> 3. Health as a commodity
> 4. Health as a personal strength.
>
> What problems can you identify with each of these four views of health?

1. *Health as an ideal state* provides a holistic and positive definition of health. It is important in showing the interrelationship of different dimensions of health. A medical diagnosis of ill health does not necessarily coincide with a sense of personal illness or feeling unwell. Equally, a person free from disease may be isolated and lonely. However, it has been argued that this definition is too idealistic and vague to provide practical guidance for health promoters. Health in this sense is probably unattainable.

2. *Health as mental and physical fitness* is a perspective developed by Talcott Parsons (1951), a functional sociologist. It suggests that health is when people can fulfil the everyday tasks and roles expected of them. The functional view of health imposes social norms without regard to individual variation. It excludes people who, owing to a chronic illness or disability, are unable to fulfil normal social roles such as that of being an employee. Using a functional definition of health, a contented and coping person who has a disability is not counted as healthy.

3. *Health as a commodity* leads to unrealistic expectations of health as something which can be purchased. Health cannot be guaranteed by paying a higher price for health care. This view also tends to compartmentalize the total experience of health or ill health into different activities which can be costed. This is at odds with how people experience health and illness.

4. *Health as a personal strength* is a view which derives from humanistic psychology and suggests that an individual can become healthy through self-actualization and discovery (Maslow 1970). This approach encourages individuals to define their own health but it does not address the social environment which creates health and ill health.

Seedhouse suggests that these four views can be combined in a unified theory of health as the foundation for human achievement. Health is thus a means to an end rather than a fixed state to which a person should aspire.

> *[Health is] the extent to which an individual or group is able, on the one hand, to realize aspirations and satisfy needs; and, on the other hand, to change or cope with the environment. Health is, therefore, seen as a resource for everyday life, not an object of living; it is a positive concept emphasising social and personal resources, as well as physical capacities (World Health Organization 1984).*

Provided certain central conditions are met, people can be enabled to achieve their potential. The task of practitioners working for health is to create these conditions for people to achieve health:

- Basic needs of food, drink, shelter, warmth
- Access to information about the factors influencing health
- Skills and confidence to use that information.

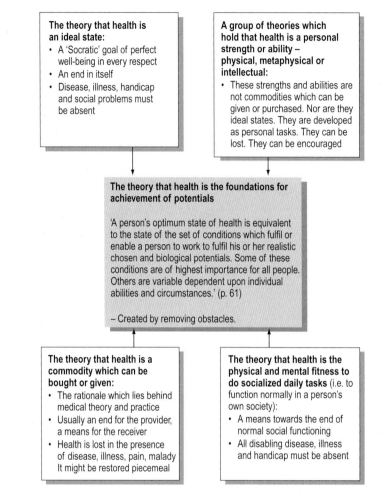

The theory that health is an ideal state:
- A 'Socratic' goal of perfect well-being in every respect
- An end in itself
- Disease, illness, handicap and social problems must be absent

A group of theories which hold that health is a personal strength or ability – physical, metaphysical or intellectual:
- These strengths and abilities are not commodities which can be given or purchased. Nor are they ideal states. They are developed as personal tasks. They can be lost. They can be encouraged

The theory that health is the foundations for achievement of potentials

'A person's optimum state of health is equivalent to the state of the set of conditions which fulfil or enable a person to work to fulfil his or her realistic chosen and biological potentials. Some of these conditions are of highest importance for all people. Others are variable dependent upon individual abilities and circumstances.' (p. 61)

– Created by removing obstacles.

The theory that health is a commodity which can be bought or given:
- The rationale which lies behind medical theory and practice
- Usually an end for the provider, a means for the receiver
- Health is lost in the presence of disease, illness, pain, malady It might be restored piecemeal

The theory that health is the physical and mental fitness to do socialized daily tasks (i.e. to function normally in a person's own society):
- A means towards the end of normal social functioning
- All disabling disease, illness and handicap must be absent

Figure 1.4 • A summary of theories of health. Adapted from Seedhouse (1986).

This definition acknowledges that people have different starting points which set limits for their potential for health. It encompasses a positive notion of health which is applicable to everyone, whatever their circumstances. However, it could be argued that this definition does not acknowledge the social construction of health sufficiently. People as individuals have little scope to determine optimum conditions for realizing their potential.

By health I mean the power to live a full, adult, living, breathing life in close contact with what I love ... I want to be all that I am capable of becoming (Mansfield 1977, p. 278).

The view of health as personal potential is attractive because it is so flexible, but this very flexibility causes problems. It leads to relativism (health may mean a thousand different things to a thousand different people), which makes it impracticable as a working definition for health promoters.

Health is regarded by the World Health Organization as a fundamental human right and there are certain prerequisites for health which include peace, adequate food and shelter and sustainable resource use.

Looking at health this way establishes it as a social as well as an individual product, and it emphasizes the dynamic and positive nature of health. Health is viewed as both a fundamental human right and a sound social investment. This view has been publicly affirmed by the Jakarta Declaration which linked health to social and economic development (World Health Organization 1997). This definition provides a variety of reasons for supporting health, which are likely to meet the concerns of a range of groups. It establishes a broad consensus for prioritizing health, and legitimizes a range of activities designed to promote health. For example, in addition to the more acceptable strategies of primary health care and personal skills development, the World Health Organization also identified in the Ottawa Charter the more radical strategies of community participation and healthy public policy as essential to the promotion of health (World Health Organization 1986). However, it could still be argued that such a broad definition makes it difficult to identify practical priorities for health promotion activities.

There is no agreement on what is meant by health. Health is used in many different contexts to refer to many different aspects of life. Given this complexity of meanings, it is unlikely that a unified concept of health which includes all its meanings will be formulated.

Conclusion

There are no rights and wrongs regarding concepts of health. Different people are likely to hold different views of health and may operate with several conflicting views simultaneously. Where people are located socially, in terms of social class, gender, ethnic origin and occupation, will affect their concept of health. The medical model has, however, dominated western thinking about health. Yet its value for health promotion is limited:

- It relies on a concept of normality that is not widely accepted.
- It ignores broader societal and environmental dimensions of health.
- It ignores people's subjective perceptions of their own health.
- The focus on pathology and malfunction leads to practitioners responding to ill health rather than being proactive in promoting health.

There is such a range of meaning attached to the notion of health that in any particular situation, it is important to find out what views are in operation. Clarifying what you understand about health, and what other people mean when they talk about health, is an essential first step for the health promoter.

Questions for further discussion

- How would you describe your own concept of health?
- What have been the most important influences on your views?

Summary

Definitions of health arise from many different perspectives. Whilst scientific medicine is the most powerful ideology in the west, it is not all-embracing. Social sciences' perspectives on health produce a powerful critique of scientific medicine, and point to the importance of social factors in the construction and meaning of health. Lay concepts of health derived from different cultures coexist alongside scientific medicine. Attempts to produce a unified concept of health appear to founder through overgeneralization and vagueness.

Further reading and resources

Barry A, Yuill C 2008 Understanding the sociology of health: an introduction, 2nd edn. Sage, London. *An accessible introduction to the sociology of health and illness exploring key concepts and the social structures that shape and pattern health.*

Lupton D 2003 Medicine as culture: illness, disease and the body in Western societies, 2nd edn. Sage, London.

An interesting account of the dependence on, and disillusionment with, medicine.

Naidoo J, Wills J 2008 Health studies: an introduction, 2nd edn. Palgrave Macmillan, Basingstoke. *An accessible introduction to different disciplinary perspectives on health including sociology, culture and anthropology and biology.*

References

Antonovsky A 1993 The sense of coherence as a determinant of health. In: Beattie A, Gott M, Jones L et al (eds) Health and wellbeing: a reader. Macmillan/Open University, Basingstoke, pp. 202–214.

Blaxter M 1990 Health and lifestyles. Tavistock/Routledge, London.

Bunton R, Nettleton S, Burrows R 1995 (eds) The sociology of health promotion: critical analyses of consumption, lifestyle and risk. Routledge, London.

Cochrane A L 1972 Effectiveness and efficiency. Nuffield Provincial Hospitals Trust, London.

Cornwell J 1984 Hard-earned lives. Tavistock, London.

Crawford R 2000 The ritual of health promotion. In: Williams S J, Gabe J, Calnan M (eds) Health, medicine and society: key theories, future agendas. Routledge, London, pp. 219–235.

Freidson F 1986 Professional powers: a study of the institutionalization of formal knowledge. University of Chicago Press, Chicago.

Goffman E 1968 Stigma: notes on the management of a spoiled identity. Penguin, Harmondsworth.

Hart G, Wellings K 2002 Sexual behaviour and its medicalisation: in sickness and in health. British Medical Journal 324: 896–900.

Illich I 1975 Medical nemesis, part 1. Calder and Boyers, London.

Lewis G 1986 Concepts of health and illness in a Sepik society. In: Currer C, Stacey M (eds) Concepts of health, illness and disease: a comparative perspective. Berg, Leamington Spa, pp. 119–135.

McKeown T, Lowe C R 1974 An introduction to social medicine. Blackwell Scientific Publications, Oxford.

Mansfield K 1977 In: Stead C K (ed) The letters and journals of Katherine Mansfield: a selection. Penguin, Harmondsworth.

Maslow A H 1970 Motivation and personality, 2nd edn. Harper and Row, New York.

Parsons T 1951 The social system. Free Press, Glencoe, IL, USA.

Robertson S 2006 Not living life in too much excess: Lay men understanding health and well-being. Health 10: 175–189.

Seedhouse D 1986 Health: foundations for achievement. John Wiley, Chichester.

Shaw M, Dorling D, Gordon D et al 1999 The widening gap: Health inequalities and policy in Britain. Policy Press, Bristol.

Stacey M 1988 The sociology of health and healing. Unwin Hyman, London.

Tarlov A R 1996 Social determinants of health: the sociobiological translation. In: Blane D, Brunner E, Wilkinson R (eds) Health and social organisation: towards a health policy for the 21st century. Routledge, London.

Wilkinson R G 1996 Unhealthy societies: the afflictions of inequality. Routledge, London.

World Health Organization 1946 Constitution. World Health Organization, Geneva.

World Health Organization 1984 Health promotion: a discussion document on the concept and principles. World Health Organization Regional Office for Europe, Copenhagen.

World Health Organization 1986 Ottawa charter for health promotion. Journal of Health Promotion 1: 1–4.

World Health Organization 1997 4th International conference on health promotion. New players for a new era – leading health promotion into the 21st century. World Health Organization, Jakarta.

2

Influences on health

Key points

- Factors influencing health
- Links between: social class and health; gender and health; and ethnicity and health
- Effects of income, housing and employment on health
- Social cohesion
- Explanations for health inequalities

OVERVIEW

Chapter 1 showed that there is a wide range of meanings attached to the concept of health, and different perspectives offered by the scientific medical model and social science. It emphasized the importance of social factors in the construction and meaning of health. This chapter shows how the major influences on mortality and morbidity are social and environmental factors. It summarizes recent research which suggests that there are inequalities in health status between groups of people which reflect structural inequalities in society such as social class, gender and ethnicity.

Determinants of health

Since the decline in infectious diseases in the 19th and early 20th centuries, the major causes of sickness and death are now circulatory disease, including coronary heart disease (CHD) and stroke (36%), cancers (27%) and respiratory disease (14%) (Office of National Statistics 2007a). In the UK increased longevity and the current life span of women to 81 years and men to 76 years account for the increase in degenerative diseases in the population as a whole. Despite the increase in life expectancy, epidemiologists who study the pattern of diseases in society have found that not all groups have the same opportunities to achieve good health and there are population patterns which make it possible to predict the likelihood that people from different groups will die prematurely.

In trying to determine what affects health, social scientists and epidemiologists will seek to compare at least two variables: firstly, a measure of health, or rather ill health, such as mortality or morbidity; and, secondly, a factor such as gender or occupation that could account for the differences in health. Of course, effects on health can be due to several variables interacting together. For example, research

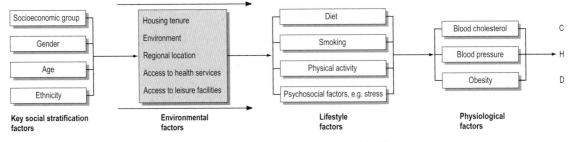

Figure 2.1 • Factors influencing the development of coronary heart disease (CHD).

into CHD has linked a large number of factors with the incidence of the disease: high levels of blood cholesterol, high blood pressure, obesity, cigarette smoking and low levels of physical activity. Other research indicates there may be links between CHD and psychosocial factors, such as stress and lack of social support, depression and anger (Stansfield & Marmot 2001). Many studies have also tried to establish whether there is a coronary-prone personality that is competitive, impatient and hostile (known as type A). We also know that mortality from CHD is higher among lower socioeconomic groups, among men rather than women, and among South Asians (Department of Health 2000). Figure 2.1 illustrates in a simple form how health status can be accounted for not by one variable, but by many factors interacting together. It shows that some factors have an independent effect on health or they may be mediated by other intervening variables. Whilst physical inactivity, smoking and raised blood cholesterol are the major risk factors for CHD (Britton & MacPherson 2000), it is important to look 'upstream' and understand the causes of these causes and their roots in the social context of people's lives.

What is clear is that ill health does not happen by chance or through bad luck. The Lalonde report, published in Canada in 1974, was influential in identifying four fields in which health could be promoted:

1. Genetic and biological factors which determine an individual's predisposition to disease

2. Lifestyle factors in which health behaviours such as smoking contribute to disease

3. Environmental factors such as housing or pollution

4. The extent and nature of health services.

Genetic factors remain largely unalterable and what limited scope there is for intervention lies in the medical field. Chapter 1 outlined McKeown & Lowe's work (1974) which showed that medical interventions in the form of vaccination had remarkably little impact on mortality rates. This suggests that factors other than the purely biological determine health and well-being and that probably the greatest opportunities to improve health lie in the environment and individual lifestyles.

 Box 2.1

Lifestyles are frequently the focus of health promotion interventions. Figure 2.2 shows a whole range of factors that may influence smoking behaviour. Take another of the factors implicated in coronary heart disease such as nutrition and identify the influences on that health behaviour.

Dahlgren & Whitehead (1991) thus talk of 'layers of influence on health' that can be modified (Figure 2.2):

• Personal behaviour and lifestyles and the knowledge, awareness and skills that can enable change in relation to, for example, diet or activity

• Support and influence within communities which can sustain or damage health

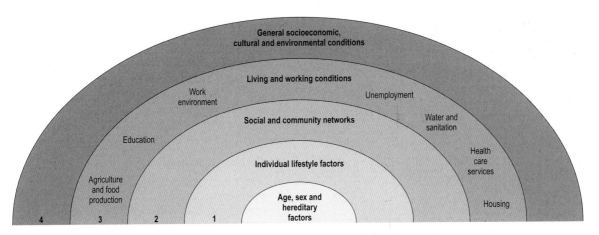

Figure 2.2 • The main determinants of health. From Dahlgren & Whitehead (1991).

- Living and working conditions and access to facilities and services
- Economic, cultural and environmental conditions such as standards of living or the labour market.

In all societies, health behaviours and physical and mental health vary between social groups. The main axes of variation include socioeconomic status, gender, ethnicity and place of residence. The specific features and pathways by which societal conditions affect health are termed the social determinants.

Social class and health

Most research which has sought to identify the major determinants of health and ill health has focused on the links between social class and health. A report was published of a Department of Health and Social Security working group on inequalities in health (Townsend & Davidson 1982). The report, which is known as the Black report, after the group's chairman, Sir Douglas Black, provided a detailed study of the relationship between mortality and morbidity, and social class.

The terms social class, social disadvantage, socio-economic status and occupation are often used interchangeably. The classification of social class derived from the Registrar General's scale of five occupational classes ranging from professionals in class I to unskilled manual workers in class V. This was largely unchanged from 1921 (class III was divided into manual and non-manual work in 1971). From 2001 the National Statistics Socio-Economic Classification (NS-SEC) has been used for all official statistics and surveys (Table 2.1).

Although social class classification is not a perfect tool, it does serve as an indicator of the way of life and living standards experienced by different groups. It correlates with other aspects of social position such as income, housing, education and working and living environments.

The Black report and a later report commissioned by the Health Education Authority, *The Health Divide* (Whitehead 1988), found significant differences in death rates between socioeconomic classes. More recent reports (Acheson 1998) draw together data which show that, far from ill health being a matter of bad luck, health and disease are socially patterned with the more affluent members of society living longer and enjoying better health than disadvantaged social groups. Although the health of the population has steadily improved, there is still a strong relationship between socioeconomic group and health status. This is evident in life expectancy, infant mortality, causes of death, prematurity and long-standing illness.

Table 2.1 Social class classification

1.	Higher managerial and professional
1.1	e.g. company directors, bank managers, senior civil servants
1.2	e.g. doctors, barristers and solicitors, teachers, social workers
2	Lower managerial and professional
	e.g. nurses, actors and musicians, police, soldiers
3	Intermediate
	e.g. secretaries, clerks
4	Small employers and own-account workers
	e.g. publicans, playgroup leaders, farmers, taxi drivers
5	Lower supervisory, craft and related occupations
	e.g. printers, plumbers, butchers, train drivers
6	Semi-routine occupations
	e.g. shop assistants, traffic wardens, hairdressers
7	Routine occupations
	e.g. waiters, road sweepers, cleaners, couriers
8	Never worked and long-term unemployed

Box 2.2

The extent and nature of health inequalities

Life expectancy

- A man in the professional group is likely to live around 7 years longer than a man in the unskilled or manual group.

Infant mortality

- Children from manual backgrounds are twice as likely to die before the age of 15 as a child born into a non-manual background.
- For babies registered by both parents infant mortality is highest for babies with fathers in semiskilled and unskilled groups.

Causes of death

- Of the 66 major causes of death in men, 62 were more common among manual groups than in other social classes.
- Lower social groups are 5.5 times more likely to die from respiratory diseases than higher social groups (Office of National Statistics 2001).

Self-reported ill health

- Nearly four times as many long-term unemployed or those who have never worked rate their health as poor compared to professional groups or managers
- Long-term illness is five times higher among this group than those in professional or managerial groups.

Figure 2.3 shows that there are substantial differences in life expectancy according to social class. Although infant deaths are declining, children from manual backgrounds are more likely to die in the first year of life or from accidental injury. Low birth weight is probably the most important predictor of death in the first month of life and this is clearly class-related, with two-thirds of babies under 2500 g born to mothers in social class V (Office of National Statistics 2007b). Although it is common to talk of 'diseases of affluence' such as CHD being the major killers in contemporary Britain, most disease categories are more common among lower socioeconomic groups. Particularly large differentials have developed for respiratory disease, lung cancer, accidents and suicide. An exception to this is death rates from breast cancer, which is evenly distributed across social groups. People from lower socioeconomic groups also experience more sickness and ill health. Measures of mental health and well-being also reflect a social gradient (Bromley et al 2005). This pattern of class and health gradient is thus visible in many ways including death rates, cause of death and reports of ill health.

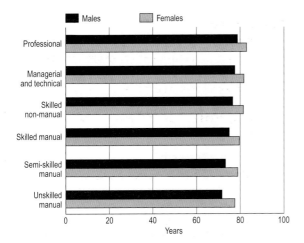

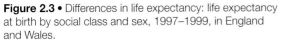

Figure 2.3 • Differences in life expectancy: life expectancy at birth by social class and sex, 1997–1999, in England and Wales.
Source: National Statistics website: www.statistics. gov.uk. Crown copyright material is reproduced with the permission of the Controller Office of Public Sector Information (OPSI).

In our companion book *Public Health and Health Promotion: Developing Practice* (Naidoo & Wills 2005) we discuss the determinants developing practice of health in more detail.

The most immediate causes of socioeconomic inequalities in health have been summarized by Macintyre (2007) as:

- Exposures, e.g. damp housing, hazardous work, adverse life events
- Behaviours, e.g. smoking, diet, exercise
- Personal strengths and capabilities (see Chapter 1).

The pathways by which members of different socioeconomic status groups are at risk of such exposures and vulnerabilities are often due to political and economic forces and social stratifications in society. Some of these pathways are discussed in the next section.

Income and health

In the UK better health is strongly associated with income. It is estimated that in the UK 10 million live in poverty, defined as having incomes below half the national average after allowing for housing costs (Department of Work and Pensions 2005). Those most likely to be in this category are the unemployed, pensioners, lone parents, families with three or more children and the low-paid.

Poverty can affect health directly by, for example, children not having enough to eat, eating a high-processed diet and limited access to food outlets. Across the UK dietary initiatives such as breakfast clubs, cookery clubs and community cafés promote healthy eating in low-income communities (for an example, see www.communityfoodandhealth.org.uk).

In low-income countries, infectious diseases such as diarrhoeal illness and malaria are associated with lack of income resulting in lack of access to clean water, food and medical services. Disease then further impoverishes the poor, preventing people from working and incurring high medical costs.

Housing and health

Frank Dobson, briefly Minister for Health in 1997, remarked: 'everyone with a grain of sense knows that it's bad for your health if you don't have anywhere to live'. The issues of housing stock, dampness, inadequate heating and energy efficiency are recognized as key determinants of health (Department of Health 1999 paras. 4.28–4.31).

For example, there are 40 000 excess winter deaths (deaths which would not be expected if the average death rate for the rest of the year applied in winter) each year in the UK. These are attributable to:

- Energy efficiency
- Level of occupancy
- Income
- Cost of fuel.

Cold and damp housing have been shown to contribute to illness. Children living in damp houses are likely to have higher rates of respiratory illness, symptoms of infection and stress (Marsh et al 1999). These will be exacerbated by overcrowding.

The high accident rates to children in social class V are associated with high-density housing where there is a lack of play space and opportunities for parental supervision. Psychological and practical difficulties accompany living in high-rise flats and isolated housing estates, which may adversely affect the health of women at home or older people.

Box 2.3

Linda visits her GP with Alex, aged 4, who has a chronic wheeze. Linda has two other children under 7 whom she is bringing up alone on a high-rise estate which is due for demolition in the next 5 years. The flats are damp with condensation running down the walls. There has been a recent infestation of cockroaches. Linda last visited her GP 6 weeks ago for her own bronchitis. The GP told her to stop smoking.
- What would you expect the GP to advise regarding Alex's health?
- How effective do you think this advice would be?

Employment and Health

Work is important to consider as a social determinant of health:
- It determines income levels.
- It affects self-esteem.
- The type of employment may itself directly affect health.

The traditional focus of occupational health has been to consider how particular types of employment carry high occupational health risks. This may be because of the risk of accidents (for example, in mining), exposure to hazardous substances or because of stress. Some occupations encourage lifestyles which may be damaging to health. Publicans, for example, are at high risk of developing cirrhosis.

Box 2.4

Consider how the following differences between manual and non-manual occupations can influence health:
- Pay
- Hours of work
- Occupational pension and sickness scheme
- Holiday entitlements
- Accidents at work
- Exposure to toxic substances and environmental hazards
- Job security
- Occupational mobility
- Prestige and status
- Autonomy.

There has been considerable interest in how the psychosocial environment of work can affect health (Marmot et al 2006). Most research has identified high demands and low control over work decisions as contributing to job stress and cardiovascular risk. These factors together with the amount of social support people get at work have been confirmed in workplace studies in many developed countries (see Chapter 14 for further discussion). There is also a considerable body of evidence, mostly gathered in the 1980s, that unemployment can damage health (McLean et al 2005). It is however uncertain whether unemployment itself can lead to a deterioration in health or whether it is the poverty associated with unemployment which contributes to the poor health of the unemployed.

Box 2.5

Consider the following evidence concerning the effects of unemployment on health. What could account for this relationship?
1. The unemployed report higher rates of mental ill health, including depression, anxiety and sleep disturbance.

2. Suicide and parasuicide rates are twice as high among the unemployed as among the employed.
3. The death rates among the unemployed are at least 20% higher than expected after adjustment for social class and age.
4. The unemployed have higher rates of bronchitis and ischaemic heart disease than the employed.
5. Over 60% of unemployed people smoke compared to 30% of employed people.

It seems that unemployment has a profound effect on mental health, damaging a person's self-esteem and social structure. Part of its effect on health must also arise from the material disadvantage of living on a low income and social isolation (McLean et al 2005).

Gender and health

Gender refers to the social categorization of people as men or women, and the social meaning and beliefs about sexual difference.

Box 2.6

What could account for the following evidence of gender differences in health?
- Women live on average 6 years longer than men, yet females report higher levels of ill health at all ages.
- 26% of those attending structured weight loss programmes at local surgeries are men, although 67% of men compared to 57% of women are overweight.
- Men are twice as likely as women to die from all the cancers affecting both sexes.
- Under the age of 45 men visit their GP only half as often as women (www.menshealthforum.org.uk).

Some of the sex differences in morbidity have been attributed as an artefact of measurement of the use of health services. Women are more likely to report illness as they are less likely to be in full-time employment and have easier access to primary care or because they are more inclined to take care of their health, resulting in increased consultation rates. However, this does not explain the sex difference in mortality. Nor is there a consistent tendency for women's greater willingness to consult: women are no more likely than men to visit their GP for musculoskeletal, respiratory or digestive problems.

The biological explanation suggests that women are more resistant to infection and benefit from a protective effect of oestrogen, accounting for their lower mortality rates. Paradoxically, female hormones and the female reproductive system are claimed to render women more liable to physical and mental ill health. Biological explanations are unable to account for the social class difference in women's health whereby women in professional and managerial social classes experience better health than women in lower socioeconomic groups. It is also important to note that greater female longevity only arose in the 20th century and is mostly attributable to the dramatic decline in infectious disease mortality and a decline in the number of births. It is also not evident in low-income countries.

Lifestyle explanations argue that women are socialized to be passive, dependent and sick. Women readily adopt the sick role because it fits with preconceived notions of feminine behaviour. Men, by contrast, are encouraged to be aggressive and risk-taking both at work and in their leisure time. The higher rates for accidents and alcoholism amongst men are cited as evidence for this.

Recent research is much more nuanced about gender, finding men and women in 'masculine' or 'feminine' roles and thus provides fewer easy answers to account for gender differences in health (Annandale & Hunt 2000).

Box 2.7

Many explanations have been offered to account for women's ill health. With which of the following do you most agree?

1. Women consult their GPs more frequently than men and so will appear to have greater morbidity.
2. Women acknowledge their feelings of illness.
3. In the same situation, a man would be told to get on with things. A woman is labelled as ill.
4. Many women are workers inside and outside the home and have care responsibilities.
5. Much of women's ill health is due to depression from their social isolation at home.
6. Much of women's ill health relates to their reproductive organs.
7. The patriarchal control of medicine has deprived women of control over natural processes such as child-bearing and child-rearing, producing more problems.
8. Women have less access to material resources than men.

Finally, it has been argued that women's social position as both carers and workers inside and increasingly outside the home is a dual burden which leads to increased stress and ill health. Some 42% of the employed workforce is female and yet women receive on average two-thirds of the male wage for equal work. Most women work part-time with less security and benefits than full-time workers, and working conditions at home and in the workplace may be hazardous, especially for poorer women in social classes IV and V (Doyal 1995). Employment outside the home does have a protective benefit for some women but this seems to be dependent on material circumstances (Arber 1990).

Health of ethnic minorities

Race is a biological marker of difference and is widely used to describe populations, e.g. 'Asian' or 'Chinese'.

Actually there is little variation in the genetic composition of different groups.

Ethnicity is a complex concept that is used to refer to those with a shared culture, social background, language or religion.

The Fourth National Survey of Ethnic Minorities in England and Wales (Nazroo 1997) notes:

- Two-fifths of Caribbean, Pakistanis and Bangladeshis have poor general health.
- Pakistanis and Bangladeshis have a greater risk of heart disease than whites.
- One in 18 people from an ethnic-minority group is diagnosed as diabetic.
- 50% of Bangladeshi men smoke.

Figure 2.4 shows the distribution of self-reported ill health amongst Black and minority ethnic groups. That particular diseases, poor perceived health or

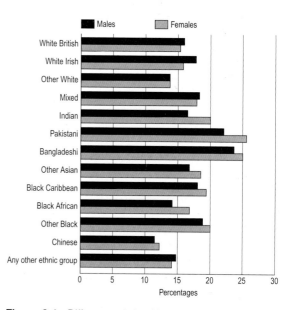

Figure 2.4 • Differences in health between ethnic groups: age-standardized long-term illness by ethnic group and sex, 1997–1999, in England and Wales.
Source: National Statistics website: www.statistics.gov.uk. Crown copyright material is reproduced with the permission of the Controller Office of Public Sector Information (OPSI).

premature death is commoner in these population groups is a complex issue. In the past explanations tended to focus on simple differences in culture.

Box 2.8

Why is coronary heart disease so common in South Asians?

In the UK the highest record rates of CHD mortality are in people born in the Indian subcontinent countries of India, Pakistan and Bangladesh (South Asians). Several factors are implicated:

- High prevalence of risk factors e.g. diabetes, low high-density lipoprotein cholesterol. But smoking, though high in Bangladeshi men, is low amongst Indian and Pakistani men.
- Greater susceptibility, e.g. unidentified genetic differences. Migration has been shown to cause rapid rises in serum cholesterol.
- Specific risk factors, e.g. lifestyle, including use of ghee and cooking oils, stress from racism, insulin resistance (British Heart Foundation 2000).

The factors influencing ethnic health inequalities have been summarized by Bhopal (2007) as:

- Culture, e.g. taboos on alcohol
- Social education and economic status, e.g. knowledge of biology and health influences, languages spoken and read
- Environmental, before and after migration
- Lifestyle, e.g. behaviours in relation to diet, alcohol and tobacco
- Accessing and concordance with health care advice, willingness to seek health and social services, use of complementary/alternative methods of care or treatment
- Genetic and biological factors, e.g. birth weight, body composition.

Socioeconomic factors have profound impact but it is important not to put all members of ethnic minorities into one disadvantaged category. More data would enable us to find out how many people from ethnic-minority groups are disadvantaged, and how. It would also then be possible to determine whether the poor health of black and ethnic-minority groups is associated with the low income, poor working conditions or unemployment, and poor housing shared by those in lower social classes, or whether there is, in addition, ill health resulting from other factors. Racism in service delivery, either directly or through the ethnocentrism of services which are based on the needs of the majority, is often invoked as the explanation for inequalities.

Box 2.9

- Why might ethnic minority patients get worse care?
- What kinds of racism have you seen?

Place and health

In the 1980s mortality rates were shown to increase steadily in the UK, moving from the south-east to the north-west, with a north–south divide present for most diseases. This seemed to be associated with poverty and disadvantage. Glasgow Shettleston, for example, has twice the average mortality rate. More recent studies have shown that there are variations within cities and regions (Dorling et al 2000). One obvious explanation for the geographic differences in death rates might be differences in social class distribution, those areas with high mortality rates being those areas with a greater proportion of people in lower socioeconomic groups. Increasingly, the effect of place on health has been seen as more complex, including not only the socioeconomic characteristics of individuals concentrated in particular places but also the local physical and social environment and the shared norms and traditions that might promote or inhibit health.

Explaining health inequalities

Inequality means a lack of uniformity, or difference. In this chapter we have noted differences in health outcomes according to gender and ethnicity. In the context of health and health care, the term inequalities is mainly used to refer to differences that arise from socioeconomic factors including income, work, housing or location of residence. Our companion volume *Public Health and Health Promotion: Developing Practice* (Naidoo & Wills 2005) explores these social determinants of health in more detail.

 Box 2.10

What explanation would you offer for the inequalities in health between social classes?

You may believe that people in the lower social classes choose more unhealthy ways of living, or you may believe that they have low incomes which prevent them adopting a healthy lifestyle and cause them to live in unhealthy conditions. There is a continuing debate over this question and no simple answer. Explanations suggested by the Black report of 1980 were of four broad types: artefact, social selection, cultural/behavioural and materialist/structural. More recently, attention has focused on psychosocial explanations and the 'life course' explanation that suggests that adverse environmental conditions at different points can lead to ill health.

Health inequalities as an artefact

The artefact explanation argues that the widening gap in mortality figures between the social classes is not real, but an effect of the way in which class and health are measured. Because there have been changes in the classification of occupations and in the structure of social classes, it is impossible to make comparisons over time. For example, the assignment of occupations to social classes has changed over several decades, as has the relative size of the classes. Using the old social classification, there is a much smaller proportion of the population in class V and comparisons between class I and class V over 30–50 years are not comparing similar-sized segments of the population. There may have been changes in the relative status of the classes also. The smaller class I before 1945 may be very different from the expanded class I in the 1980s when the Black report was published. It is also argued that the mortality rates of lower socioeconomic groups are skewed because, as social mobility continues, this class contains a greater proportion of older people at risk from dying.

Establishing a relationship between social class and health, particularly over time, is difficult. However, a considerable amount of research supports the view that the relationship is a real phenomenon and not merely an artefact of the data. When other indicators of disadvantage are used, such as housing, access to a car, education, household possessions and income, they all show a similar pattern of health inequalities between the top and bottom of the social scale.

Health inequalities as a selection process

Social selection theory argues that the relationship between class and health is a causal one, but that it is health which determines people's class, and not vice versa. The healthy experience upward social mobility and mortality rates are kept low in the upper classes. People with higher levels of illness drift down the social scale and thus inflate the rates of death and disability among lower social groups. There is some evidence that health can affect social status. A study of women in Aberdeen found that those who were taller tended to marry into a higher social class. As height may be taken as an indicator of health, this evidence suggests some sort of health selection taking place at marriage (Illsley 1986). Chronic illness can also account for downward social mobility. Manual workers with failing health are often moved into other jobs because of sickness and are more likely to have difficulty finding new work.

The argument suggests that health is a static property rather than a shifting state of being which is influenced by social and economic circumstance. Thus some people, because of their genetic health potential, are able to overcome disadvantage and 'climb out of poverty'. Although this may be true for some people, the extent of social mobility is not sufficient to account for the overall scale of social class differences in health (Wilkinson 1986).

Health inequalities as a result of lifestyles

This argument suggests that the social distribution of ill health is linked with differences in risk behaviours. These behaviours – smoking, high alcohol consumption, lack of exercise, high-fat and high-sugar diets – are more common among lower socioeconomic groups.

For example, although smoking has decreased in all social classes over the last 20 years, there are still major differences in the proportion of smokers in classes I–V, as shown in Figure 2.5.

Behaviour cannot, however, be separated from the social context in which it takes place. Graham (1992), in many studies on smoking, has shown how the decision to smoke by many working-class women

is a coping strategy to deal with the stress associated with poverty and isolation. The decision to smoke *is* a choice but it is not taken through recklessness or ignorance; it is rather a choice between 'health evils' – stress versus smoking.

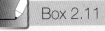

Box 2.11

Smoking is the biggest single cause of the differences in death rates between rich and poor people. Which of the following comes closest to your own view?

'Poor people bring ill health upon themselves. They don't care about their health. If they are so poor how can they afford to smoke and drink and eat junk food?'

'People's use of tobacco and alcohol is to a large extent determined by their social relations and networks, which in turn affects their self-esteem and levels of stress. Tobacco offers a prop of sorts.'

Some writers claim that there are cultural differences between social groups in their attitudes towards health and protecting their health for the future. Thus giving up cigarettes, as a form of deferred gratification, is more likely to appeal to middle-class people who, as we saw in Chapter 1, may have a stronger locus of control and may believe that they determine the course of their life. Working-class people who may have to struggle to get by each day do not make long-term plans and have a fatalistic view of health, believing it to be a matter of luck. Thus attitudes are passed on from generation to generation. This phenomenon is referred to as the 'culture of poverty' or 'cycle of deprivation'. According to such views, ill health can be explained in terms of the characteristics of poor people themselves and their inadequacy and incompetence. In 1986, Edwina Currie, a newly appointed health minister, caused a storm of controversy by suggesting that the high levels of premature death, permanent sickness and low birth weights in the northern regions were due to ignorance and people failing to realize that they had some control over their lives.

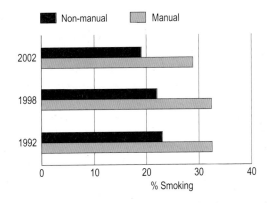

Figure 2.5 • Prevalence of cigarette smoking by sex and socioeconomic group, England, 1992, 1998 and 2002.

A behavioural explanation which sees lifestyles and cultural influences determining health has considerable appeal to any government that is concerned to reduce public expenditure. If individuals are seen as responsible for their own health, government inactivity is legitimized. Such viewpoints, which are particularly associated with neoliberal governments (see Chapter 7) have been widely criticized as victim-blaming, in that people are seen as being responsible for factors which disadvantage them but over which they have no control.

Health inequalities as a consequence of the life course

This explanation for health inequalities suggests that early life circumstances predict future morbidity and mortality rates. Parental income and education determine housing conditions, food quality and employment and thus the future socioeconomic position of the child.

There is some evidence that intrauterine conditions affect birth outcomes and low birth weight has been shown to be associated with health outcomes many years later in respect of CHD, stroke and respiratory disease.

Box 2.12

Chart your own life course in relation to health.
- Are there any external factors which influenced you and your family's health?
- Were there any personal events which affected your physical and psychological well-being?

Health inequalities as a consequence of psychosocial factors

There is a growing body of evidence demonstrating that it is *relative* inequalities in income and material

resources, coupled with the resulting social exclusion and marginalization, which are linked to poor health (Blane et al 1996; Wilkinson 1996). The key evidence on this comes from international data on income distribution and national mortality rates. In high-income countries it is not the richest countries which have the best health but the most egalitarian, such as Sweden. Whilst the exact mechanisms linking social inequality to ill health are uncertain, it is likely that relative inequality in relation to others can provoke distrust and stress, resulting in increased risk of disease (Wilkinson 1996; Wilkinson and Marmot 2003). Healthy, egalitarian societies are more socially cohesive and have a stronger community life with greater social capital.

Box 2.13

The quality of the social life of a society is one of the most powerful determinants of health (and this, in turn, is very closely related to the degree of income equality) (Wilkinson 1996, p. 5).

Which of the following, in your view, reflects the characteristics of life of a healthy society?
- High level of civic activities
- High gross national product
- Low crime rates
- High percentage of adults receiving a university education
- Availability and accessibility of information exchange mechanisms
- High levels of employment
- Narrow differences in income
- Sense of social solidarity and cohesion.

The degree to which an individual is integrated into society and has a social support network has been shown to have a significant impact on health. Research has shown that those with few friends or family are more likely to die early and less likely to survive a heart attack. Social exclusion is a term now widely used to describe those unable, usually because of low income, to participate in everyday social activities.

Box 2.14

Which groups in society do you regard as 'socially excluded'?

Box 2.15

Health is an important dimension of social exclusion which involves not only social but also economic and psychological isolation. Although people may know what affects their health, they can find it difficult to act on what they know, setting up a downward spiral of deprivation and poor health (Department of Health 1999, p. 44).

The negative emotional experience that arises from living in an unequal society is illustrated in the Whitehall II study (Marmot 2006), a longitudinal study of civil servants and their experience of ill health. Irrespective of health behaviour, those in control of their working lives (those in higher grades) are less likely to suffer from CHD, diabetes and metabolic syndrome.

Health inequalities as a result of material disadvantage

This explanation argues that the distribution of health and ill health in the population reflects a profoundly unequal distribution of resources in society. Thus those who experience ill health are those who are lower in the social hierarchy, who are least educated, who have least money and fewest resources. Low income may be the result of unemployment or ill-paid hazardous occupations; it can lead to poor housing in polluted and unsafe environments with few opportunities to build social support networks; and in turn such conditions lead to poor health. Lack of money can make it difficult for households to implement what they may know to be healthy choices.

A common response to the evidence of health inequalities is to see it as a consequence of restricted access to services. The intention of the National Health Service – to provide a universal service freely available to all – might have been expected to reduce inequalities in health status. Yet in the early 1970s a GP writing in *The Lancet* put forward a radical view that good health care tends to vary inversely with the need of the population (Tudor Hart 1971).

In areas with most sickness and death, GPs have more work, larger lists, less hospital support and inherit more clinically ineffective traditions of consultation than in the healthiest areas; and the hospital doctors shoulder heavier caseloads with less staff and equipment, more obsolete buildings and suffer recurrent crises in the availability of beds and replacement of staff. These trends can be summed up as the Inverse Care Law: that the availability of good medical care tends to vary inversely with the needs of the population served (Tudor Hart 1971).

Box 2.16

Consider the following evidence on the nature and extent of childhood accidents:
- Accidents are the leading cause of death among children aged 1–4.
- Children from lower social classes are twice as likely to suffer a fatal accident as children from professional groups.

To what do you attribute this?
- Children from lower social classes are more accident-prone or more reckless.
- Parents from lower social classes do not exercise due care in safeguarding their home and supervising their children.
- The physical environment in which poor children play has less space and is less likely

to have safety features such as stairgates and fireguards. Poor children are more likely to have to play outside in environments lacking safety features.

 Box 2.17

Even in the UK, where services are universally available and not dependent on the ability to pay, some groups are more adept at accessing services than others. Why is this?

There is evidence of variation in the quality and quantity of care available to people in different social groups, between regions and between different ethnic groups. However, since medical care has had little impact on the overall death rate from heart disease or cancers, and probably only about 5% of deaths are preventable through medical treatment, it must be concluded that differences in health status are not wholly attributable to variations in the amount and type of care received.

Tackling inequalities in health

Life expectancy, health and health-related behaviours have shown a steady improvement over the last 50 years but there are gross inequalities in health between countries. Life expectancy at birth, for example, ranges from 34 in Sierra Leone to 81.9 in Japan (World Health Organization 2004). Within countries, too, there are inequalities. In the USA Native Americans from South Dakota can expect to live only 58 years whilst Asian-American women from New Jersey have the highest national life expectancy of 91 years (Murray et al 2005). Mortality statistics can reveal a social gradient in disease in *all* countries.

Such disparities are linked to chronic non-communicable diseases related principally to tobacco, alcohol, diet and obesity; to poverty; to violence; to access to health services; and to the circumstances in which people live and work.

There is also wordwide a considerable burden of non-fatal disease and, in particular, mental illness. The Ottawa Charter (World Health Organization 1986) identified key action areas.

- *Strengthening individuals.* This means ensuring that people have information and skills so that they are supported and enabled to make informed choices. It means taking account of different material circumstances and constraints on choice, e.g. parenting programmes, assertiveness skills for problem drinkers.

- *Strengthening communities.* This means supporting people in their communities to make decisions about health issues affecting them, e.g. training and education programmes and neighbourhood regeneration.

- *Improving access to facilities and services.* This involves mediating between people and service providers in order to ensure that needs are met, e.g. providing outreach services in local or community settings, supporting advocacy and linkworker agencies which advocate on behalf of client groups, such as people with learning difficulties or those for whom English is not their mother tongue, who find accessing services difficult.

- *Encouraging a healthy public policy.* A healthy public policy underpins other areas. Wider social and economic change reduces poverty and ensures that the environment and living conditions are conducive to health, e.g. progressive taxation, income support, integrated transport systems, food safety.

Box 2.18

Saving Lives: Our Healthier Nation

To achieve its aims [of improving the health of the population as a whole and improving the health of the worst-off in society and narrowing the health gap] the government is setting out its third way between the old extremes of individual victim-blaming on the one hand and nanny-state social engineering on the other …

Connected problems require joined-up solutions. This means tackling inequality which stems from poverty, poor housing, pollution, low educational standards, joblessness and low pay. Tackling inequalities generally is the best means of tackling health inequalities in particular (Department of Health 1999, pp. 5, 12).

Tackling inequalities requires both 'upstream' and 'downstream' interventions – those that create an environment in which the healthier choice is easier *and* those that support people to change.

Education, employment and income are the key to reducing health inequalities. Education increases employability and ability to cope with many issues. Employment provides income and thus access to health-promoting resources such as food, housing and heating. Addressing inequalities in the UK has thus included early education initiatives such as Sure Start and neighbourhood renewal programmes.

Interventions to reduce inequalities in health, e.g. in relation to diet, could address:

- The structural level, e.g. trade policy, food-labelling regulations, food fortification.
- The local/community level, e.g. food gardens, free fruit and vegetables in school, food outlets.
- The individual/family level, e.g. nutrition education in school or during pregnancy. Mass media campaigns such as that to reduce salt, weight loss programmes.

Although many health promoters may feel power-less to effect change at a macro structural level, it is possible to address health inequalities in planning health promotion interventions, as the above examples illustrate. One of the central tasks for health promoters is to acknowledge socioeconomic factors as crucial in determining individual and population health (Naidoo & Wills 2005).

Conclusion

Health promotion is not a purely technical activity. As we have seen, even identifying the causes of ill health will lead to political judgements being made.

Box 2.19

Consider the following points of view about the causes of health and illness. Which comes closest to your own?

- Ill health is the result of people's unhealthy lifestyles. No one makes people live this way and so it is up to individuals to take responsibility for their own health. The role of the health promoter is to provide information to encourage people to be concerned about their health and make healthier decisions.

- Ill health is the result of the social and economic conditions in which people live. It is not people's fault if they become ill. People may have unhealthy lifestyles but this is because it is difficult to make healthy choices on a low income. The role of the health promoter is to try to empower people to take charge of their lives by raising awareness of the factors that influence their health. Health promoters need to draw the attention of policy-makers to the influence of social and economic conditions on their clients' health.

In any area of work or discipline, there will always be debate about what constitutes good practice. It is important to clarify your thinking and where you stand because it will affect your views on the purpose of health promotion and what would be appropriate health promotion activities. It is also important that you share these thoughts with colleagues and clients to reach a common understanding of the ideals upon which health promotion activities are based.

In practice, behavioural and structural explanations are often aligned to the right or left of the political spectrum, and have become linked with very different policies and approaches to health promotion. The behavioural approach, which focuses on individual lifestyles, has informed much of health education because it suggests that information, advice or mass media messages can change behaviours such as smoking or sexual activity. A structural approach, which sees health as determined by social and economic conditions, and reflecting the unequal distribution of power and resources in society, requires the health promoter to become involved in political activity.

Questions for further discussion

- Is it fair or effective to encourage individuals to change their health behaviour?
- Good health depends on adequate income. Do you agree?
- What long-term social policy initiatives would most bring about an improvement in the health of your clients?

- What are the implications for professional practice of the links between health and wealth?

Summary

This chapter has reviewed the evidence concerning health differences in the population and the physical, social and environmental variables that are implicated in ill health: poverty, unemployment, inadequate housing, stressful and dangerous working conditions, lack of social support, air and water pollution. It goes on to consider the ways in which risk factors associated with personal behaviour – smoking, nutrition, exercise – are influenced by the social environment.

Several explanations for inequalities in health have been discussed. None offers a complete explanation, but the chapter concludes that there is sufficient evidence to point to social and economic factors determining health. It argues that disadvantage can give rise to or exacerbate health-damaging behaviours such as smoking or poor nutrition, and so health behaviours should not be separated from their social context.

Further reading

Acheson D 1998 Independent inquiry into inequalities in health: a report. Stationery Office, London. *Brings together recent research on continued inequalities in health and identifies a number of key areas for action to tackle inequalities in health.*

Marmot M, Wilkinson R G 2006 (eds) Social determinants of health, 2nd edn. Oxford University Press, Oxford. *An overview of the factors known to affect health including unemployment, work and social support.*

Wilkinson R, Marmot M 2003 Social determinants of health: the solid facts. World Health Organization,

Copenhagen. *www.who.dk/document/e81384.pdf. This online document summarizes some of the arguments linking health status to social determinants. The actions of the World Health Organization Commission on the Social Determinants of Health can be found at http://www.who.int/social_determinants/en/.*

Useful websites include: www.poverty.org.uk

The Black Report can be downloaded from http://www.sochealth.co.uk/history/black.htm

References

Acheson D 1998 Independent inquiry into inequalities in health: a report. Stationery Office, London.

Annandale H, Hunt K (eds) 2000 Gender inequalities in health. Open University Press, Buckingham.

Arber S 1990 Opening the black box: inequalities in women's health. In: Abbott P, Gilbert N (eds) New directions in the sociology of health. Falmer, Basingstoke.

Bhopal R S 2007 Ethnicity, race and health in multicultural societies. Oxford University Press, Oxford.

Blane D, Brunner E, Wilkinson R (eds) 1996 Health and social organisation: towards a health policy for the 21st century. Routledge, London.

British Heart Foundation 2000 South Asians and heart disease. Available online at: www.bhsoc.org/bhf_factfiles

Britton A, McPherson K 2000 Monitoring the progress of the 2010 target for coronary heart disease mortality: consequences on CHD incidence and mortality from changing prevalence of risk factors. National Heart Forum, London.

Bromley C, Sprosten K, Shelton N (eds) 2005 The Scottish health survey 2003, vol. 2: Adults. Scottish Executive, Edinburgh.

Dahlgren G, Whitehead M 1991 Policies and strategies to promote social equity in health. Institute for Future Studies, Stockholm.

Department of Health 1999 Saving lives: our healthier nation. Stationery Office, London.

Department of Health 2000 National Service Framework: coronary heart disease. Stationery Office, London.

Department of Work and Pensions 2005 Households below average income statistics. Department of Work and Pensions, London.

Dobson F 1997 Healthy houses for healthy lives: address to National Housing Federation 16/10/97. Department of Health press release 97/282.

Dorling D, Mitchell R, Shaw M et al 2000 The ghost of Christmas past: health effects of poverty in London in 1896 and 1991. British Medical Journal 321: 1547–1551.

Doyal L 1995 What makes women sick? Gender and the political economy of health. Macmillan, Basingstoke.

Graham H 1992 Smoking among working class mothers with children. Department of Applied Social Studies, University of Warwick, Warwick.

Illsley R 1986 Occupational class, selection, and the production of inequalities. Quarterly Journal of Social Affairs 2: 151–165.

Lalonde M 1974 A new perspective on the health of Canadians. Ministry of Supply and Services, Ottawa, Canada.

Macintyre S 2007 Inequalities in health in Scotland: what are they and what can we do about them? Occasional

paper 17. MRC Social and Public Health Sciences Unit, Glasgow.

McKeown T, Lowe C R 1974 An introduction to social medicine. Blackwell Science, Oxford.

McLean C, Carmona C, France C et al 2005 Worklessness and health: what do we know about the causal relationship?. Health Development Agency, London.

Marmot M, Siegrist J, Theorell T 2006 Health and the psychosocial environment at work. In: Marmot M, Wilkinson R (eds) The social determinants of health, 2nd edn. Oxford University Press, Oxford.

Marsh A, Gordon D, Pantazis C et al 1999 Home sweet home? The impact of poor housing on health. Policy Press, London.

Murray C, Kulkarni S, Ezzati M 2005 Eight Americas: new perspectives on US health disparities. American Journal of Preventive Medicine 29: 4–10.

Naidoo J, Wills J 2005 Public health and health promotion: developing practice. Baillière Tindall, London.

Nazroo J 1997 The health of Britain's ethnic minorities. Policy Studies Institute, London.

Office of National Statistics 2001 Census. Longitudinal study. Available online at: www.statistics.gov.uk

Office of National Statistics 2007a Health statistics quarterly, spring 2007 no. 33. ONS, London.

Office of National Statistics 2007b Childhood, infant and perinatal mortality statistics. HD3. ONS, London.

Stansfield S, Marmot M 2001 Stress and the heart: psychosocial pathway to coronary heart disease. BMJ Books, London.

Townsend P, Davidson N 1982 Inequalities in health: the Black report. Penguin, Harmondsworth.

Tudor Hart J 1971 The inverse care law. Lancet 1: 405.

Whitehead M 1988 The health divide. HEC, London.

Wilkinson R 1986 Class and health: research and longitudinal data. Tavistock, London.

Wilkinson R 1996 Unhealthy societies: the afflictions of inequality. Routledge, London.

Wilkinson R, Marmot M 2003 Social determinants of health: the solid facts. World Health Organization, Copenhagen.

World Health Organization 1986 Ottawa charter for health promotion. Journal of Health Promotion 1: 1–4.

World Health Organization 2004 World health report: changing history. World Health Organization, Geneva.

Chapter **Three**

3

Measuring health

Key points

- Sources of health information:
- Mortality rates
- Morbidity rates
- Objective health measures
- Measuring deprivation
- Subjective health measures
- Epidemiology and health promotion

OVERVIEW

We have seen in Chapter 1 how people define health in different ways and in Chapter 2 how there are different determinants of health. This would suggest that measuring health is not a simple task. This appears to be borne out by the existence of a number of ways of measuring health and a lack of clear agreement about which are the best ways to measure health and which sources of information are most useful. This chapter looks first at why we might want to measure health. It goes on to investigate the different means of measuring health currently in use and unpacks some of the assumptions underlying their use. Finally, the uses of the different kinds of measures are explored. The practical uses of measuring health are discussed further in Chapters 18 and 19 on needs assessment and programme planning, and in Chapter 20 on evaluation.

Why measure health?

Finding a means to measure health is an important practical task for health promoters. There are several reasons why this is so.

1. *To establish priorities.* Collecting and evaluating information about the health status and health problems of a community are important ways of identifying needs.

2. *To assist planning.* Health promoters need information to assist the planning and evaluation of health promotion programmes. It is important to establish baseline data in order to plan priorities and to have a standard against

which health promotion interventions can be evaluated.

3. *To justify resources.* Health promotion is often in competition with other activities for scarce resources. To make a claim for resources and to prove that their activities are effective, health promoters need information on the health status of populations.

4. *To assist the development of the profession.* Measurements of health gain are important to the professional development of health promoters. Unless there is a means of measuring the effect of our actions, health promotion work will remain invisible, underfunded and low-priority. By demonstrating the efficacy of health promotion interventions, it is possible to argue for resources, credibility and funding.

Ways of measuring health

Depending on the purpose, different measures of health may be used or developed. The means of measuring health depend primarily on the view of health which is held. If health is basically about physical functioning, then measures of physical fitness will be an adequate measure of health. If health is defined as having no disease, then measures of the extent of disease may be used (in reverse) as measures of health. However, if health is defined as including social and mental aspects and as meaning something other than being not ill, specific measurements of health will need to be developed.

Box 3.1

If you wanted to describe the health of the people where you live or work, what information would you need?

It is likely that you included:

- Information about the health status of the community (e.g. the number of deaths and the main causes of death; the number of episodes of illness and the main types of illness)
- Information on the determinants of health (e.g. people's lifestyles; the quality of housing; levels of employment; the adequacy and accessibility of health services)
- Information about the community itself (e.g. the age, gender, ethnic and socioeconomic breakdown of the population).

Community health workers who profile their communities have many different ways of building a picture of their area. Some of these are described in Chapter 18 on needs assessment. In this chapter we look at sources of information available to describe a community's health. A great deal of information is available online. For example, in the UK you can find out about your local area by visiting http://neighbourhood.statistics.gov.uk and, for those living in Scotland, www.gro-scotland.gov.uk/statistics.

We shall look next at the contribution of epidemiology through the measurement of health as a negative variable, and move on to consider the measurement of health as a positive variable. Measuring health as a negative variable means measuring the opposite to health (e.g. disease or death) and using these results to infer the degree of health. Health is therefore being defined as a negative (health is not being ill or dead), not as a positive (health as positive well-being).

Measuring health as a negative variable (e.g. health is not being diseased or ill)

Epidemiology is the study of the occurrence and spread of diseases in the population. It is concerned with the health status (or, more usually, the ill-health status) of populations. Health promoters use epidemiological evidence to identify health problems, at-risk groups and the effectiveness of preventive measures. The most common means of assessing a population's health are through mortality and morbidity rates. This reflects the reductionist model of health which sees health as a simple matter of illness or its absence. Thus data on deaths and illnesses are often used as surrogate measures of health. There are clearly shortcomings to this approach. Measuring conditions which limit health, such as illness, is not the same as measuring health itself. Measuring mortality rates does not reflect the extent of illness in the population, nor does it say anything about the quality of health experienced by people when they were alive. Conditions such as arthritis or schizophrenia cause considerable suffering and pain but do not lead to premature death and so are not reflected in mortality rates.

Box 3.2

If you wished to develop a health promotion intervention to improve food hygiene, why would mortality rates be a poor indicator of its priority?

- How else could you find out about the extent of poor food hygiene in your area?
- Why might mortality statistics be a good indicator in a low-income country of the necessity of health promotion around food hygiene?

On the plus side, statistics concerning mortality are readily obtainable in developed countries. A death certificate is taken to the Registrar of Births, Deaths and Marriages and the Director of Public Health in every health authority and the total number of deaths, the geographic and population variations and the causes of death are all collated in each district's annual public health report. The statistics can also be used in international comparisons because most countries hold some form of database on deaths and disease rates.

All countries have systems of collecting data on the health status of the population and the use of services. Although these statistics are often presented as if they were objective facts, it is important to remember that statistics are devised by people in a social context, subject to assumptions, bias and error. At every stage of the data-collecting process, decisions are taken which help shape the ultimate form of information presented.

Box 3.3

In low-income countries mortality statistics may not be complete. Can you think of reasons why this might be the case?

- In rural areas the infrastructure for recording may not exist.
- Particular causes of mortality may be easier to recognize or be less stigmatized than others.
- People in higher socioeconomic groups are more likely to have sought medical care prior to death and thus have a detailed cause of death recorded.

Box 3.4

The *International Classification of Diseases, Injuries and Causes of Death* (ICD) classifies death according to diagnosed diseases which cause death, e.g. cancer of the lung. Death certificates which use the ICD thus give no information about contributory risk factors such as smoking or diet.

- What impact do you think this has on our perception of risk factors and causes of disease, and on suitable strategies for prevention and treatment?
- Is it likely to foster understanding of social, environmental or biological causes of disease?

Mortality statistics

There are several different ways of expressing death rates. The crude death rate is the number of deaths per 1000 people per year. However, this figure is affected by the age structure of the population, which may vary over time and region. An area with a high proportion of older people, such as a south-coast retirement town, would have consistently higher death rates than a more deprived area with a higher percentage of premature deaths, such as an inner-city area. The standardized mortality ratio (SMR) measures the death rate, taking into account differences in age structure. It is the number of deaths experienced within a population group (which may be defined by geographic or socioeconomic factors) compared to what would be expected for this group if national averages applied, taking age differences into account. The overall average for England and Wales is 100, so SMRs of below 100 indicate a lower than average mortality rate, whereas SMRs of more than 100 indicate higher than average mortality rates.

The infant mortality rate (IMR) is another commonly used statistic. The IMR is the number of deaths in the first year of life per 1000 live births. The IMR is strongly associated with adult mortality rates. It reflects maternal health, particularly nutrition, and the provision of social care and child welfare. The IMR is therefore capable of being used as an indicator of the general health of the population, particularly when comparisons between countries are being drawn. The perinatal mortality rate (PMR) is the number of stillbirths and deaths in the first 7 days after birth per 1000 births. The neonatal death rate is the number of deaths occurring in the first 28 days after birth per 1000 live births. Both the SMR and the IMR are readily available statistics, and therefore easy to use as surrogate measures of health. Table 3.1 (p. 39) compares key health indicators for different countries worldwide.

Box 3.5

- Which country has the highest life expectancy for women and men?
- Which country has the lowest life expectancy for women and men?
- Which country has the highest IMR?
- What reasons can you give to explain these findings?

Death rates are also available broken down by gender, social class and cause. In the UK, it is well established that death rates are related to social class and gender (Department of Health 2005; Lantz et al 2001; Townsend et al 1998). People in the lower social classes have higher than average death rates at all ages and for virtually all causes. These social class differences show no sign of diminishing. Indeed, social class inequalities in IMRs and life expectancy continue to grow, although there are some signs of progress, e.g. in child poverty and housing indicators (Department of Health 2005). It may well take some time for any strategies currently being implemented to have an impact on mortality indicators. Women in developed countries live longer on average than men, so their premature death rate is lower than that of men. This is discussed in greater detail in Chapter 2.

Reductions in mortality for selected causes among targeted groups in the population constitute the majority of targets in public health strategies.

Box 3.6

Targets of *Saving Lives: Our Healthier Nation*

By 2010, reductions in mortality in the following areas:

1. Heart disease and stroke: reduce the death rate in people under 75 years by at least two-fifths.
2. Accidents: reduce the death rate by at least a fifth and serious injury by at least a tenth.
3. Cancers: reduce the death rate amongst people under 75 years by at least a fifth.
4. Mental illness: reduce the death rate from suicide and undetermined injury by at least a fifth.

   Baseline: 1996 (Department of Health 1999).

Morbidity statistics

Statistics measuring illness and disease are more difficult to obtain. This is due in part to the difficulty in establishing a hard and fast line between health and disease. There is no one source of data for the

Table 3.1 Key health indicators worldwide (2005)

Country	Life expectancy (years)		Adult mortality rate (probability of dying age 15–60) per 1000 population		Infant mortality rate (per 1000 live births)
	Men	Women	Men	Women	
Belgium	M 76	F 82	M 120	F 64	4
Canada	M 78	F 83	M 90	F 56	5
UK	M 77	F 81	M 101	F 62	5
USA	M 75	F 80	M 137	F 81	7
Zimbabwe	M 43	F 42	M 771	F 789	60
China	M 71	F 74	M 155	F 98	23
Argentina	M 72	F 78	M 162	F 86	14
Sweden	M 79	F 83	M 78	F 50	3
India	M 62	F 64	M 280	F 207	56
Australia	M 79	F 84	M 84	F 47	5

Taken from World Health Statistics 2007 part 2 Mortality http://www.who.int/whosis/whostat2007/en/

whole population concerning disease and illness. Instead, there are a number of different sources of relevant information. These are summarized below.

Box 3.7

Sources of health information in the UK
These sources of data may be accessed from public health departments, hospital-based data sets, the Health Protection Agency, primary care consultation rates, local delivery plans, local surveys and the Office for National Statistics. Useful websites include: www.statistics.gov.uk (Office for National Statistics); www.hpa.org.uk (Health Protection Agency); www.apho.org.uk (Association of Public Health Observatories); www.rcgp.org.uk (Royal College of General Practitioners); and www.hse.gov.uk (Health and Safety Executive).

Mortality
- Death by cause, age, sex and area of residence

- Infant deaths (in children under 1 year)
- Perinatal deaths (after 28th week of pregnancy and in the first 7 days after birth)
- Neonatal deaths (within first 28 days of birth)

Morbidity
- General Household Survey (annual survey of health behaviour and experience of illness)
- Health service records on consultation and treatment episodes in hospital and general practice, e.g. hospital episodes and statistics (HES)
- Registers for specific conditions such as cancers, disability, blindness and partial sight, people at risk of harm, drug addiction
- Notification systems for infectious (communicable) diseases from the Health Protection Agency and the Communicable Diseases Surveillance Centre (Wales)
- National General Practice Morbidity Survey conducted by the Office for National Statistics together with the Royal College of General Practitioners

- Surveys on mental health and pyschiatric morbidity (for England, Scotland and Wales, since 1993)

  Reporting of Injuries, Diseases and Dangerous Occurrences (RIDDOR) regulations data available from the Health and Safety Executive (HSE)
- Data regarding incidence of disease obtained from screening programmes, e.g. for cervical cancer
- Notifiable congenital malformations.

Information on health status and behaviour

GP records on diagnoses, communicable and respiratory disease monitoring, e.g. PRIMIS + (primary care information services)
- Dental health records
- Child health surveillance records
- National surveys for the Office for National Statistics, e.g. the annual Health Survey for England, the annual National Food Survey, Children and Smoking and Infant Feeding survey and occasional surveys, e.g. Active People Survey (Sport England)

Demographic data

- Census information on the whole population is collected every 10 years (information includes numbers in household by age, sex, marital status, place of birth, occupation, ethnicity (since 1991), educational level, house type and tenure, accommodation and facilities). Information on self-reported health is collected
- Register of births, including birth weight and mother's occupation
- Claimants of unemployment benefit, free school meals, housing benefit, income support

Environmental indicators and deprivation indices

- Services available
- Levels of pollution: air, water and noise
- Crime statistics
- Type of housing
- Leisure facilities
- Road traffic accidents
- Education, skills and training
- Employment

The health services collect routine data on the use of their services and activity rate. These data can be used to express the disease experience of different populations but there are several problems with adopting this approach. The main problem with using many of the health authority measurements is that they were developed primarily for administrative, planning or management tasks, and reflect available services and use of these services rather than health itself. Health authority data are primarily collected as a management tool. To some extent, this determines what data are collected. Routinely available morbidity data represent only the tip of the illness iceberg. Many people who are ill do not seek help from primary care services or hospitals. However, the advantage of using data of this kind is that they are routinely collected, are consistent across regions and are easily accessed.

Box 3.8

Hospital episodes statistics (HES) is a patient-based data set that contains all finished episodes of hospital care by diagnosis and treatment (www.hesonline.nhs.uk):
- What will these data tell you about the health status of the local population?
- What do they not tell you?
- Why do you think they are collected in this way?

The General Household Survey (GHS) is a continuous government survey of a sample of the population. The GHS includes questions on people's experience of illness, both long-term (chronic) and within the last fortnight (acute). GHS data are difficult to use comparatively over time as the wording of the questions changes occasionally. The following are examples of questions used in the GHS:
- Over the last 12 months would you say your health has on the whole been good, fairly good or not good?
- Do you have any long-standing illness, disability or infirmity? By long-standing I mean anything

that has troubled you over a period of time or that is likely to affect you over a period of time.

- Now I'd like you to think about the 2 weeks ending yesterday. During those 2 weeks, did you have to cut down on any of the things you usually do (about the house/at work or in your free time) because of (any chronic condition cited earlier in the interview) or some other illness or injury?

The GHS is useful in providing information on people's subjective experience of illness, because it relies on people's self-reported illness rather than use of services. It also collects information on people's health-related behaviour such as smoking, drinking and exercise. For example, one question asks: 'Do you smoke cigarettes at all nowadays?'

A number of proxy measures of health are used such as the number of days at work lost due to sickness. However, such data are only available for people in paid employment. The large section of the population who are not in paid employment, and their experience of illness, is therefore invisible.

Box 3.9

Two areas of equal size and population structure experience very different unemployment rates. Area A has 40% unemployment whereas area B has 10%. The sickness rate for employed people is the same.

- Numerically, which area will have the greatest ill health if days lost at work due to sickness is the measure used?
- Will this reflect the likely extent of ill health in the two areas?

Area B will have the highest sickness rate, but it is likely that the actual extent of ill health will be greater in area A, because unemployment is associated with increased ill health (Moser et al 1990; White 1991; Bethune 1997).

Various government research studies have developed measures to assess disability and to produce estimates of the number of people with disabilities

in the population. The Office for National Statistics (ONS) uses questions based on the World Health Organization's *International Classification of Impairments, Disabilities and Handicaps* (1980). These disability indices are based on the results of questionnaires asking people what, if any, difficulty they experience in daily life. The onus is therefore placed on the individual being unable to perform certain tasks such as taking a bath or walking unaided up flights of stairs. The reason for these difficulties could be located in housing design and might be capable of being remedied by modifying the home environment. However, by treating disability as an inherent individual attribute, the effect of the social environment in generating and maintaining disability is rendered invisible. This approach has been criticized by proponents of the social model of disability, who argue that the social production of disability should be recognized and challenged (Shakespeare & Watson 1997). The revised World Health Organization (2001) *International Classification of Functioning, Disability and Health* separates impairments of body functions from restrictions in the ability to perform social roles and participate.

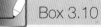

Box 3.10

A typical question from disability surveys is: 'Does this illness or disability limit your activities in any way?'
- How many different reasons can you think of for someone answering 'yes' to this question?
- How many of these reasons refer to physical diseases?
- How many of these reasons refer to mental illnesses?
- How many of these reasons refer to social factors?
- How many of these reasons refer to environmental factors?

Epidemiological studies examine the distribution and patterns of health and disease in populations. Epidemiological data help to build up a picture by:

1. Showing the scale of the problem
2. Showing the natural history and aetiology of the condition
3. Showing causation and association
4. Identifying risk.

Scale of the problem

- *Incidence.* The number of people developing a disease over a specified period, e.g. in 2004 there were 44 659 newly diagnosed cases of breast cancer in the UK (www.info.cancerresearchuk.org).
- *Prevalence.* The number of people with a condition or characteristic at a specified time, e.g. in 2004 25% of the adult population were regular smokers (www.statistics.gov.uk/ghs).
- How the condition is distributed by gender, age, socioeconomic class, ethnicity, etc., e.g. women in lower social classes are almost twice as likely to be obese as women in higher social classes (in 2001 30% of women in routine occupations were classified as obese compared to 16% in higher managerial and professional occupations (www.statistics.gov.uk/ghs).

Natural history and aetiology of the condition

- Indicates if primary prevention is possible
- Shows severity of the problem and ways in which individuals, families or communities may be affected.

Causation and association

- Shows if there is evidence that exposure to a particular environmental, lifestyle or socioeconomic factor contributes to ill health. There is a difference between causation (without which the ill health would not have occurred) and association.

Box 3.11

Lung cancer and smoking

Most patients with lung cancer have smoked. The proportion of smokers who develop lung cancer is much higher than the proportion of non-smokers. Does smoking *cause* lung cancer?

Not all smokers will develop lung cancer, and some non-smokers will develop lung cancer. That someone smokes is not a sufficient or necessary cause to develop lung cancer, but it is a very strong risk factor and the more an individual smokes, the greater the risk. The Bradford Hill criteria for determining causation are discussed in Crichton (2008) and Unwin et al (1997).

Identifying risk

- Assessing the chance or probability of a disease or condition occurring
- Assessing how much illness is due to a particular factor (the *attributable risk*).

Epidemiologists assess risk in terms of the statistical probability of adverse events or death occurring. The link between these events and identified contributory factors varies from negligible to high. Lay people, by contrast, assess risk in the light of their personal experience. This difference in focus (whole populations versus specific individuals at a specific time) is problematic for health promoters. Rose (1981) called this the 'prevention paradox': for one person to benefit, many people have to change their behaviour, even though they will not benefit from so doing. Public awareness of this paradox can become a barrier to behaviour change.

Epidemiological studies of mortality, illness, disease and disability are often used to talk about health. Such usage reinforces, albeit in an indirect way, the definition of health as 'not disease'. But the advantage of such statistics is that they are already collected, are relatively consistent and are readily available. Recognizing the limitations of such measures has prompted health promoters to develop new means of measuring health as an independent phenomenon distinct from illness or disease. These measures may be conveniently divided into those describing health as an objective quality which is an attribute of people or environments, and those describing health as a subjective reality which is socially produced.

Measures of health as an objective attribute

There are a number of ways of measuring health as an objective factor, including:

- Health measures
- Health behaviour indicators
- Environmental indicators
- Socioeconomic or deprivation indicators.

Health measures

There are a number of measures of the health status of people, including vital statistics such as height and weight, and dental health status (the decayed, missing and filled teeth, or DMF, index). Floud (1989) argues that the average height of a population may be taken as a measure of health, as it represents a proxy for nutritional status and therefore welfare. The *Health Survey for England 2003* (Department of Health 2004) included height and weight measurements for this reason. In the same way, Townsend et al (1987) use the percentage of low-birth-weight babies as an indicator of health.

Health behaviour indicators

Increasingly common are measurements of people's behaviour which are then used as a measure of health. For example, the number of people smoking, drinking alcohol, using drugs, taking regular exercise, eating a healthy diet, practising safer sex or planned fertility may all be used to describe different populations, and to make comparisons between them regarding relative health status. This information may be routinely collected, such as smoking prevalence in young people, or it may be obtained from commissioned surveys. For example, Cancer Research UK commissioned the ONS to carry out a sun protection survey in 2003 (http://cancerresearchuk.org). These lifestyle measures are sometimes narrowed down to more specific behaviour in relation to the health services. For example, the percentage of children immunized against childhood illnesses, or the percentage of women screened for cervical and breast cancer, may be used to describe the health status of a population.

Environmental indicators

The same method may be applied to physical and social environments. Measurements of the physical environment include air and water quality, and housing type and density. These measures are routinely collected by the environmental health departments of local authorities. The European Happy Planet Index combines measures of carbon footprints, life expectancy and life satisfaction (Thompson et al 2007).

Socioeconomic indicators

Socioeconomic status (SES), including educational attainment, occupational status and income, is related to health in developed countries, with higher SES being associated with better health (Adler et al 2007). The social environment may also be measured in terms of its 'healthiness'. One of the measures most commonly used to assess the social environment is wealth. The gross domestic product (GDP – the value of all goods and services produced within a nation in a given year) measures economic well-being, but this forms only part of social well-being (also called quality of life or social welfare). Happiness and life satisfaction are only weakly related to GDP for the developed Organization for Economic Cooperation and Development (OECD) countries (Allin 2007). Factors that are more strongly associated with health include well-developed primary health care systems (Macinko et al 2003), redistributive and egalitarian policies (Navarro et al 2006) and more equal income distribution, high levels of female education and reduced ethnic fragmentation and conflict (Filmer & Pritchett 1999).

The United Nations Development Programme has introduced a new way of measuring development that incorporates health. The human development index (HDI) is a single statistic that combines indicators of life expectancy, educational attainment and income and was first used in 1990 (http://hdr.undp.org/en/humandev/hdi/). Since then, gender inequalities have also been added into the equation, leading to the gender-related development index.

Objective measurements of people's health status, health-related behaviour and the environment may be combined to provide an overall picture of health. The health of different populations, from neighbourhoods to nations, may be assessed and compared using this method. Targets for improvements in health may also be set using these measurements.

Improvements in the social and physical environment, such as an increase in the number, accessibility and safety of play areas and sports centres, or improvements in housing amenities and density, may also be added into the equation (Catford 1983; World Health Organization 1985). People's health-related beliefs and attitudes, and the extent to which they conform to professional beliefs, have also been considered to be a measure of health (Catford 1983). For example, the percentage of the population seeking to make recommended lifestyle changes, or having an understanding of basic health issues, has been suggested as a positive health measure. Subjective social status (SSS), a judgement of one's socioeconomic position taking into account education, income and occupation, has also been linked to health status (Adler et al 2007). Combining a number of discrete elements to measure health is attractive because it gives a more rounded picture of health, and provides a clear basis and direction for health promoters.

Box 3.12

How might you set about doing a health impact assessment of a proposal to build flats on an area of open ground currently used informally for exercise and recreation by the local community?

Health impact assessment

Health impact assessment (HIA) has emerged as a systematic means of assessing health and measuring the health outcomes of policies and interventions on defined populations (Lock 2000). HIAs are often used to evaluate the impact of policies that focus on factors other than health. HIA includes qualitative and quantitative methodologies and collaboration with interested partners, including workers, clients and other stakeholders. This allows for a multidisciplinary definition of health to evolve. Some examples may be found via the HIA gateway at www.apho.org.uk. A rapid HIA of the proposed Olympic Games was conducted for London (www.londonshealth.gov.uk/PDF/Olympic_HIA.pdf). It concluded that hosting the Olympic Games would provide net benefits to local communities due to increased employment, greater physical activity and enhanced community cohesion.

Measuring deprivation

Box 3.13

How would you measure deprivation?

Much of the evidence which finds that people who are most disadvantaged experience more illness and premature death has derived from the link between occupational class and health status. Occupational class is still the main measure of SES, although other factors such as gender, age and ethnicity are also recognized as having an important impact on SES. The limitations of using occupational categories are discussed in Chapter 2. The classification of socioeconomic classes is derived from census information on type of employment. Since 2001 eight socioeconomic classes have been used (see Chapter 2 for further details).

The index of multiple deprivation (IMD) combines seven discrete domains of deprivation at a local area level to form a single score. The seven domains of deprivation are: income; employment; health and disability; education, skills and training; housing and services; living environment; and crime (www.communities.gov.uk). Each domain includes several different indicators. For example, the income domain includes:

- Adults and children in Income Support households (2001)
- Adults and children in Income-Based Job Seekers Allowance households (2001)
- Adults and children in Working Families Tax Credit households whose equivalized income (excluding housing benefits) is below 60% of median before housing costs (2001)
- Adults and children in Disabled Person's Tax Credit households whose equivalized income (excluding housing benefits) is below 60% of median before housing costs (2001)
- National Asylum Support Service supported asylum seekers in England in receipt of subsistence only and accommodation support (2002).

In addition indices for income deprivation affecting children and older people have been developed.

Explanations of health inequalities are discussed in Chapter 2 and may be divided into four categories: psychosocial (social stress); behavioural (lifestyle choices); lifecourse (cumulative cross-generational factors); and neomaterialist explanations (wider socioeconomic and psychosocial environments) (Bartley 2004).

Subjective health measures

The previous section has outlined means of measuring health as if it were an objective property of beings, societies, or environments, capable of scientific scrutiny. However, it is apparent that health is not such a simple or uncontested attribute. Chapter 1 highlighted the importance of subjective interpretations of health and the multiple meanings health may have in different contexts. This has led some researchers to attempt to devise measurements of health which incorporate subjective reporting of

health. Herzlich (1973) identified three different aspects to people's accounts of health:

1. Health as a vacuum (not being ill)
2. Health as a reserve (of strength and resilience)
3. Health as equilibrium (balance and well-being).

Bowling (1997) identifies five dimensions of subjective health:

1. Functional ability
2. Health status
3. Psychological well-being
4. Social networks and social support
5. Life satisfaction and morale.

This is very similar to the Blaxter's (1990) earlier classification, with the one difference being the last category, where Blaxter identified physical fitness and vitality instead of life satisfaction and morale.

Box 3.14

Jeff is 78 years old. His wife died last year after several years of Alzheimer's disease, during which he cared for her. He has one son who visits rarely. Jeff has been in good physical health and used to walk to the local shops every day. He lives in the same terraced house in which he was born. The area is now full of young working couples. Jeff has been to see his GP for the first time in 8 years because he is suffering from acute headaches.

What indicators could be used to assess Jeff's:

- Physical well-being?
- Psychological well-being?
- Social well-being?
- Quality of life?

Physical well-being, functional ability and health status

Most measures of functional ability use people's self-reports of physical activity, such as the ability to perform everyday activities, e.g. personal care, degree of mobility, domestic activities. A widely used tool to measure health is the short-form 36-item (SF-36) health survey (Ware & Sherbourne 1992). The SF-36 is a multi-item scale that assesses the following eight health concepts:

1. Limitations in physical activities because of health problems
2. Limitations in social activities because of physical or emotional problems
3. Limitations in usual role activities because of physical health problems
4. Bodily pain
5. General mental health
6. Limitations in usual role activities because of emotional problems
7. Vitality
8. General health perceptions.

Box 3.15

What are the advantages and disadvantages of the SF-36 health survey?

The SF-36 measures people's subjective assessment of their physical, mental and social health. It does not measure physical health in an objective manner, e.g. screening for markers of disease. The main criticism of such measures is that people may become accustomed to limitations of bodily function and not perceive them as such.

Psychological well-being

Several questionnaires have been developed to measure psychological well-being, including Goldberg's general health questionnaire (GHQ) (Goldberg et al 1997). Goldberg's GHQ, which measures minor psychological distress and social dysfunction, has been validated for use worldwide and includes items such as:

• Able to concentrate
• Enjoy normal activities

• Capable of making decisions
• Feeling unhappy and depressed
• Lost much sleep.

Social health

Health includes the dimension of social health, which may be defined as the degree to which people function adequately as members of the community. A key characteristic of social health is social support, incorporating both the extent of a person's social networks and perceived adequacy (Antonovsky 1987). More recently, the concept of 'social capital' has been used to describe these networks and the trust which links people together in a community (Wilkinson 1996). Higher levels of social capital are associated with better health, less violent crime, better schooling, more tolerance and more economic and civic equality (Putnam 2001). Attempts to measure social capital have used data regarding membership of voluntary organizations, clubs and committees as well as data on informal networking and questions about trust to assess the degree of civic participation (Paldam 2001; Putnam 2001). It has been argued that a reduction or disinvestment in social capital, triggered by increased income inequality, leads to increased mortality (Kawachi et al 1997).

Box 3.16

What examples can you think of where social support may have an effect on health?

Quality of life

Quality of life has been used by some researchers to encompass the broader notion of health. Research amongst older people found quality of life included the following components (Brown et al 2004):

• Physical health and functioning
• Psychosocial well-being

- Psychological outlook
- Psychological and social role functioning
- Social support and resources
- Independence, autonomy and perceived control over life
- Material and financial circumstances
- Community social capital
- The external environment, including the political environment.

Quality of life is therefore a complex concept, including several different multilevel interacting influences. Veenhoven (1996) has identified the concept of happy life expectancy (HLE), a combination of life expectancy plus appreciation of life. HLE scores are highest in north-west European countries and lowest in Africa.

 Box 3.17

What might account for the high scores for happy life expectancy in north-west European countries and the low scores for African countries?

Seventy percent of the statistical variance in HLE scores is explained by four characteristics: affluence, freedom, education and tolerance.

QALYs

The desire to include a measurement of health in evaluating health care outcomes has led to the development of quality-adjusted life years (QALYs). QALYs are an explicit attempt to include not just years of life saved but also the quality of life, when making resource allocation decisions regarding different medical procedures. The quality of life includes things such as freedom from pain and discomfort, and the ability to live independently. The assessment of quality of life is made by both health professionals and lay people. The QALY is the arithmetic product of life expectancy and an adjustment for the quality of the remaining life years gained (Baldwin et al 1990). These two components are quite separate. QALYs are an important tool in making decisions about how to ration health care resources.

There is much theoretical and methodological confusion in attempts to measure different aspects of positive health and a lack of consensus in how this may best be achieved. It is an area which is currently being refined and researched, and is undoubtedly important to any adequate conceptualization and measurement of health.

Conclusion

Measuring health is an important activity for health promoters, and is integral to the planning and evaluation of health promotion programmes. Yet there is no consensus on the best means to measure health, and a wide variety of methods have been used. Some are opportunistic, relying on data already collected and available, such as the annual Health Survey for England and QALYs. The drawback of using these methods is that they use data which have been collected for specific reasons, often managerial or administrative. Other methods, such as the SF-36, have arisen from research which has addressed the issue of how to measure health. The fact that the concept 'health' can have so many different meanings, as outlined in Chapter 1, also contributes to the variety of different methods used. Some methods focus on one dimension of health, whereas others try to span different dimensions. It is also the case that different measures may suit different purposes. It is unlikely that any one method will ever prove to be a comprehensive measure of health, even if it combines different measurements within a weighted index. What is important then is to be specific about *why* you wish to measure health, and then to go on to select the most appropriate means of doing so, bearing in mind constraints on the time and money you have at your disposal.

Box 3.18

You are putting together a proposal to justify a health promotion intervention around the following conditions. In each case, what sorts of information would you need? Where would you obtain this information?

- Childhood obesity
- Parenting for lone mothers
- Young people, alcohol and drug use and accident prevention.
- Neighbourhood regeneration and renewal-maximizing the role of active healthy older people

Questions for further discussion

- What are the advantages and disadvantages of measuring health as:
  A negative variable (health is not being ill)?

A positive variable (health is positive well-being)?

- What are the dilemmas of measuring health as an objective or a subjective phenomenon?
- Thinking of your own work, how can you most usefully measure health?

Summary

This chapter has examined the reasons for attempting to measure health, and demonstrated that the most commonly used measures of health are in fact measures of ill health, disease and premature death. Recently there has been more activity directed towards trying to find ways of measuring health as an independent positive variable in its own right. Different approaches have been taken, including attempts to combine the measurement of health as an objective property of people or environments with the measurement of health as it is subjectively experienced and interpreted by people. These different approaches have been identified and described.

Further reading

Bowling A 2005 Measuring health: a review of quality of life measurement scales, 3rd edn. Open University Press, Milton Keynes. *A detailed and comprehensive account of the different ways of measuring health and their comparative validity and reliability. Health measures include subjective measures of function, health status and psychological health as well as social health, life satisfaction and quality of life.*

Crichton N 2008 Epidemiology. In: Naidoo J, Wills J (eds) Health studies: an introduction. Palgrave Macmillan, Basingstoke. *A concise and readable introduction to epidemiological theories and methods, including features designed to help the reader reflect on the material and relate it to their own concerns.*

Sidell M, Lloyd CE 2007 Studying the population's health. In: Earle S, Lloyd CE, Sidell M et al (eds) Theory and research in promoting public health. Sage/Open University, London, chapter 8. *A thorough and comprehensive account of how knowledge about the health of human populations is produced, focusing particularly on quantitative data, demography and epidemiology.*

Unwin N, Carr S, Leeson J et al 1997 An introductory study guide to public health and epidemiology. Open University Press, Buckingham. *A basic introduction to epidemiology which explains core concepts in a simple and readable form.*

References

Adler N, Singh-Manoux A, Schwartz J et al 2007 Social status and health: A comparison of British civil servants in Whitehall-11 with European- and African-Americans in CARDIA. Social Science and Medicine 66: 1034–1045.

Allin P 2007 Measuring societal wellbeing. Economic and Labour Market Review 1: 10.

Antonovsky A 1987 Unravelling the mystery of health: how people manage stress and stay well. Jossey-Bass, San Francisco.

Baldwin S, Godfrey C, Propper C 1990 Quality of life: perspectives and policies. Routledge, London.

Bartley M 2004 Health inequality – an introduction to theories, concepts and methods. Polity, Cambridge.

Bethune A 1997 Unemployment and mortality. In: Drever F, Whitehead M (eds) Health inequalities: decennial supplement. Stationery Office, London.

Blaxter M 1990 Health and lifestyles. Routledge, London.

Bowling A 1997 Measuring health: a review of quality of life measurement scales. Open University Press, Buckinghamshire.

Brown J, Bowling A, Flynn T N 2004 Models of quality of life: a taxonomy and systematic review of the literature. Report commissioned by the European Forum on Population Ageing Research/Quality of Life. University of Sheffield, Sheffield.

Catford J 1983 Positive health indicators – towards a new information base for health promotion. Community Medicine 5: 125–132.

Crichton N 2008 Epidemiology. In: Naidoo J, Wills J (eds) Health studies: an introduction. Palgrave Macmillan, Basingstoke.

Department of Health 1999 Saving lives: Our healthier nation (white paper). Stationery Office, London.

Department of Health 2004 The health survey for England 2003. Stationery Office, London.

Department of Health 2005 Tackling health inequalities: status report on the programme for action. Stationery Office, London.

Filmer D, Pritchett L 1999 The impact of public spending on health: does money matter? Social Science and Medicine 49: 1309–1323.

Floud R 1989 Measuring European inequality: the use of height data. In: Fox J (ed) Health inequalities in European countries. Gower, Aldershot, pp. 231–249.

Goldberg D P, Gater R, Sartorius N et al 1997 The validity of two versions of the GHQ in the WHO study of mental illness in general health care. Psychological Medicine 27: 191–197.

Herzlich C 1973 Health and illness. Academic Press, London.

Kawachi I, Kennedy B P, Lochner D et al 1997 Social capital, income inequality and mortality. American Journal of Public Health 87: 1491–1498.

Lantz P M, Lynch J W, House J S et al 2001 Socioeconomic disparities in health change in a longitudinal study of US adults: the role of health-risk behaviours. Social Science and Medicine 53: 29–40.

Lock K 2000 Health impact assessment. British Medical Journal 320: 1395–1398.

Macinko J, Starfield B, Shi L 2003 The contribution of primary care systems to health outcomes within Organization for Economic Cooperation and Development (OECD) countries 1970–1998. Health Services Research 38: 831–865.

Moser K A, Goldblatt P, Fox J et al 1990 Unemployment and mortality. In: Goldblatt P (ed) Longitudinal study: mortality and social organization. OPCS series LS no. 6. HMSO, London.

Navarro V, Muntaner C, Borrell C et al 2006 Politics and health outcomes. Lancet 368: 1033–1037.

Paldam M 2001 Social capital: one or many? Definition and measurement. In: Sayer S (ed) Issues in new political economy. Blackwell, Oxford, pp. 117–143.

Putnam R 2001 Social capital: measurement and consequences. Isuma, Canadian Journal of Policy Research 2: 41–51.

Rose G 1981 Strategy of prevention: lessons from cardiovascular disease. British Medical Journal 282: 1847–1851.

Shakespeare T, Watson N 1997 Defending the social model. In: Barton L, Oliver M (eds) Disability studies: past, present and future. The Disability Press, Leeds, pp. 263–273.

Thompson S, Abdallah S, Marks N et al 2007 The European happy planet index: an index of carbon efficiency and well-being in the UK. New Economic Foundation/ Friends of the Earth. Available online at: www.foe.co.uk/ resource/reports/euro_happy_planet_index.pdf

Townsend P, Phillimore P, Beattie A 1987 Health and deprivation: inequality and the North. Croom Helm, London.

Townsend P, Davidson N, Whitehead M 1988 Inequalities in health: the Black report and the health divide. Penguin, Harmondsworth.

Unwin N, Carr S, Leeson J et al 1997 An introductory study guide to public health and epidemiology. Open University Press, Buckingham.

Veenhoven R 1996 Happy life-expectancy. Social Indicators Research 39: 1–58.

Ware J E, Sherbourne C D 1992 The MOS 36-item short-form health survey (SF-36): 1: conceptual framework and item selection. Medical Care 30: 473–483.

White M 1991 Against unemployment. Policy Studies Institute, London.

Wilkinson R G 1996 Unhealthy societies: the afflictions of inequality. Routledge, London.

World Health Organization 1980 International classification of impairments, disabilities and handicaps. WHO, Geneva.

World Health Organization 1985 Targets for health for all. WHO Regional Office for Europe, Copenhagen.

World Health Organization 1992 The international classification of diseases, injuries and causes of death (ICD-10), 10th edn. WHO, Geneva.

World Health Organization 2001 International classification of functioning, disability and health. WHO, Geneva.

Defining health promotion

Key points

- The development of health promotion
- Definitions of health education and health promotion and the relationship between them
- Definition of public health
- The role of the World Health Organization in health promotion

OVERVIEW

The process of attempting to promote health may include a whole range of interventions including:

- Those which foster healthy lifestyles
- Those which encourage access to services and involvement in health decisions
- Those which seek to promote an environment in which the healthy choice becomes the easier choice
- Those which educate about the body and keeping healthy.

Until the 1980s most of these interventions were referred to as 'health education' and the practice was almost exclusively located within preventive medicine or, to a lesser extent, education. In recent years, the term health promotion has become widely used. There is no agreed consensus on what health promotion is or what health promoters do when they try to promote health, nor what a successful outcome

might be. Many professions, including nursing, have found health promotion to be part of an expanding job description. This development reflects the arguments presented in this book, that it is health and not illness or disease which should underpin health care work. Yet what practitioners do in the name of health promotion varies enormously. This chapter outlines the historical development of health promotion and considers different views on the purpose, the nature and the scope of health promotion practice.

Foundations of health promotion

The term health promotion is a recent one used for the first time in the mid-1970s (Lalonde 1974) and the Alma Ata conference (World Health Organization 1978) is cited as setting the agenda for health promotion. Its foundations are complex and differ between countries and regions but in general arose from:

- A change in perceptions of the determinants of health and shift away from the tendency to equate health simply with health care services
- The shift from communicable to chronic diseases attributable to people's lifestyles
- An awareness of the potential of primary health care as a first line for prevention and treatment.

The term health promotion is used in a number of different ways, often without any clarification of meaning. In 1985 when the term was becoming widely adopted, Tannahill (1985) described it as a meaningless concept because it was used so differently. Over a decade later, Seedhouse (1997) describes the field of health promotion as muddled, poorly articulated and devoid of a clear philosophy. These early understandings reflect the origins of health promotion and range from:

- 'Slick salesmanship of health' (Williams 1984)
- 'Attempts to persuade, cajole or otherwise influence individuals to alter their lifestyle' (Gott & O'Brien 1990)
- 'Any combination of education and related legal, fiscal, economic, environmental and organisational interventions designed to facilitate the achievement of health and the prevention of disease' (Tones 1990)
- 'An approach and philosophy of care which reflects awareness of the multiplicity of factors which affect health and which encourages everyone to value independence and individual choice' (Wilson-Barnett 1993).

More recently, health promotion is defined by building on the Ottawa Charter (World Health Organization 1986) definition, as Nutbeam (1988, pp. 1–2) explains:

Health promotion represents a comprehensive social and political process. It not only embraces actions directed at strengthening the skills and capabilities of individuals, but also actions directed towards changing social, environmental and economic conditions so as to alleviate their
impact on public and individual health. Health promotion is the process of enabling people to take control over the determinants of their health and thereby improve their health.

Box 4.1

- What do you consider to be the main features of health education?
- And what do you consider the main features of health promotion?
- Is your work mostly health education or health promotion?

A shared understanding of the meaning and purpose of health promotion is elusive. A diversity of disciplinary and ideological perspectives and policy changes has resulted in apparently conflicting conceptualizations. Health promotion as a concept can thus be understood as:

- A discrete discipline that draws from other disciplines (e.g. psychology, education, sociology) to understand a particular problem (Naidoo & Wills 2008)
- A process or way of working that seeks to empower individuals and groups by enabling them to address their own needs and valuing their experience (Naidoo & Wills 2005)
- A field of activity that includes supporting people to develop personal health skills, fostering public participation, building partnerships, coordinating policy and strategy (Department of Health/ Welsh Assembly 2005).

Origins of health promotion in the UK

The first phase of health promotion development is known as the 'social hygiene period' with roots in both public health and health education. Its origins of health promotion lie in the 19th century when epidemic disease eventually led to pressure for sanitary reform for the overcrowded industrial towns. Alongside the public health movement emerged the idea of educating the public for the good of its health. The Medical Officers of Health appointed to each town under the Public Health legislation of 1848 frequently disseminated every-day health advice on safeguards against 'contagion'. Voluntary associations were also formed, including the London Statistical Society (1839), the Health of Towns Association (1842) and the Sanitary Institute (1876). The temperance movement held Band of Hope mass meetings, and through schools and churches lectured to young people on the virtue of abstinence. By the 1920s health education had become associated with diarrhoea, dirt, spitting and venereal disease! The evidence that between 10% and 20% of soldiers in the First World War had con-tracted venereal disease led to propaganda, one-off lectures and the first of 'shock-horror' techniques in which soldiers were shown lurid pictures of diseased genitals to dissuade them from having sex (Blythe 1986; Welshman 1997).

The second phase of health promotion devel-opment is known as the 'personal services' period. Changing patterns of morbidity and mortality shifted attention away from disease to personal behaviour. The Central Council for Health Education was established in 1927, paid for by local authority pub-lic health departments, and public health doctors formed the majority of its membership. An extract from some of the tasks listed as important reflects an emphasis on information, and education to bring about change in personal habits and behaviour:

- The provision of better and cheaper posters and leaflets
- The provision of exhibits for exhibition
- The production of a readable monthly bulletin
- The provision of a panel of lecturers who really could lecture and hold an audience.

The Central Council was principally concerned with propaganda and instruction. During the Second World War it delivered 3799 lectures on sex education and venereal disease which were attended by 340 000 people (Amos 1993). A database of health education film synopses is held by the British Film Institute (at http://www.ftvdb.bfi.org.uk/sift/organization/9345http://ftvdb.bfi.org.uk/sift/organi-zation/9345) and confirms the emphasis on propa-ganda and instruction.

> **Box 4.2**
>
> **Health education**
> - Health education slogans were produced in the 1920s by insurance companies keen to reduce health insurance claims:
>   - 'Have a hot bath at least once a week'
>   - 'Moderation in all things – every hour you steal from digestion will be reclaimed by indigestion'
>   - 'Cultivate cheerfulness, hopefulness of mind and evenness of temper which are the most wonderful of remedial agencies'
>   - 'Do not spit – it dries in the dust and other people breathe it in'.

The Health Education Council (HEC), which was set up in 1968 as a quango – a quasi-autonomous non-governmental organization – reflected the Department of Health and Social Security's, as it then was, medical model of health. The members were drawn from public health, and the medical and dental professions, with the inclusion of advertising and consumer affairs representatives. Its brief was to create a 'climate of opinion generally favourable to health education, develop blanket programmes of education and selected priority subjects' (Cohen Committee 1964). Similar health education agen-cies were set up in Wales, Scotland and Northern Ireland.

The HEC came to be associated with mass pub-licity campaigns such as Look After Yourself (LAY) which was launched in 1978. LAY reflected the view that people could be encouraged to adopt lifestyles which would lead to better health. The lead agency for health education in England consistently emphasized such mass campaigns and short-term initiatives. Sutherland, the first director of education and training at the HEC, has vividly described the pressures and lobbying which led the HEC away from confrontation with vested interests, such as agriculture or tobacco, and kept it confined to mass-media campaigns despite evidence of their limited effect (Sutherland 1987).

By the 1970s there was an increasing recognition that health policy could not continue to be confined to clinical and medical services, which were both proving expensive and not improving the health status of the population. Health education and the prevention of disease represented a means of cutting costs and an ideology which could place the onus of responsibility on the individual.

 Box 4.3

Health as an individual responsibility
The government document *Prevention and Health: Everybody's Business* (Department of Health and Social Security 1976) was published in 1976 and encapsulated a behavioural approach which saw health problems as the result of individual lifestyles.

> *To a large extent though, it is clear that the weight of responsibility for his own health lies on the shoulders of the individual himself. The smoking-related diseases, alcoholism and other drug dependencies, obesity and its consequences, and the sexually transmitted diseases are among the preventable problems of our time and, in relation to all of these, the individual must decide for himself (Department of Health and Social Security 1976).*

The message of the document is that improving health depends on individuals changing the way they live in order to avoid 'lifestyle' diseases. A decade later, in 1987, a similar message was put forward

by the White Paper *Promoting Better Health* which suggested that the major killer diseases could be avoided if people took greater responsibility for their own health (Department of Health 1987). The *Health of the Nation* strategy was also permeated by a philosophy of individualism despite the acknowledgement in the strategy that 'responsibilities for action are widely spread from individuals to government' (Department of Health 1992). Later White Papers in England, *Saving Lives: Our Healthier Nation* (Department of Health 1999) and *Choosing Health: Making Healthier Choices Easier* (Department of Health 2004) similarly look to individuals to make informed decisions about their health. The latter document highlighted the following behavioural priorities:

- Reducing the numbers who smoke
- Tackling obesity
- Improving sexual health
- Improving mental health and well-being
- Reducing alcohol-related harm and encouraging sensible drinking.

Alongside this government response, however, was the awareness that poor health was linked to poverty. In 1980 the Black report, commissioned by the government, showed how those in lower social classes had a far higher risk of dying prematurely than more advantaged groups (Townsend & Davidson 1982). The HEC commissioned a further study on inequality, *Inequalities in Health: The Black Report and the Health Divide* (Townsend et al 1992). The report was published on a national holiday in August, ostensibly to avoid publicity, so damning was its evidence on the extent of poverty and deprivation. The last three decades have seen a re-emergence of public health measures and a recognition of the need to address the social, economic and environmental determinants of health. The Acheson report (HM Government 1998), commissioned by an incoming Labour government, recommended that as part of health impact assessment, all policies likely to have an impact on health should be formulated in such a way to favour the less well-off. In all countries, making the connection between the social determinants of health and health promotion policy and action is a major task, as discussed by the international Commission on the Social Determinants of Health (http://www.who.int/social_determinants/en/). Developing healthy public policy is the subject of Chapter 11. In many countries however, much of health promotion remains 'downstream', focusing on the behavioural determinants of ill health such as smoking rather than the material factors and sociostructural conditions outlined in Chapter 2.

Public health

In 1920, Winslow Professor of Public Health at Yale University described public health as:

> *The Science and Art of preventing disease, prolonging life, and promoting health and efficiency through organized community effort for:*
> - *The sanitation of the environment*
> - *The control of communicable diseases*
> - *The organization of medical and nursing services for the early diagnosis and preventative treatment of disease*
> - *The development of social machinery to ensure everyone a stand of living adequate for the maintenance of health, so organizing these benefits so as to enable every citizen to enjoy his birthright of health and longevity.*

In the UK health promotion and public health are terms that are often used interchangeably. Health promotion is sometimes distinguished as one of the processes in securing public health. In many countries there is understood to be a clear distinction: public health is the practice of public health medicine with an emphasis on the prevention and control of disease. This distinction is explored in greater detail in our companion volume, *Public Health and Health Promotion: Developing Practice* (Naidoo & Wills 2005).

Historically, public health has been driven by social policy as much as by medicine. The early

public health movement in the 19th century in the UK used a medical scientific model to explain the disease process. The gathering of information and interpretation of quantitative data (epidemiology) was employed to underpin decisions. Social policy interventions were deployed to protect the public and prevent disease (see Chapter 11).

Box 4.4

Many practitioners now have public health included in their job remit, e.g. specialist community nurses, occupational health nurses. How is your role in public health defined?

The UK Faculty of Public Health identifies three domains of public health practice: health improvement, service improvement and health protection. The term health promotion is not included. Instead, the term multidisciplinary public health has become widely adopted, signalling environmental, social and individual health dimensions. Our companion volume (Naidoo & Wills 2005) discusses the similarities and differences between public health and health promotion in more detail.

The World Health Organization and health promotion

The World Health Organization has played a key part in proposing a broader agenda for health promotion. In 1977 the World Health Assembly at Alma Ata committed all member countries to the principles of *Health for All 2000* (HFA 2000: World Health Organization 1977) that there 'should be the attainment by all the people of the world by the year 2000 of a level of health that will permit them to lead a socially and economically productive life'. The World Health Organization made explicit five key principles for health promotion in a discussion paper commonly referred to as the Copenhagen document:

1. It involves the population as a whole in the context of their everyday life, rather than focusing on people at risk for specific diseases.

2. It is directed towards action on the causes or determinants of health to ensure that the total environment which is beyond the control of individuals is conducive to health.

3. It combines diverse, but complementary, methods or approaches, including communication, education, legislation, fiscal measures, organizational change, community development and spontaneous local activities against health hazards.

4. It aims particularly at effective public participation supporting the principle of self-help movements and encouraging people to find their own ways of managing the health of their community.

5. Although health promotion is basically an activity in the health and social fields and not a medical service, health professionals – particularly in primary health care – have an important role in nurturing and enabling health promotion (World Health Organization 1984).

The context for the development of broad-based health strategies thus needed to be based on equity, community participation and intersectoral collaboration, The World Health Organization also identified that improvement in lifestyles, environmental conditions and health care will have little effect if certain fundamental conditions are not met. These include:

• Peace and freedom from the fear of war
• Equal opportunity for all and social justice
• Satisfaction of basic needs, including food and income, safe water and sanitation, housing, secure work and a satisfying role in society
• Political commitment and public support (World Health Organization 1985).

The World Health Organization launched a programme for health promotion in 1984, and conferences at Ottawa (1986), Adelaide (1988), Sundsvall (1991), Jakarta (1997), Mexico (2000) and Bangkok (2003) have further outlined areas for action. The practice and principles of health promotion developed in the Ottawa Charter (World Health Organization 1986) are still widely used to provide a framework for practice:

1. Building a healthy public policy
2. Creating supportive environments
3. Developing personal skills, including information and coping strategies
4. Strengthening community action, including social support and networks
5. Reorienting health services away from treatment and care and improving access to health services.

Box 4.5

What activities might be encompassed in each of these action areas?

Each of these health promotion actions is the subject of a chapter in Part 2 of this book.

The processes of mediation, advocacy and enablement were identified as ways in which health could be promoted. These processes are discussed further below.

Defining health promotion

Disease prevention

In Chapter 1 we saw that there are many different meanings attached to the concept of health but the notion that health is the 'absence of disease' is a dominant one. Different perceptions about the nature of health and the factors contributing to it underpin interpretations of health promotion. The shift from infectious and communicable disease to chronic diseases in the 20th century highlighted the role of people's lifestyles in disease causation. Prevention therefore became much more important, often through targeting high-risk groups who have an increased likelihood of developing a specific disease.

Health promotion is often categorized as concerned with primary, secondary or tertiary prevention.

- Primary prevention seeks to avoid the onset of ill health by the detection of high-risk groups and the provision of advice and counselling. Examples of primary prevention include immunization and cervical cytology as well as health education in schools or workplaces.
- Secondary prevention seeks to change health-damaging behaviour to shorten episodes of illness and prevent the progression of ill health. Examples include education about medication, advice on healthy eating for a diabetic person and relaxation for cardiac patients.
- Tertiary prevention seeks to limit disability or complications arising from a chronic or irreversible condition and enhance quality of life. Examples include education about the use of a disability aid and rehabilitation therapy.

Medical support and symptom control are important to those living with life-threatening illness but so too is enhancing their quality of life.

For those working in a clinical setting, this is the usual interpretation of health promotion. It can differ little from the education of patients about the condition that brought them to the health service. Its aim is for patients to avoid a recurrence by following a treatment regime or some change in their lifestyle and to enhance quality of life when living with a chronic condition. Disease prevention does not, however, look beyond the risk factors or groups to the origins of ill health.

Box 4.6

McKinlay (1979), in persuading us of the need to refocus upstream, tells a story:

There I am standing by the shore of a swiftly flowing river and I hear the cry of a drowning man. So I jump into the river, put my arms around him, pull him to shore and apply artificial respiration. Just when he begins to breathe, there is another cry for help. So

I jump into the river, reach him, pull him to shore, apply artificial respiration, and then just as he begins to breathe, another cry for help. So back in the river again, without end, goes the sequence. You know I am so busy jumping in, pulling them to shore, applying artificial respiration, that I have no time to see who the hell is upstream pushing them all in.

The concept of refocusing upstream is a powerful and persuasive argument for health promotion. It can help us to reorient our thinking from a belief that medical care can, or will, solve most health problems towards prevention.

Box 4.7

- What examples can you think of in your own work of short-term problem-specific activity?
- What would a reorientation upstream involve?
- Who or what do you think is pushing people in?

Figure 4.1 illustrates some specific examples of downstream interventions tackling health behaviours that give rise to problems and upstream interventions tackling the causes of such behaviours.

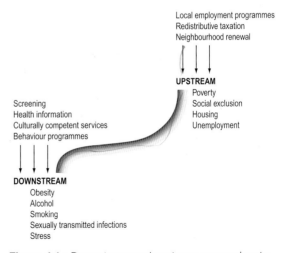

Figure 4.1 • Downstream and upstream approaches to promoting health.

Box 4.8

What would health-promoting palliative care look like?

You might have included the fostering of hope and support, prevention of depression, home help, death education (Kellehear & O'Connor 2008).

Health education

Educating people about their health is commonplace but 'health education' as a formalized activity only emerged in the 1980s. The recognition of the need to diffuse information about the physical and moral 'evils' of squalor and drink can however be dated to the mid 19th century. An awareness that individuals make health choices which can contribute to the development of disease led to the view that it was possible to inform people about the prevention of disease, to motivate them to change their behaviour, through persuasion and mass communication techniques, and to equip them through education with the skills for a healthy lifestyle.

'Traditional' health education was often criticized for its narrow focus on information provision based on the assumption of a simple causation relationship between knowledge and behaviour. The emphasis on individual responsibility for health led to accusations of victim-blaming. Victim-blaming makes individuals feel guilty, although it may be factors beyond their control (poverty, social and environmental factors) that prevent them from making health changes.

Box 4.9

Is health in your hands?

Health education may be defined as planned opportunities for people to learn about health and make changes in their behaviour. It includes:
- Raising awareness of health issues and factors contributing to ill health

- Providing information
- Motivating and persuading people to make changes in their lifestyle for their health
- Equipping people with the skills and confidence to make those changes.

This might be seen as a limited interpretation of a health promotion role confining activity to information, education and communication, as discussed in Chapter 9.

One of the paradoxes of health education and a prevailing professional dilemma is the degree of voluntarism or free choice. Health education is based on an expert authority model derived from both medicine and education. It is the health educator or doctor who decides if there is a health need and the adequacy of an individual's lifestyle, who decides the nature of the intervention and the most effective means of communication, who tries to ensure compliance, and who will decide if the intervention has 'worked'. When we look at the practice of health education, we might be led to believe that health education is the *giving* of information and success in promoting health is when the client follows the advice. For other health educators education is a means of *drawing out*. Clients are not 'empty vessels' who will rationally change their behaviour once provided with the relevant information, advice or guidance. After all, information about the risks to health from smoking has been known since 1963 and information about human immunodeficiency virus (HIV) transmission since 1986, yet people continue to smoke and not use condoms. These health educators seek neither to coerce nor to persuade, both because this is unlikely to be effective but also because it is unethical. The health educator is a facilitator and enabler rather than an expert. Rather than telling clients what to do, the health educator works with them to identify their needs and work towards an informed choice, even when this may lead to health-damaging behaviour. The goal is to empower individuals to take health-related decisions by developing health literacy, self-efficacy, self-esteem and coping skills (Nutbeam 2000; Kickbusch 2001).

Box 4.10

Health literacy may be defined as the capacity of an individual to obtain, interpret and understand basic health information and services in ways that are health enhancing (US Department of Health and Health Services 2000).

Who might be disadvantaged by efforts to improve health literacy?

The concept of health literacy is not new or radical and can be identified in many of the definitions of empowerment. However, it contains a central message that, although knowledge alone is insufficient to achieve change, not understanding the conditions that determine health or knowing how to change them is also de-powering (Abel 2007). We are faced with a society in which there is more choice of foods and other products, more health information from many sources, more choice in patient treatments, more choice of providers. In such a consumer society, Kickbusch (2006) argues active health citizenship is a critical empowerment strategy that enables people to make sense of and discriminate between such choices.

Box 4.11

John is a labourer on the roads. He is 47 and single and his social life revolves around the pub. He drinks a few pints at lunchtime with his sandwiches and usually four pints on the way home. He visits his GP with backache. The GP takes his blood pressure and finds it dangerously high. Do you:

1. Tell him that the recommended drinking limit for adult males is 28 units per week. Stress the damage to his heart and liver and that he risks a heart attack.

2. Discuss the reasons for his drinking behaviour and whether he sees it causing problems.

3. Prescribe medicine to lower his blood pressure and tell him to see the practice nurse in 2 weeks to see if his blood pressure has come down.

This scenario illustrates some of the key tensions in health education:

- Should health education be about telling people what is best for them?
- Are health educators failing in their role if they accept their clients' health-damaging behaviour?
- Who should determine what constitutes a healthy life – practitioner or client?
- Should health behaviour and its effects be seen as a matter of individual choice?

These issues are discussed further in Chapter 6 on ethical issues and Chapter 11 on developing healthy public policy.

The two strands of voluntarism and authoritarianism reflect the historical development of health education, as educationists and social scientists challenged the mainstream of preventive medicine by contesting the assumption that health education could, or indeed should, seek to bring about behaviour change through information or persuasion. Thus emerged the principle of self-empowerment which many argue is central to the practice of health education (Tones & Tilford 2001). Empowerment is an approach which enables people to take charge of their lives, including changing their behaviour if they so wish. Tones (1986) argues that an essential element of health education is 'critical consciousness-raising' to raise people's awareness of the fundamental causes of ill health, a notion first espoused by the Brazilian priest Paolo Freire. Only through this process can the structural influence on health be addressed (see Chapter 5 for a discussion of Tones' model of health promotion) and policy change be pursued and accepted.

Box 4.12

Is enabling people to make informed choices the goal of health promotion?

The underlying principle of health education is to facilitate people to make their own choices about health behaviour. For those who believe the roots of ill health lie in social structures, this emphasis on choice is merely illusory. In Chapter 6 we shall explore further the limits to freedom of choice and how far an ethical principle such as the promotion of autonomy can govern our practice as health educators.

The range of approaches to health education are outlined and discussed in the following chapter. They range from the medical model, focusing on health surveillance and achieving behaviour change, to the educational model, which relies on the exploration of attitudes and values. Alongside these are the approaches more closely aligned to health promotion, such as community development, which emphasizes the need to take collective action for health, and a social model which focuses on the need to influence decision-makers at local and national level.

Health promotion

The World Health Organization has moved the definition of health promotion away from prevention of specific diseases or the detection of risk groups towards the health and well-being of whole populations. Instead of experts and professionals diagnosing problems, the people themselves define health issues of relevance to them in their local community. Teachers, primary health care workers, workplace managers, social and welfare workers can all be involved in promoting health. Instead of health being seen as the responsibility of individuals alone, the social factors determining health are taken into account, and health is viewed as a collective responsibility of society which needs to be prioritized by organizations and government in their decision-making.

Box 4.13

Consider these descriptions of the work of a nurse on an acute medical ward and a health promotion adviser working with young people. Would you consider them to be practising health education or health promotion? What criteria do you use to make your judgement?

- 'Patient education for coronary care is carried out one to one with information booklets. The overall aim is to alleviate anxiety, promote recovery and educate about the cause of the attack to get the patient back to normal and even healthier. Patients may be given factual information about the working of the heart, be taught relaxation exercises and encouraged to talk about concerns such as sex after a heart attack. They will be educated about their medication, how to eat healthily, keeping their weight down and curbing their cholesterol intake, and ways to increase physical activity.'

- 'Health education in schools passes on knowledge, allows for discussion and leads to understanding. It gives young people the freedom to choose and make health decisions and at the same time it asserts an appreciation and respect for the choices of others. The end result should lead to positive pleasure for the young person whilst enabling him or her to remain healthy and disease-free'.

A key difference between these two interventions is their aims. In the coronary care unit, the nurse is actively engaged in disease prevention – to prevent a further heart attack. In the school, the health promotion adviser aims to equip young people with the information and skills for a healthy lifestyle. In both cases, the health promoter aims for behaviour change, more obviously so in the coronary care unit. Both use similar educational methods of providing information, encouraging clients to reflect on their attitudes and experience, and providing opportunities to practise skills.

The terms health education and health promotion are often used interchangeably but, whilst health promotion can be seen as an umbrella term incorporating aspects of health education, it is much broader in concept.

Health promotion incorporates all measures deliberately designed to promote health and handle disease ... A major feature of health promotion is undoubtedly the importance of 'healthy public policy' with its potential for achieving social change via legislation, fiscal, economic and other forms of 'environmental engineering' (Tones 1990).

There are, as we saw in Chapter 2, a range of factors which influence people's health. Some are material–structural and some are behavioural. These need to be addressed other than by education alone. Health promotion thus involves public policy change and community action to enable people to make changes in their lives. A phrase first coined by Milio (1986) has come to encapsulate health promotion – 'making the healthy choice the easier choice' – and was adopted as the strapline for the Public Health Strategy for England (Department of Health 2004). As we have seen, it is easy for practitioners to confine their health promotion role to offering information and advice on how to adopt a healthier lifestyle. However, for people to make such changes, the factors and situations which led them to adopt 'unhealthy' behaviours need to be addressed. People may smoke because of stress, even though they know it is bad for their health. Others may use an illegal drug because it is widely used by their peer group and is part of their social life. Equally, it is easier for some people to make healthy choices than it is for others. It is easy to eat a diet with fresh fruit and vegetables for people with reasonable incomes who have easy access to supermarkets or high-street

shopping. Some factors affecting individual health are outside individual control: inadequate housing, busy roads, lack of child care.

Box 4.14

School nurses were concerned that a high proportion of children's packed lunches contained fizzy drinks, jam sandwiches, crisps and a chocolate bar. How can the healthy choice be made an easier choice?

Schools are cautious about giving advice to parents as they don't want to be seen as interfering. Advice can be given in leaflets and children encouraged to prepare food in cook–eat sessions. Personal social and health education (PSHE) sessions could include discussions of what makes a healthy lunch and why it is important.

Nutritional standards for school meals were introduced in 2006 in all UK countries and 'junk food' was removed from vending machines. The 'healthy choice' thus became a necessary one. The dilemma of whether policy measures such as this are coercive is discussed in Chapter 6.

Box 4.15

The new methods of health promotion are introducing new forms of social regulation which are not ostensibly oppressive or obviously controlling. In these, often innocuous-looking forms, they nevertheless enter and regulate our lives in new ways and bring with them new concerns for our civil liberties and rights (Bunton 1992).

Think of some examples of social regulation aimed to promote health. Do you share this concern at the extension of health promotion into areas beyond 'health'?

An integrated definition of health promotion

Although health promotion is part of national efforts to improve health, its rejection of a disease-oriented pathogenic model of health differentiates it from medical approaches. Its goals derive from a positive, salutogenic concept of health and well-being (as discussed in Chapter 1). Its methods are empowering, 'enabling individuals and groups to have a say in how their health is promoted and valuing their perspective; supporting people to acquire the skills and confidence to take greater control over their health' (Naidoo & Wills 2005, p. 14).

In practice, health promotion encompasses different political orientations which can be characterized as the individual versus structural approaches. For some, health promotion is a narrow field of activity which seems to explain health status by reference to individual lifestyles and is a process largely determined by an expert who advises on beneficial changes. In its emphasis on personal responsibility it sees a minimal role for the state and, thus, has come to be associated with a conservative viewpoint. For others, including the World Health Organization, health promotion recognizes that health and wealth are inextricably linked, and seeks to address the root causes of ill health and problems of inequity using radical and challenging approaches (www.who.int/social_determinants/en/).

It is not helpful to debate whether one form of activity is better or worse than the other: both are necessary. Health promotion may involve lobbying and political advocacy, but it may just as easily involve working with individuals and groups to enhance their knowledge and understanding of the factors affecting their health.

Health education has become equated with persuasive attempts to manipulate behaviour but this is a narrow interpretation and ignores its importance as a core element of health promotion. Tones & Green (2004) propose the term new health education to refocus understanding and activity to education that enables individuals and communities to achieve greater control over their health.

Many practitioners believe that their role is limited in achieving the social changes necessary to eliminate health inequalities or the community change necessary to provide social support. Yet there are ways in which individual practitioners can promote health over and beyond merely informing, advising or listening. The World Health Organization identifies three ways in which practitioners can promote health through their work: advocacy, enablement and mediation.

Advocacy

Advocacy in health promotion is the process of defending or promoting a cause. It may mean representing the interests of disadvantaged groups and may mean speaking on their behalf or lobbying to influence policy. It may also mean action to gain political commitment, policy support, social acceptance and systems support for a particular goal or cause. For example, health promotion networks in Australia, New Zealand, the USA and Canada have long advocated for a focus on the health of indigenous peoples.

Box 4.16

- To what extent do you work 'on behalf of' clients or the public?
- Do you regard advocacy as part of your health promotion role?

Enablement

Enabling means that health promotion practitioners take action in partnership with others to promote health by identifying needs and developing networks and resources in the community; assisting people to develop knowledge and skills; and helping people identify and address the determinants of their own health. Enablement is an essential core skill for health promoters since it requires them to act as a catalyst and then stand aside, giving control to the community (see Chapter 10 for further discussion of working with communities).

Mediation

Health promoters mediate between different interests by providing evidence and advice to local groups and by influencing local and national policy through lobbying, media campaigns and participation in working groups.

In the definitions of health promotion so far, health promotion has been interpreted as a process of improving the health of individuals or community. It can also be seen as a set of values or principles. The World Health Organization identifies these as empowerment, equity, collaboration and participation. These values should be incorporated in all health and welfare work for it to be health-promoting (Naidoo & Wills 2005).

 Box 4.17

To what extent do you encourage participation and enable your clients to take more control over their health?

Health promotion is thus an integrating approach to identifying and doing health work. Cribb & Dines (1993) argue that 'the central question is not what is the domain of health promotion but is this being done in a health-promoting way? And this is a question that can be asked about any and every example of practice, not merely those which are clearly aimed at disease prevention or health education.'

To accept such a definition means there can be no boundaries to health promotion since any situation or event between client and practitioner has the potential to be health-promoting.

 Box 4.18

What would you define as health-promoting aspects of your contact with clients? You might have included:
• Listening in an open way to a client's views and using as a starting point his or her knowledge, attitudes and beliefs

• Taking opportunities to be positive about the client's achievements and abilities
• Making links between the client's situation and those of others in the community
• Providing information about informal support available in the community
• Negotiating future action with the client to ensure that it is reasonable, appropriate and realistic.

Conclusion

Many health workers are strongly committed to health education and the promotion of health. However, this has often been manifested in one-to-one programmes limited to providing information. Many may be daunted by the broad definition of health promotion and feel that this broad approach is beyond their professional remit. Indeed, it would not be possible for any one worker or group to bring about the changes needed for a health-promoting society. It is important that we remind ourselves of the World Health Organization view which describes the process of promoting health as not only involving political change and interagency collaboration, but also enabling people to take more control over their own health and equipping them with the means for well-being. Health promotion thus includes increasing individual knowledge about the functions of the body and ways of preventing illness, raising competence in using the health care system, and raising awareness and strengthening community action about the political and environmental factors that influence health.

 Box 4.19

Britain has one of the highest rates of teenage pregnancy in Europe. The under-18 conception rate dropped by 11.8% between 1998 and 2005 and now is at its lowest for 20 years.

The conception rate for under-16s in 2005 was 7.8 per 1000 which means 7462 girls under 16 getting pregnant each year: 57% of these led to legal termination (Teenage Pregnancy Unit 2007).

Which of the following aims for a health promotion intervention around teenage pregnancy would come closest to your own?

- Reduce teenage pregnancy rates.
- Educate young people about the risks of under-age sex.
- Support and advise young mothers.
- Improve access to services and contraceptive advice.
- Raise awareness of sexual health among teenagers.
- Enable young people to make informed and confident choices about their sexual health.

Which of the following activities would you consider a priority for a health promotion intervention? Why?

- Run a youth counselling drop-in service.
- Work with teachers to develop a sex education curriculum.
- Give talks at local schools.
- Open a young people's session at the family planning clinic.
- Write a leaflet on contraception.
- Research the pattern and trends of teenage pregnancies in the area.
- Set up a teenage mothers' group.
- Set up an information stall on the local market.
- Set up an interagency group with employers, housing, education and leisure services to discuss young people's needs.
- Lobby the health authority to provide free condoms for all clubs and leisure centres.

- Run a training course for doctors on counselling young people (Health Development Agency 2003).

Questions for further discussion

- Is it useful to try to distinguish between health education and health promotion? Which term would you choose to describe your work in improving people's health?

- How do you explain the emphasis on health promotion in contemporary health care work?

Summary

This chapter has looked at the origins of health promotion and shown how different interpretations arise from different origins. It has shown that health promotion is a broad term encompassing interventions which differ in aims and purpose and in the role accorded to the practitioner. It may be seen as a set of activities clearly intended to prevent disease and ill health, to educate people to a healthier lifestyle, or to address the wider social and environmental factors which influence people's health. It may also be seen as a set of principles to orient health work towards addressing inequality and promoting collaboration and participation. Health promoters thus need to be clear in their understanding of what health is, what aspect of health is being promoted and the ways in which health is affected by wider influences than individual behaviour.

Further reading

Bunton R, Macdonald G 2002 Health promotion: disciplines and diversity, 2nd edn. Routledge, London. *An interesting collection of contributions which traces the theoretical roots of health promotion through the disciplines of psychology, sociology, education and epidemiology.*

Keleher H, MacDougall C, Murphy B 2007 Understanding health promotion. Oxford University Press, Melbourne. *An interesting Australian textbook that applies equity approaches to health promotion.*

MacDonald T H 1998 Rethinking health promotion: a global approach. Routledge, London. *A discussion of the relationship between biomedicine and health promotion. Not easy reading, but stimulating.*

Nutbeam D 1998 A health promotion glossary. Available at http://www.who.int/hpr/NPH/docs/hp_glossary_en.pdf

Scriven A, Garman S (eds) 2005 Promoting health global perspectives. Palgrave Macmillan, Basingstoke. *A collection of views on the challenges facing the promotion of health around the globe.*

Seedhouse D 1997 Health promotion: philosophy, prejudice and practice. Wiley, Chichester. *A stimulating, personal analysis of the conceptual roots of health promotion.*

Tones K, Green J 2004 Health promotion planning and strategies. Sage, London. *A useful textbook which includes thoughtful and provocative discussion on the goals and methods.*

National health promotion agencies or associations can provide useful insight into health promotion work. See for example:

Northern Ireland: www.healthpromotionagency.org.uk

Scotland: www.healthscotland.com

Wales: www.wales.gov.uk/subsite/healthchallenge

Australia: www.healthpromotion.org.au

New Zealand: www.hpforum.org.nz

Canada: www.canadian-health-networks.ca

USA: odphp.osophs.dhhs.gov

Journals can also be helpful. For example:

American Journal of Health Promotion

Critical Public Health

Health Education Research

Health Promotion International

Health Promotion Journal of Australia

Scandinavian Journal of Health Promotion

The Ottawa charter can be donloaded from the WHO website at: http://www.who.int/hpr/NPH/docs/ottawa_charter_hp.pdf

References

Abel T 2007 Cultural capital in health promotion. In: McQueen D V, Kickbush I (eds) Health and modernity: the role of theory in health promotion. Springer, New York.

Amos A 1993 In her own best interests: women and health education, a review of the last 50 years. Health Education Journal 52: 3.

Blythe M 1986 A century of health education. Health and Hygiene 7: 105–115.

Bunton R 1992 More than a woolly jumper: health promotion as social regulation. Critical Public Health 3: 4–11.

Cohen Committee 1964 Health education. Report of a joint committee of the Central and Scottish Health Services Councils. HMSO, London.

Cribb A, Dines A 1993 What is health promotion? In: Dines A, Cribb A (eds) Health promotion: concepts and practice. Blackwell Scientific, Oxford.

Department of Health 1987 Promoting better health. HMSO, London.

Department of Health 1992 The health of the nation. HMSO, London.

Department of Health 1999 Saving lives: our healthier nation (White paper). Stationery Office, London.

Department of Health 2004 Choosing health: making healthier choice easier. Stationery Office, London.

Department of Health and Social Security 1976 Prevention and health; everybody's business. HMSO, London.

Department of Health/Welsh Assembly 2005 Shaping the future of public health. Promoting health in the NHS: delivering Choosing Health and Health Challenge Wales. Stationery Office, London.

Gott M, O'Brien M 1990 Attitudes and beliefs in health promotion. Nursing Standard 5: 30–32.

Health Development Agency 2003 Teenage pregnancy and parenthood: a review of reviews. Evidence based briefing. HDA, London.

Health Education Authority (HEA) 1998 Reducing the rate of teenage conceptions: an overview of the effectiveness of interventions and programmes aimed at reducing unintended conceptions in young people. HEA, London.

HM government 1998 Independent inquiry into inequalities in health (Acheson report). Stationery Office, London.

Kellehear A, O'Connor D 2008 Health promoting palliative care. Critical Public Health 18: 111–115.

Kickbusch I 2001 Health literacy: addressing the health and education divide. Health Promotion International 16: 289–297.

Kickbusch I 2006 Ottawa – challenges we face. Presentation. Available at www.specialisedhealthpromotion.org.uk/downloads/kickbuschlondonnov2006.ppt

Lalonde M 1974 A new perspective on the health of Canadians. Government of Canada, Ottawa.

McKinlay J B 1979 A case for refocussing upstream: the political economy of health. In: Jaco E G (ed) Patients, physicians and illness. Macmillan, Basingstoke.

Milio N 1986 Promoting health through public policy. Canadian Public Health Association, Ottawa.

Naidoo J, Wills J 2005 Public health and health promotion: developing practice. Baillière Tindall, London.

Naidoo J, Wills J 2008 Health studies: an introduction, 2nd edn. Palgrave Macmillan, Basingstoke.

Nutbeam D 1998 Health promotion glossary. World Health Organization, Geneva.

Nutbeam D 2000 Health literacy as a public health goal: a challenge for contemporary health education and communication strategies into the 21st century. Health Promotion International 15: 259–267.

Seedhouse D 1997 Health promotion: philosophy, prejudice and practice. Wiley, Chichester.

Sutherland I 1987 Health education: half a policy. National Extension College, Cambridge.

Tannahill A 1985 What is health promotion? Health Education Journal 44: 4.

Teenage Pregnancy Unit 2007 Teenage conception statistics for England 1998–2005. TPU, London.

Tones B K 1986 Health education and the ideology of health promotion: a review of alternative approaches. Health Education Research 1: 3–12.

Tones K 1990 Why theorise: ideology in health education. Health Education Journal 49: 1.

Tones K, Green J 2004 Health promotion planning and strategies. Sage, London.

Tones K, Tilford S 2001 Health education: effectiveness, efficiency, equity, 3rd edn. Nelson Thornes, Cheltenham.

Townsend P, Davidson N 1982 Inequalities in health: the Black report. Penguin, Harmondsworth.

Townsend P, Whitehead M, Davidson N 1992 (eds) Inequalities in health: the Black Report and the Health Divide, 2nd edn. Penguin, London.

US Department of Health and Human Services 2000 Healthy people 2010. Available at http://www.healthypeople.gov/default.htm

Welshman J 1997 Bringing beauty and brightness to the back streets: health education and public health in England and Wales 1890–1940. Health Education Journal 56: 199–209.

Williams G 1984 Health promotion – caring concern or slick salesmanship. Journal of Medical Ethics 10: 191–195.

Wilson-Barnett J 1993 The meaning of health promotion: a personal view. In: Wilson-Barnett J, Macleod Clark K (eds) Research in health promotion and nursing. Macmillan, Basingstoke.

Winslow C E A 1920 The untilled field of public health. Modern Medicine 2: 183–191.

World Health Organization 1977 Health for all by the year 2000. World Health Organization, Geneva.

World Health Organization 1978 Declaration of Alma Ata, international conference on primary health care, Alma Ata, 6–12 September. World Health Organization, Geneva.

World Health Organization 1984 Health promotion: a discussion document on concepts and principles. World Health Organization, Geneva.

World Health Organization 1985 Targets for health for all. World Health Organization, Geneva.

World Health Organization 1986 Ottawa charter for health promotion. World Health Organization, Geneva.

Chapter Five

Models and approaches to health promotion

Key points

- Different approaches to health promotion:
  - Medical
  - Behaviour change
  - Educational
  - Empowerment
  - Social change
- Aspects of these approaches:
  - Aims
  - Methods
  - Means of evaluation
- The importance of theory in health promotion
- Different models of health promotion

OVERVIEW

The diversity in concepts of health, influences on health and ways of measuring health lead, not surprisingly, to a number of different approaches to health promotion. Chapter 4 began to explore the concepts of health education and health promotion. In this chapter, five different approaches will be discussed:

1. Medical or preventive
2. Behaviour change
3. Educational
4. Empowerment
5. Social change.

These approaches will be examined in terms of their different aims, methods and means of evaluation. These approaches have different objectives:

- To prevent disease
- To ensure that people are well informed and able to make health choices
- To help people to acquire the skills and confidence to take greater control over their health
- To change policies and environments in order to facilitate healthy choices.

All of the approaches reflect different ways of working. Identifying the different approaches is primarily a descriptive process. The framework is descriptive – it does not indicate which approach is best, nor why a practitioner might adopt one approach rather than another. A number of theoretical frameworks or models of health promotion are outlined, discussed and assessed in relation to practice in the latter part of the chapter.

It is common for a practitioner to think that theory has no place in health promotion and that action is determined by work role and organizational objectives rather than values or ideology. We have argued elsewhere that practitioners should be aware of the values implicit in the approach they adopt: 'Values thus determine the way in which the world is seen and the selection of activities and priorities and how strategies are implemented' (Naidoo & Wills 2005, p. 13).

Models of health promotion are not guides to action but attempts to delineate a contested field of activity and to show how different priorities and strategies reflect different underlying values. They are useful in helping practitioners think through:

- Aims
- Implications of different strategies
- What would count as success
- Own role as a practitioner.

The medical approach

Aims

This approach focuses on activity which aims to reduce morbidity and premature mortality. Activity is targeted towards whole populations or high-risk groups. This kind of health promotion seeks to increase medical interventions which will prevent ill health and premature death. This approach is frequently portrayed as having three levels of intervention:

1. *Primary prevention* – prevention of the onset of disease through risk education, e.g. immunization, encouraging non-smoking.

2. *Secondary prevention* – preventing the progression of disease, e.g. screening and other methods of early diagnosis.

3. *Tertiary prevention* – reducing further disability and suffering in those already ill; preventing recurrence of an illness, e.g. rehabilitation, patient education, palliative care.

The medical approach to health promotion is popular because:

1. It has high status because it uses scientific methods, such as epidemiology (the study of the pattern of diseases in society).

2. In the short term, prevention and the early detection of disease are much cheaper than treatment of people who have become ill. Of course, in the long term, this may not be the case as people live longer and experience degenerative conditions and draw pensions for a longer period.

3. It is an expert-led, or top-down, type of intervention. This kind of activity reinforces the authority of medical and health professionals who are recognized as having the expert knowledge needed to achieve the desired results.

4. There have been spectacular successes in public health as a result of using this approach, for example the worldwide eradication of smallpox as a result of the vaccination programme.

As we have seen in Chapter 1, the medical approach is conceptualized around the absence of disease. It does not seek to promote positive health and can be criticized for ignoring the social and environmental dimensions of health. In addition, the medical approach encourages dependence on medical knowledge and removes health decisions from lay people. Thus, health care workers are encouraged to persuade patients to cooperate and comply with treatment.

Public health medicine is the branch of medicine which specializes in prevention, and most day-to-day preventive work is carried out by the community health services which include specialist community public health nurses and district nurses.

Methods

The principle of preventive services such as immunization and screening is that they are targeted to groups at risk from a particular condition. Whilst immunization requires a certain level of take-up for it to be effective, screening is offered to specific groups. For example, in the UK cervical screening every 3–5 years is offered to all women aged 25–64.

For screening to be effective for the condition or disease:

- The disease should have a long preclinical phase so that a screening test will not miss its signs.
- Earlier treatment should improve the outcomes.
- The test should be sensitive, i.e. it should detect all those with the disease.
- The test should be specific, i.e. it should detect *only* those with the disease.
- It should be cost-effective, i.e. the number of tests performed should yield a number of positive cases, making it an economically sound intervention.

The UK National Screening Committee oversees screening policies and gives advice based on available evidence. For more details visit www.nsc.nhs.uk/uk_nsc.

Preventive procedures need to be based on a sound rationale derived from epidemiological evidence. The medical approach also relies on having an infrastructure capable of delivering screening or an immunization programme. This includes trained personnel, equipment and laboratory facilities, information systems which determine who is eligible for the procedure and record uptake rates, and, in the case of immunization, a vaccine which is effective and safe. It can be seen then that the medical approach to health promotion can be a complex process, and may depend on the establishment of national programmes or guidelines.

Box 5.1

Consider the example of amniocentesis – the testing of the amniotic fluid around a fetus to detect chromosomal abnormalities. Does this test meet the criteria for effective screening outlined above?

In most districts, amniocentesis is only offered to women over the age of 35 and those with a family history of chromosomal abnormality. Yet 80% of children with Down's syndrome are born to mothers under 35 simply because more women in this age group have babies. Amniocentesis is not a simple test. It carries a risk of miscarriage. It can also only be performed after 14–16 weeks of pregnancy when a possible termination is more difficult. It is less than 100% sensitive and therefore some women may go away falsely reassured. A termination and/or counselling is the only intervention available.

Having screening or immunization facilities available is only effective if people can be persuaded to use them.

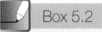

Box 5.2

What methods can you think of that are used to increase the uptake of preventive screening services?

Mass media campaigns can raise awareness but an additional personalized trigger is often needed for people to access screening services. Personal invitations and appointments, telephone calls, telephone counselling and reminders from health care professionals have all been identified as helpful in increasing screening uptake. Removing economic barriers, such as transport or postage costs, can increase uptake in lower-income groups (Jepson et al 2000).

Evaluation

Evaluation of preventive procedures is based ultimately on a reduction in disease rates and associated mortality. This is a long-term process and a more popular measure capable of short-term evaluation is, for example, the increase in the percentage of the target population being screened or immunized.

Although there appears to be a close correlation between immunization uptake and a decline in disease rates, the example of whooping cough suggests some caution is needed. In 1974 80% of children were vaccinated against whooping cough. Following media publicity about the safety of the vaccine, immunization rates fell and did not reach 80% population coverage again until 1987. There were major whooping cough epidemics in 1977–1979 and 1981–1983, suggesting that immunization had contributed to the decline in notifications. However, the overall decline in mortality from whooping cough was occurring before the vaccine was introduced in 1957, suggesting that better nutrition, living conditions and medical care may also be significant.

Box 5.3

The medical approach is not always successful. Recently, whooping cough has re-emerged in countries with high vaccination coverage and low mortality rates (*British Medical Journal* 2002). What could account for this?
You probably included some of the following:
- Underdiagnosis because whooping cough has mild forms and clinicians may not consider whooping cough in older children or adults
- Inadequate methods of diagnosis
- More virulent forms of the bacteria
- Inability to reach infants most at risk, e.g. migrants, travellers, refugees.

Behaviour change

Aims

This approach aims to encourage individuals to adopt healthy behaviours, which are seen as the key to improved health. Chapter 9 shows how making health-related decisions is a complex process and, unless a person is ready to take action, it is unlikely to be effective. As we saw in Chapter 4, seeking to influence or change health behaviour has long been part of health education.

This approach is popular because it views health as a property of individuals. It is then possible to assume that people can make real improvements to their health by choosing to change their lifestyle. It also assumes that if people do not take responsible action to look after themselves then they are to blame for the consequences.

Box 5.4

Consider the reasons why people may not be able to put a healthy diet into practice. Reasons include:
- Lack of information
- Lack of cooking skills
- Lack of money
- Family preferences
- Lack of availability and affordability of healthy foods in local shops ('food deserts')
- Lack of cooking facilities.
Evidence supports some factors, e.g. lack of money (Morris et al 2000). Other factors, e.g. 'food deserts', are more speculative (Cummins & Macintyre 2002).

It is clear that there is a complex relationship between individual behaviour and social and environmental factors. Behaviour may be a response to the conditions in which people live and the causes of these conditions (e.g. unemployment, poverty) are outside individual control.

Methods

The behaviour change approach has been the bedrock of activity undertaken by the lead agencies for health promotion. Campaigns persuade people to desist from smoking, adopt a healthy diet and undertake regular exercise. This approach is targeted towards individuals, although mass means of communication may be used to reach them. It is most commonly an expert-led, top-down approach, which reinforces the divide between the expert, who knows how to improve health, and the general public who need education and advice. However, this is not inevitable. Interventions may be directed according to a client's stated needs when these have been identified. For example, social marketing techniques (see Chapter 12) focus on finding out what consumers want and need, and then providing it.

Many health care workers educate their clients about health through the provision of information and one-to-one counselling. Patient education about a condition or medication may seek to ensure compliance, in other words, a behaviour change, or it may be more client-directed and employ an educational approach.

Evaluation

Evaluating a health promotion intervention designed to change behaviour would appear to be a simple exercise. Has the health behaviour changed after the intervention? But there are two main problems: change may only become apparent over a long period, and it may be difficult to isolate any change as attributable to a health promotion intervention.

 Box 5.5

A recent systematic review of interventions using behaviour change methods to prevent weight gain found mixed results. Only one randomized controlled trial, that included various methods

including a correspondence programme, goal setting, self-monitoring and being prepared for contingencies, reported significant positive results. The review concluded that progress in this field would be facilitated by:

- The explicit use of methods of behaviour change that have been successful in other contexts (e.g. individual goal setting, the use of incentives, feedback on behaviour change)
- Explicit description of interventions in write-ups
- A longer follow-up of the behaviour being targeted, to assess if any changes made are adhered to in the long term (Hardeman et al 2000).

The educational approach

Aims

The purpose of this approach is to provide knowledge and information, and to develop the necessary skills so that people can make an informed choice about their health behaviour. The educational approach should be distinguished from a behaviour change approach in that it does not set out to persuade or motivate change in a particular direction. However, education *is* intended to have an outcome. This will be the client's voluntary choice and it may not be the one the health promoter would prefer.

The educational approach is based on a set of assumptions about the relationship between knowledge and behaviour: that by increasing knowledge, there will be a change in attitudes which may lead to changed behaviour. The goal of a client being able to make an informed choice may seem unambiguous and agreed upon. However this ignores not only the very real constraints that social and economic factors place on voluntary behaviour change, but also the complexities of health-related decision-making (see Chapter 9).

Methods

Psychological theories state that learning involves three aspects:

1. Cognitive (information and understanding)
2. Affective (attitudes and feelings)
3. Behavioural (skills).

An educational approach to health promotion will provide information to help clients to make an informed choice about their health behaviour. This may be through the provision of leaflets and booklets, visual displays or one-to-one advice. It may also provide opportunities for clients to share and explore their attitudes to their own health. This may be through group discussion or one-to-one counselling. Educational programmes may also develop clients' decision-making skills through role plays or activities designed to explore options. Clients may take on roles or practise responses in 'real-life' situations. For example, clients taking part in an alcohol programme may role-play situations where they are offered a drink. Educational programmes are usually led by a teacher or facilitator, although the issues for discussion may be decided by the clients. Educational interventions require the practitioner to understand the principles of adult learning and the factors which help or hinder learning (Ewles & Simnett 2003).

Evaluation

Increases in knowledge are relatively easy to measure. Health education through mass-media campaigns, one-to-one education and classroom-based work have all shown success in increasing information about health issues, or the awareness of risk factors for a disease. Information alone is, however, insufficient to change behaviour and, as we shall see in Chapter 9, even the desire and ability to change behaviour are no guarantee that the individual will do so.

Empowerment

Aims

The World Health Organization (1986) defined health promotion as enabling people to gain control over their lives. This approach helps people to identify their own concerns and gain the skills and confidence to act upon them. It is unique in being based on a 'bottom-up' strategy and calls for different skills from the health promoter. The health promoter needs to become a facilitator whose role is to act as a catalyst, getting things going and freeing up resources, and then to withdraw from the situation.

Box 5.6

- What do you understand by the term 'empowerment'?
- Can a practitioner empower a client?
- Are there health promotion actions which can disempower someone?

When we talk of empowerment, we need to distinguish between *self*-empowerment and *community* empowerment. Self-empowerment is used in some cases to describe those approaches to promoting health which are based on counselling and which use non-directive, client-centred approaches aimed at increasing people's control over their own lives. For people to be empowered they need to:

- Recognize and understand their powerlessness
- Feel strongly enough about their situation to want to change it
- Feel capable of changing the situation by having information, support and life skills.

Empowerment is also used to describe a way of working which increases people's power to change their 'social reality'. Chapter 10 includes a discussion of community development as a way of working which seeks to create active participating communities who are *empowered*, and able to challenge and change the world about them. This may or may not include political consciousness-raising such as that advocated by the radical educationist Paulo Freire (1972).

Methods

Many health, education and social care practitioners use empowerment strategies, which may be referred to as client-centred approaches, advocacy or self-care. Laverack (2005) states that the challenge for practitioners is to use their own power (power-over) to help clients to gain power (power-from-within).

Box 5.7

Empowering though reminiscence

Reminiscence is an example of a communication strategy which encourages older people to tell their story and recall past events. This provides opportunities for them to say what kind of care they want. It shifts the balance of the relationship to the client or patient and helps build trust and understanding. In dementia care, older people can be encouraged to retrieve their past experience and maintain their personhood. Some ethnic groups with strong oral traditions use reminiscence to preserve their cultural identity (Coleman & O'Hanlon 2004).

Community development is a similar way of working to empower groups of people by identifying their concerns and working with them to plan a programme of action to address these concerns. Some health promoters have a specific remit to undertake community development work; most do not. Community development work is time-consuming and most health promoters have clearly defined priorities which take up all their time. Funding for this kind of work is invariably insecure and short-term. The communication, planning and organizational skills necessary for this approach may not be included in professional training. For many health promoters, relinquishing the expert role may be difficult and uncomfortable. Ways of working with communities are discussed more fully in Chapter 10.

Box 5.8

Examples of health promotion through community development

1. Community development workers working with tenants on a housing estate to improve play space
2. Health promotion practitioners using a variety of methods to identify health needs of residents in a particular area
3. Setting up groups to meet specific needs, e.g. a girls' group at a youth centre
4. Linkworkers or advocates acting as 'care navigators' for Asian women.

Evaluation

Evaluation of such activity is problematic, partly because the process of empowerment and networking is typically long-term. This makes it difficult to be certain that any changes detected are due to the intervention and not some other factor. In addition, positive results of such an approach may appear to be vague and hard to specify, especially when compared to outcomes used by other approaches, such as targets or changes in behaviour which are capable of being quantified. Evaluation includes the extent to which specific aims have been met (outcome evaluation) and the degree to which the group has gelled, or been empowered as a result of the intervention (process evaluation). Evaluation therefore needs to include qualitative methods that reveal people's perceptions and beliefs as well as quantitative methods that demonstrate outcomes such as behaviour change.

Social change

Aims

This approach, which is sometimes referred to as radical health promotion, acknowledges the importance of the socioeconomic environment in determining health. Its focus is at the policy or environmental level, and the aim is to bring about changes in the physical, social and economic environment which will have the effect of promoting health. This may be summed up in the phrase 'to make the healthy choice the easier choice'. A healthy choice is available, but to make it a realistic option for most people requires changes in its cost, availability or accessibility. Chapter 11 discusses the processes involved in creating healthy public policies.

Box 5.9

Several studies have shown that a healthy diet which includes fruit and vegetables costs more than the typical diet of a low-income family (Cade et al 1999). What should be the focus of health promotion interventions on healthy eating?
You may have included some of the following:

- Changes in pricing structures such as reducing the price of wholemeal bread compared to white bread
- Working with food manufacturers and distributors to promote food labelling, making it easier for customers to identify low-fat, low-sugar foods
- Farming subsidies which encourage the production of lean meat
- The provision of healthy food in workplaces and hospitals

- The reintroduction in 2006 of nutritional standards for school meals which promote healthy food
- Widening the number and type of food outlets in local communities.

Methods

The social change or radical approach is targeted towards groups and populations, and involves a top-down method of working. Although there may be widespread consultation, the changes being sought are generally within organizations, and require commitment from the highest levels. Chapter 11 discusses developing healthy public policy and how legislation has had an enormous impact on the nation's health. The successful implementation of policy and legislation requires the support of the public which is achieved through education, lobbying and social marketing. Chapter 12 discusses social marketing in greater detail.

For most health promotion workers, the scope for this type of activity will be more limited than for the traditional medical or behaviour change approaches. The necessary skills for working in this way, such as lobbying, policy planning, negotiating and implementation, may not be included in professional training. Working in such a way may be interpreted as beyond the brief of the job, too political or someone else's remit. There is however scope for professional organizations to become involved as stakeholders in social change processes. For example, health practitioners' professional bodies were involved in lobbying for a total smoking ban in public places, alongside pressure groups such as Action on Smoking and Health (ASH) (Ford 2005).

Evaluation

Evaluation of the social change approach includes outcomes such as legislative, organizational or regulatory changes which promote health, e.g. regulations governing food labelling, a ban on tobacco sponsorship and advertising or a ban on smoking in public places.

The extent of partnership working and the profile of health issues on common agendas may also be used to demonstrate a greater degree of commitment to social change for health. These outcomes are typically long-term, complex processes where it would be difficult to prove a link to particular health promotion interventions.

Box 5.10

Are there parts of your work which are aimed at social change? Have you sought to influence policies and practices which affect health?

Organizational development, environmental health measures, economic or legislative activities and public policies on housing, education or the provision of services may all be examples of health promotion aimed at social change.

Partnership working with other agencies enables the socioeconomic and environmental determinants of health to be targeted, e.g. health, education and environment practitioners may work together to lobby for the provision of safe outdoor recreation areas.

Practitioners may seek to address the root causes of ill health by developing health profiles, conducting health equity audits, working in partnerships with other agencies, social commentary and research.

Box 5.11

Table 5.1 uses the example of healthy eating to show how different approaches to health promotion will have different aims and use different methods, The public health White Paper *Choosing Health: Making Healthier Choices Easier Choices* has the following priorities: reducing smoking, reducing obesity and improving diet,

encouraging sensible drinking, improving sexual health and improving mental health (Department of Health 2004). Consider how health promotion interventions in one of these areas will be affected by working with the five identified approaches to health promotion: medical, behaviour change, educational, empowerment and social change.

In each case what would working within this approach entail in terms of:

- Aims or focus?
- Methods?
- Worker–client relationship?

How would you evaluate your success using each approach?

With which approach would you feel most comfortable (Table 5.1)?

Models of health promotion

The above schema of different approaches to health promotion is primarily descriptive. It is what health promoters do, and it is possible to move in and out of different approaches depending on the situation. A more analytical means of identifying types of health promotion is to develop models of practice. All models, be they building models, diagrammatic maps or theoretical models, seek to represent reality in some way and try to show in a simplified form how different things connect. Implicit in the use of models is a theoretical framework that explains how and why the elements in the model are connected. Theory is defined as 'systematically organized knowledge applicable in a relatively wide variety of circumstances devised to analyze, predict or otherwise explain the nature or behaviour of a specified set of phenomena that could be used as the basis for action' (Van Ryn & Heany 1992). Models of health promotion may help to:

- Conceptualize or map the field of health promotion
- Interrogate and analyse existing practice
- Plan and chart the possibilities for interventions (Naidoo & Wills 2005).

Table 5.1 Approaches to health promotion: the example of healthy eating

Approach	Aims	Methods	Worker/client relationship
Medical	To identify those at risk from disease	Screening, individual risk assessment e.g. measurement of body mass index	Expert-led Passive, conforming client
Behaviour change	To encourage individuals to take responsibility for their own health and choose healthier lifestyles	Persuasion through one-to-one advice and information; mass-media campaigns, e.g. 5-a-day dietary messages	Expert-led Dependent client; possible victim-blaming ideology
Educational	To increase knowledge and skills about healthy lifestyles	Information and exploration of attitudes through individual or small group work Development of skills, e.g. cooking healthy meals	May be expert-led May also involve client in negotiation of issue for discussion
Empowerment	To work with clients or communities to meet their perceived needs	Advocacy; negotiation; networking; facilitation, e.g. community horticulture projects	Health promoter is facilitator; client becomes empowered
Social change	To address inequalities in health based on class, race, gender, geography, adopting a population perspective	Development of organizational policy, e.g. hospital catering policy Public health legislation, e.g. food labeling Lobbying Fiscal controls, e.g. subsidy to farmers to produce lean meat	Entails social regulation and is top-down

Using a model can be helpful because it encourages you to think theoretically, and come up with new strategies and ways of working. It can also help you to prioritize and locate more or less desirable types of interventions.

There has been a proliferation of models in health promotion literature, with large areas of overlap but little consensus on terminology or underlying criteria. Thus we find that Beattie (1991) uses criteria of 'mode of intervention' (authoritative-negotiated) and 'focus of intervention' (individual–collective) to generate four models (see Figure 5.2 below). Caplan & Holland (1990) use 'theories of knowledge' and 'theories of society' (see Figure 5.1 below). The terminology for models also varies. For example, French (1990) calls a social change approach 'politics of health', whilst Caplan & Holland (1990) distinguish between a radical model and a Marxist model. This can be extremely confusing for the reader.

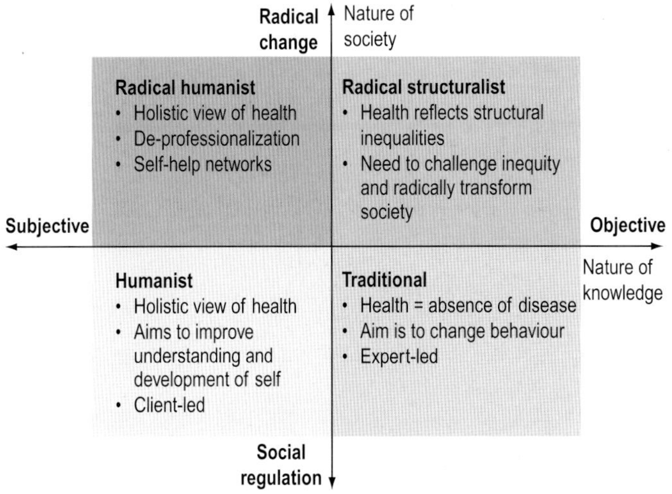

Figure 5.1 • Four paradigms or perspectives of health promotion. Adapted from Caplan & Holland (1990).

The following two models derive from sociological and social policy frameworks. They adopt a structural analysis which draws attention to the material and social influences on health and the social structures which contribute to inequalities in health. They show how health promotion approaches are influenced by political ideology and different value positions about power, responsibility and autonomy.

Caplan & Holland (1990)

This model suggests that there are essentially four paradigms or ways of looking at health promotion. These paradigms can be generated from two dimensions (Figure 5.1). The first dimension is concerned with the nature of knowledge. Knowledge is seen as based along a continuum which ranges from subjective approaches to understanding through to objective approaches. Objective explanations deriving from science (e.g. health is the absence of disease) are only part of the picture. Emphasis may also be given to lay accounts and people's own unique interpretations of what their health means to them.

The second dimension relates to assumptions concerning the nature of society. These range from theories of radical change to theories of social regulation. When these two dimensions are put together it suggests four paradigms or perspectives of health promotion, as illustrated in Figure 5.1.

Each quadrant represents a major approach to the understanding of health and the practice of health promotion. They are not necessarily exclusive but there will be situations when to hold one position or approach precludes the adoption of other approaches. Each quadrant incorporates different theoretical and philosophical assumptions about society, concepts of health and the principal sources of health problems.

1. The *traditional* perspective relates to the medical and behaviour change approaches described earlier. Knowledge lies with the experts and the emphasis is on information-giving to bring about behaviour change.

2. The *humanist* perspective relates to the educational approach. Individuals are enabled to use their personal resources and skills to maximize their chances of developing what they consider to be a healthy lifestyle.

3. The *radical humanist* perspective relates to the empowerment approach. Health promotion is concerned to raise consciousness and part of the emphasis is on the exploration of personal

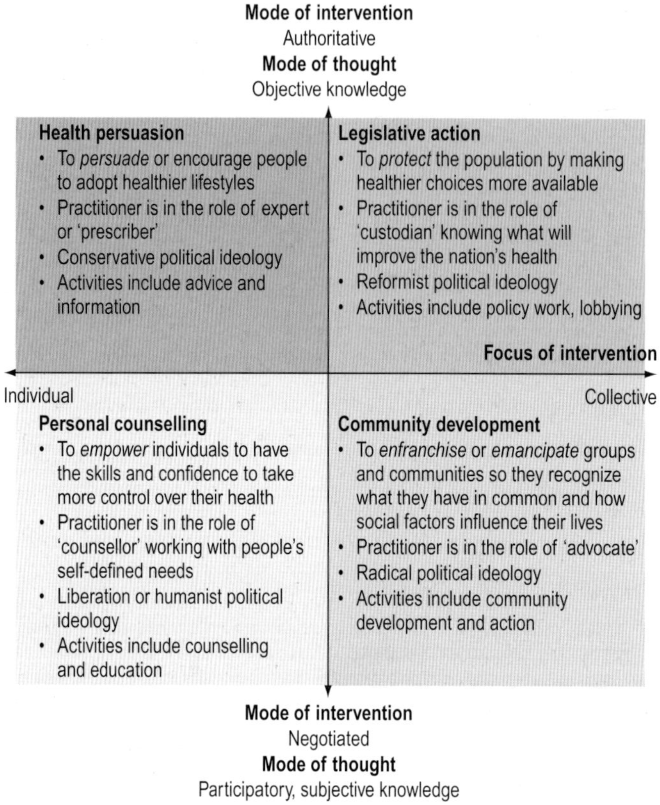

Mode of intervention
Authoritative
Mode of thought
Objective knowledge

Health persuasion	**Legislative action**
• To *persuade* or encourage people to adopt healthier lifestyles • Practitioner is in the role of expert or 'prescriber' • Conservative political ideology • Activities include advice and information	• To *protect* the population by making healthier choices more available • Practitioner is in the role of 'custodian' knowing what will improve the nation's health • Reformist political ideology • Activities include policy work, lobbying

Focus of intervention

Individual   Collective

Personal counselling	**Community development**
• To *empower* individuals to have the skills and confidence to take more control over their health • Practitioner is in the role of 'counsellor' working with people's self-defined needs • Liberation or humanist political ideology • Activities include counselling and education	• To *enfranchise* or *emancipate* groups and communities so they recognize what they have in common and how social factors influence their lives • Practitioner is in the role of 'advocate' • Radical political ideology • Activities include community development and action

Mode of intervention
Negotiated
Mode of thought
Participatory, subjective knowledge

Figure 5.2 ● Using Beattie's model to analyse practice. Based on Beattie (1991, 1993).

responses to health issues. Alongside this, individuals are encouraged to form social, organizational and economic networks.

4. The *radical structuralist* perspective holds that structural inequalities are the cause of many health problems, and the role of health promotion is to address the relationship between health and social inequalities.

The model is useful in showing that practice is the outcome of deeper social conflicts and values.

Beattie (1991)

Beattie offers a structural analysis of the health promotion repertoire of approaches. He suggests

that there are four paradigms for health promotion (Figure 5.2). These are generated from the dimensions of mode of intervention, which ranges from authoritative (top-down and expert-led) to negotiated (bottom-up and valuing individual autonomy). Much health promotion work involving advice and information is determined and led by practitioners. Equally, policy work may also be expert-led, the priorities determined by epidemiological data. The other dimension relates to the focus of the intervention which ranges from a focus on the individual who is responsible for his or her own health to a focus on the collective and the roots of ill health.

Beattie's typology generates four strategies for health promotion.

1. *Health persuasion.* These are interventions directed at individuals and led by professionals. An example is a primary health care worker encouraging a pregnant woman to stop smoking.

2. *Legislative action.* These are interventions led by professionals but intended to protect communities. An example is lobbying for tighter controls on food labelling.

3. *Personal counselling.* These interventions are client-led and focus on personal development. The health promoter is a facilitator rather than an expert. An example is a youth worker working with young people who helps them to identify their health needs and then works with them one to one or through group work to increase their confidence and skills.

4. *Community development.* These interventions, in a similar way to personal counselling, seek to empower or enhance the skills of a group or local community. An example is a community worker working with a local tenants' group to increase opportunities for further education and active leisure pursuits.

Figure 5.2 shows how Beattie's model can point up the following aspects:

- Goals and activities
- Client–practitioner relationship
- Political ideologies.

Each of the four strategies corresponds to a different political perspective. Thus conservative reformist perspectives see health promotion as attempting to correct or repair what is seen as a deficit in the conservative perspective (e.g. lack of information) or an aspect of deprivation in the reformist perspective (e.g. difficulties of access). These perspectives give rise to authoritative and prescriptive approaches. Libertarian and radical perspectives both see health promotion as seeking to empower or enfranchise individuals. The radical perspective, in addition, seeks to mobilize and emancipate communities. Each of these perspectives also casts the practitioner in a different role in relation to clients.

Beattie's model is a useful one for health promoters because it identifies a clear framework for deciding a strategy, and yet reminds them that the choice of these interventions is influenced by social and political perspectives.

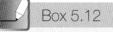 Box 5.12

Take one of the following programme objectives and using Beattie's model plot the different strategies which might be employed to reduce:
- Smoking in pregnant women
- Drinking in young people
- Accidents in older people.

Tannahill (Downie et al 1996)

This model of health promotion is widely accepted by health care workers. Tannahill talks of three overlapping spheres of activity: health education; prevention; and health protection.

1. *Health education* – communication to enhance well-being and prevent ill health through influencing knowledge and attitudes.

2. *Prevention* – reducing or avoiding the risk of diseases and ill health primarily through medical interventions.

3. *Health protection* – safeguarding population health through legislative, fiscal or social measures.

Tannahill's diagrammatic representation (Figure 5.3) shows how these different approaches relate to each other in an all-inclusive process termed health promotion.

The model is primarily descriptive of what goes on in practice. It is useful for the health promoter to see the potential in other areas of activity, and to see the scope of health promotion. It does not, however, give any insight into why a practitioner may choose one approach over another. It suggests that all approaches are interrelated but, as we have seen, they reflect distinctive ways of looking at health issues.

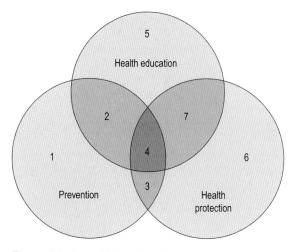

Figure 5.3 • Tannahill's model of health promotion. From Downie et al (1996).

1. Preventive services, e.g. immunization, cervical screening, hypertension case-finding, developmental surveillance, use of nicotine chewing gum to aid smoking cessation
2. Preventive health education, e.g. smoking cessation advice and information
3. Preventive health protection, e.g. fluoridation of water
4. Health education for preventive health protection, e.g. lobbying for seat-belt legislation
5. Positive health education, e.g. life skills work with young people
6. Positive health protection, e.g. workplace smoking policy
7. Health education aimed at positive health protection, e.g. lobbying for a ban on tobacco advertising.

Tones (Tones & Tilford 2001)

The following model claims to be an empowerment model which has as its cardinal principle the goal of enabling people to gain control over their own health. It prioritizes empowerment, which is seen as both the core value and the core strategy underpinning and defining the practice of health promotion.

Tones makes a simple equation that health promotion is an overall process of healthy public policy × health education (Figure 5.4).

Tones considers education to be the key to empowering both lay and professional people by raising consciousness of health issues. People are then more able to make choices and to create pressure for healthy public policies. We have seen how there is a distinction between self-empowerment and community empowerment. Tones argues that there is a reciprocal relationship between the two. Changes in the social environment achieved through healthy public policies will facilitate the development of self-empowered individuals. People who have the skills to participate effectively in decision-making are better able to access resources and shape policy to meet their needs. The support of individuals is also necessary for implementing change. Empowerment, as opposed to prevention or a radical political approach, is the main aim of health promotion in Tones' model. Working for empowerment enhances individual autonomy and enables individuals, groups and communities to take more control over their lives.

Conclusion

A number of quite different activities are subsumed under the label 'health promotion'. Attempts to organize these activities into different categories have generated a plethora of models and typologies. The most obvious starting point is to describe the variety of current practice and this is the approach taken at the beginning of this chapter.

Box 5.13

Examples of approaches to tackling teenage pregnancy

- Medical approach: providing contraception
- Behavioural approach: contraceptive advice
- Educational approach: sex education

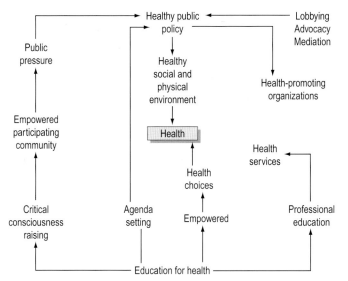

Figure 5.4 • The contribution of education to health promotion. Adapted from Tones & Tilford (1994).

- Empowerment approach: life skills, including negotiation, assertiveness and communication
- Social change approach: review of services and benefits (education and training, financial, housing) available to young women.

However, there are limitations to this method and it may be criticized as being insufficiently analytical. Theorists who have taken this one step further have identified key criteria which serve to locate different forms of practice, both existing and potential. Adopting a more analytical approach enables judgements to be made about more and less desirable forms of practice, and opens up these judgements for debate. If health promotion is to progress as a discipline and an activity in its own right, a strong theoretical framework is necessary.

The search to clarify models and typologies of practice may appear to be academic and unrelated to the 'here and now' of your activities to promote health. However, we would argue that for practice to grow beyond a reactive response to demands

made by others, practitioners need to have an idea of all available options and reflect on which approaches are most congruent with their own beliefs and values. It is only when we can contemplate different ways of promoting health that we can make judgements as to what is possible and what is preferable. Recognizing that the two are not always synonymous may be frustrating in the short term, but must in the long term contribute towards the effectiveness and efficiency of health promotion.

Questions for further discussion

- Which approach(es) to health promotion do you adopt in your work?

- What are the most important reasons for adopting your approach(es)?

- Which typology or model of health promotion do you find most helpful in providing a theoretical framework with which to analyse your health promotion activities?

Box 5.14

The smoking rate among women on low income increases with:

- Greater disadvantage
- More children to care for
- Children in poorer health
- Caring alone
- Carrying extra responsibility for family members.

Using one of the models discussed earlier, map those health promotion interventions which you would regard as:

1. Most appropriate for women smokers on a low income
2. Most likely to be adopted
3. Ones you would use.

- If the answers to 1, 2 and 3 are different, what might account for this?
- What factors influence your choice of strategies (e.g. professional training, job remit, organizational constraints, personal values, local priorities)?

Summary

This chapter has examined five different approaches to health promotion: the medical or preventive approach; the behaviour change or lifestyles approach; the educational approach; the empowerment and community development approach; and the social change or radical approach. In practice, the edges between them may be blurred. However, they do differ in significant ways. They encompass different assumptions concerning the nature of health society and change. The preferred methods of intervention, necessary skills and means of evaluation all differ. Many health promoters will find that the approach they adopt is dictated, in part at least, by their job role and functions. This chapter stresses the importance of examining your approach to health promotion and identifying any changes you may wish to make.

Further reading

Ewles L, Simnett I 2003 Promoting health: a practical guide, 5th edn. Baillière Tindall, Edinburgh. *Chapter 3 provides a short and straightforward guide to approaches to health promotion and identifies their aims and values.*

Laverack G 2005 Public health: power, empowerment and professional practice, Palgrave Macmillan, Hampshire. *This book explores the concept of power and discusses the potential and dilemmas for professional practitioners seeking to empower their clients, in both individual and community settings.*

Naidoo J, Wills J 2005 Public health and health promotion: developing practice, 2nd edn. Baillière Tindall, London. *Chapter 1 examines the body of health promotion theory, the key principles which inform practice and why their application may be difficult.*

Tones K, Tilford S 2001 Health education: effectiveness, efficiency and equity, 3rd edn. Nelson Thornes, Cheltenham. *Chapter 1 explores the values underpinning three different models of health promotion: radical-political model; self-empowerment; and preventive model.*

References

Beattie A 1991 Knowledge and control in health promotion: a test case for social policy and social theory. In: Gabe J, Calnan M, Bury M (eds) The sociology of the health service. Routledge, London.

Beattie A 1993 The changing boundaries of health. In: Beattie A, Gott M, Jones L (eds) et al Health and wellbeing: a reader. Macmillan/Open University, Basingstoke.

British Medical Journal 2002 Editorial: Whooping cough – a continuing problem: pertussis has re-emerged in countries with high vaccination coverage and low mortality. British Medical Journal 324: 1537–1538.

Cade J, Upmeier H, Calvert C et al 1999 Costs of a healthy diet: analysis from the UK women's cohort study. Public Health Nutrition 2: 505–512.

Caplan R, Holland R 1990 Rethinking health education theory. Health Education Journal 49: 10–12.

Coleman P G, O'Hanlon A 2004 Ageing and development. Arnold, London.

Cummins S, Macintyre S 2002 'Food deserts' – evidence and assumption in health policy making. British Medical Journal 325: 436–438.

Department of Health 2004 Choosing health: making healthy choices easier choices. HMSO, London.

Downie R S, Tannahill C, Tannahill A 1996 Health promotion: models and values, 2nd edn. Oxford Medical Publications, Oxford.

Ewles L, Simnett I 2003 Promoting health: a practical guide, 5th edn. Baillière Tindall, Edinburgh.

Ford J A 2005 Editorial: Protecting workers in licensed premises from the effects of secondhand smoke. Occupational Medicine 55: 583–585.

Freire P 1972 Pedagogy of the oppressed. Penguin, Harmondsworth.

French J 1990 Models of health education and promotion. Health Education Journal 49: 1.

Hardeman W, Griffin S, Johnston M et al 2000 Interventions to prevent weight gain: a systematic review of psychological models and behaviour change methods. International Journal of Obesity 24: 131–143.

Jepson R, Clegg A, Forbes C et al 2000 The determinants of screening uptake and interventions for increasing uptake: a systematic review. Health Technology Assessment 4: i–vii, 1–133.

Laverack G 2005 Public health: power, empowerment and professional practice. Palgrave Macmillan, Hampshire.

Morris J N, Donkin A J M, Wonderling D et al 2000 A minimum income for healthy living. Journal of Epidemiology and Community Health 54: 885–889.

Naidoo J, Wills J 2005 Public health and health promotion: developing practice, 2nd edn. Baillière Tindall, London.

Tones K, Tilford S 1994 Health education: effectiveness, efficiency and equity. Chapman and Hall, London.

Tones K, Tilford S 2001 Health education; effectiveness, efficiency, equity, 3nd edn. Nelson Thornes, Cheltenham.

Van Ryn M, Heany C A 1992 What's the use of theory? Health Education and Behaviour 19: 315–330.

World Health Organization 1986 Ottawa charter for health promotion. WHO, Geneva.

6

Ethical issues in health promotion

- The philosophy of health promotion
- Duties in health promotion
- The individual and the common good
- Ethical principles:
  - Beneficence (doing good)
  - Non-maleficence (doing no harm)
  - Autonomy
  - Justice and equity
  - Telling the truth

OVERVIEW

Health promotion involves working to improve people's health. This requires a series of value judgements: about what better health means for the individual and society; and about whether, when and how to make a health promotion intervention. This book has used the perspectives of social science to help you explore your role and aims in health promotion. In this chapter we consider some of the prevailing problems for a health promoter from a philosophical perspective:

- The extent to which individuals can be held responsible for their own health

- Whether it is justified to institute health promotion interventions which have not been sufficiently evaluated
- The extent to which health promotion should influence the public to choose what is deemed to be the healthy (and by implication correct and good) choice
- The legitimacy of the state to influence the environment to encourage healthy behaviour.

In particular, the chapter focuses on the limits to individual freedoms and how these are balanced against the health of the community. The chapter outlines the key ethical principles of beneficence (doing good), non-maleficence (doing no harm), justice, telling the truth and respect for people and their autonomy.

The need for a philosophy of health promotion

Debate in health promotion has centred on discussion of practice and some attempts to develop a theoretical base. However, according to Seedhouse (1988), there has been little discussion concerning the philosophy of health and yet it is an essential part of the way in which we understand the world.

Health promotion involves decisions and choices that affect other people which require judgements to be made about whether particular courses of action are right or wrong. There are no definite ways to behave. Health promotion is, according to Seedhouse (1988), 'a moral endeavour'. Philosophical debate helps to clarify what it is that one believes in most and how one wants to run one's life. It can and does help practitioners to reflect on the principles of practice, and thus to make practical judgements about whether to intervene and which strategies to adopt.

Philosophy has three main branches:

1. Logic – the development of reasoned argument

2. Epistemology – enquiry into the nature and grounds of knowledge and meanings

3. Ethics – the enquiry into how we ought to act and conduct ourselves.

Morals refer to those beliefs about how people 'ought' to behave. These debates about right and wrong, good and bad, and duty are part of everyday discourse. Is it wrong to tell a lie? Is it justified to kill another? Is it our duty to look after ageing parents? Judgement about the morality of these actions may derive from our personal values and moral beliefs which derive from: religion, culture, ideology, professional codes of practice or social etiquette, the law or our life experience. The function of ethical theory is not to provide answers but to inform these judgements and help people work out whether certain courses of action are right or wrong, and whether one ought to take a certain action.

Western philosophy has been shaped by two theories of ethics – deontology and consequentialism. Deontology comes from the Greek word *deonto* meaning duty. Deontologists hold that we have a *duty* to act in accordance with certain universal moral rules. Consequential ethics are based on the premise that whether an action is right or wrong depends on its end result.

Duty and codes of practice

Deontologists hold that there are universal moral rules that it is our duty to follow. Many of the philosophical discussions about the nature of duty are based on the theories of Immanuel Kant. The essence of Kant's thinking is encapsulated in the categorical imperative which can help us to discover, through reason, if a rule or moral principle exists (Kant 1909).

The major features of Kant's theory are:

1. Act as if your action in each circumstance is to become law for everyone, yourself included, in the future. In other words, if everyone always behaved this way, would the overall effect be good? If it would, then this is the rule to apply in all similar situations. The biblical 'Do unto others as you would they do unto you' becomes a universal moral imperative.

2. Always treat human beings as 'ends in themselves' and never merely as 'means'. A moral rule then is one that respects all people.

Deontological theories make decision-making apparently easy because, as long as we obey the rules, then we must be doing the right thing, regardless of the consequences.

Box 6.1

Screening for antenatal disorders

This screening programme is in place to reduce the birth prevalence of a chromosomal disorder. The assumption underlying screening for conditions such as Down's syndrome is that parents with a positive result will decide to terminate the pregnancy. Some positive-testing parents who do not choose termination may indirectly benefit from the test because they will be better able to adjust to the condition of their baby.

The Kantian objection is that the screened population becomes a mere means to achieve the public health goal of reducing chromosomal disorders in the population.

The ethical dilemma is pointed up, as Holland (2007, p. 182) puts it: 'how feasible it is to use antenatal and screening and termination to combat a disability on the one hand, whilst maintaining a positive societal attitude towards extant disabled people on the other'.

Box 6.2

This example centres on the duty to respect life and highlights some of the difficulties that can arise from carrying out this duty.

There is in medical care a commonly accepted doctrine of 'acts and omissions' which states that if a person fails to perform an action that would prevent negative consequences he or she is morally less blameworthy than if he or she performed an action that resulted in the same consequence.

In 2005 Dr Michael Irwin accompanied a terminally ill widow, Mrs May Murphy to Switzerland. She took a lethal dose of barbiturates while he was in the room. Assisted suicide, defined as doctors giving patients the means to kill themselves, is legal in Switzerland.

In 1992 medical staff stopped feeding Tony Bland, a young man crushed into a permanent vegetative state by the Hillsborough football disaster. This action was regarded as withholding life-saving treatment and morally acceptable.

Both acts had brought about the same consequence – the death of a patient. Is there a moral distinction, in your view, between killing and letting die? Must human life be preserved regardless of its quality?

Many health care workers have codes of practice which set out guidelines for the fulfilment of duties. For example, doctors take the Hippocratic oath which requires them as a first principle to avoid doing harm. The Nursing and Midwifery Council (2004) states the duty to respect life, the duty to care, and the duty to do no harm. Kant would have added 'the duty to be truthful in all declarations is a sacred, unconditional command of reason, and not to be limited by any expediency' (Kant 1909). The Society of Health Education and Promotion Specialists (SHEPS) includes these principles in its code of conduct:

Practitioners have a:

- Duty to care
- Duty to be fair
- Duty to respect personal and group rights
- Duty to avoid harm
- Duty to respect confidentiality
- Duty to report (SHEPS 1997).

But, as Sindall (2002) has argued, health promotion has not engaged in the kind of debate necessary to agree the principles, duties and obligations to which health promoters would need to agree to work in the field. Codes of conduct are simply devices offering a framework in which to practise. They do not help practitioners involved in the messy and complex everyday world of health care (Duncan 2008). For example, Article 3 of the nursing code (Nursing and Midwifery Council 2004) declares that the registered nurse, midwife or specialist community public health nurse must obtain consent before any treatment or care but the concept of informed consent is complex.

Box 6.3

What do you understand by the concept of informed consent? What difficulties might there be in complying with this aspect of the code of practice?

Patients have different capacities to understand the nature of treatment or intervention. Patients may feel they will be judged or withheld from other interventions if they refuse. Consent is so obviously presumed in many cases, e.g. in the 'invitation' to screen or test, that refusal can seem impossible. Practitioners may also not communicate risk clearly such that patients are not fully informed when they consent.

Consequentialism and utilitarianism: the individual and the common good

The other classical school of ethics is known as consequentialism, of which utilitarianism is its best-known branch. Consequentialism differs from deontological theories because it is concerned with ends and not only means. The utilitarian principle is that a person should always act in such a way that will produce more good or benefits than disadvantages. Utilitarians such as John Stuart Mill and Jeremy Bentham aimed for the greatest good or pleasure for the greatest number of people. Utilitarians can thus respond to all moral dilemmas by reviewing the facts and weighing up the consequences of alternative courses of action. This can, of course, prove difficult. What exactly is a good end? How does one predict whether an outcome will be favourable? One of the main problems with utilitarianism is that, if the aim of all actions is to achieve the greatest good,

does this justify harm or injustice to a few if society benefits? Smoking restrictions offer an example, where the health of society takes precedence over the right of the individual to smoke.

Health promotion raises many questions over its ends and means:

- Good health is a relative concept, so whose definition should take precedence? Is it ethical for a practitioner to persuade someone to adopt his or her perception of a healthier lifestyle?
- What means are justifiable to promote population good health? Should the interests of the majority always prevail?
- Since most ill health is avoidable, should those who adopt unhealthy behaviours be refused treatment?

In Chapter 4 we saw that some writers have expressed concern over 'social engineering' in health promotion and think that government intervention has risked becoming government intrusion. Many interventions are justified as being in the interests of a 'healthy society', yet they may not have been requested or desired.

Box 6.4

Consider these examples of healthy public policies and whether, in your view, they are ethical.

- Fluoridation of tap water
- Subsidy of lead-free petrol
- Ban on smoking in public places
- Complete ban on drinking and driving
- Compulsory testing of all visitors to the UK for human immunodeficiency virus (HIV) infection
- Ban on the use of mobile phones in cars
- Government subsidy of child-minding places
- Reintroduction of nutritional standards for all school meals
- Compulsory immunization for all children entering education.

Some of these actions are intended to protect the population from possible harm. Others are promoting evidence-based health interventions, although their universal application can restrict the actions of others. For example, the use of public funds to support child care is not relevant for those without children.

Ethical principles

Ethical principles can help to clarify the decisions that have to be taken at work. Sometimes decisions may be guided by trying to do the best for the most number of people; at other times they may be guided by an overriding concern for people's right to determine their own lives; and sometimes decisions may be guided by other ethical principles or a professional code of conduct.

There are four widely accepted ethical principles (Beauchamp & Childress 1995):

1. Respect for autonomy (a respect for the rights of individuals and their right to determine their lives)

2. Beneficence (the commitment to do actions that are of benefit)

3. Non-maleficence (the obligation not to harm patients or clients. If there is doubt, precaution should prevail)

4. Justice (the obligation to act fairly when dealing with competing claims for resources or rights).

These principles provide a framework for consistent moral decision-making. However, situations rarely involve a single option, but can encapsulate increasingly complex and sometimes conflicting choices between these principles. Seedhouse (1988) has developed these principles into an ethical grid which helps provide health promoters with an easy-to-follow guide on which to ground their work on moral principles (Figure 6.1).

The ethical grid

This provides a tool for practitioners, helping them to question basic principles and values, and be clear about what they mean and intend to do. The grid suggests ways in which practitioners can work through proposed actions. In any situation we should be asking ourselves:

1. Central conditions in working for health
   - Am I creating autonomy in my clients, enabling them to direct their own lives?
   - Am I respecting the autonomy of my clients whether or not I approve of their chosen direction?
   - Am I respecting all people as equal?
   - Do I work with people on the basis of needs first?

2. Key principles in working for health
   - Am I doing good and avoiding harm?
   - Am I telling the truth and keeping promises?

3. Consequences of ways of working for health
   - Will my action increase the individual good?
   - Will it increase the good of a particular group?
   - Will it increase the good of society?
   - Will I be acting for the good of myself?

4. External considerations in working for health
   - Are there any legal implications?
   - Is there a risk attached to the intervention?
   - Is the intervention the most effective and efficient action to take?
   - How certain is the evidence on which this intervention is based?
   - What are the views and wishes of those involved?
   - Can I justify my actions in terms of all this evidence?

Health promotion involves working to improve people's health. This requires a series of value judgements about what health means for the individual and society and about whether, when and how to intervene.

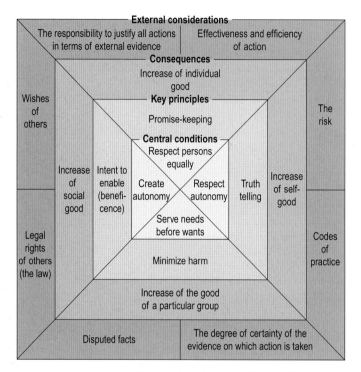

Figure 6.1 ● The ethical grid. The limit to the use of the grid is that it should be used honestly to seek to enable the enhancing potentials of people. From Seedhouse (1988).

Box 6.5

In the USA a charity has offered young women addicted to heroin or crack cocaine and who have frequent pregnancies resulting in abortions, stillbirths or addicted babies a sum of money to be sterilized.

Use Seedhouse's ethical grid illustrated in figure 6.1 to consider whether or not such action is morally justified.

You probably concluded that offering money as an inducement for sterilization is a coercive measure that does not respect the autonomy of the individual. Although it may give women greater control over

their reproduction, having more money may result in increased drug use. Sterilization is an irreversible procedure about which women need to be fully and freely informed. This action is not, then, one which increases morality. It is a quick-fix solution which fails to deal with the root causes of drug addiction.

Box 6.6

In the following scenarios, decide what ethical issues are involved and what action you would take and why.

1. You are nursing a 50-year-old who has chronic obstructive pulmonary disease. The patient has smoked 40 cigarettes a day since

he was 17. He has become very distressed by advice to stop smoking.

2. A vocal group of residents has asked for your support in a campaign against drug-taking and prostitution in your area. A local agency, working on harm minimization strategies with young people, has also requested your support.

3. A child has recently died from glue-sniffing at a local secondary school. The community police officer is keen to visit all local schools to show a video depicting a group of children who sniff glue and get into all kinds of trouble.

4. As part of a local mental health strategy, a general practice has introduced questionnaires to detect early indicators of mental health problems at all its clinics. A middle-aged, single, unemployed man regularly attends the diabetic clinic. His questionnaire indicates that he has sleep disturbance and high levels of anxiety.

Autonomy

Autonomy derives from the Greek word *autonomous* meaning self-rule. It refers to people's capacity to choose freely for themselves and be able to direct their own life. Since people do not exist in isolation from each other, there will be restrictions on individual autonomy and autonomous people have a sense of responsibility: they cannot do entirely as they like. Thus, people do not have complete freedom of choice. The limits to an individual's autonomy are when that individual's action affects others in a negative way. Beyond this, traditional notions of liberal individualism see autonomy as essential to all human beings. It is only constrained by:

- Reason and the ability to make rational choices
- The ability to understand one's environment
- The ability to act on one's environment.

In addition, a person needs to be free from pressures such as fear and want, and have the personal and social circumstances to make any chosen action possible.

Autonomy must, therefore, be thought of not as an absolute but as attainable, to a greater or lesser extent. Not everyone has autonomy. When people's capacity for rationality is affected in some way, decisions are often taken on their behalf on the basis that 'they do not know what's best for them'. Thus people with a learning disability or mental illness, young children and older people with mental confusion are often assumed to be unable to make a rational choice. It was not until the 20th century that women were deemed able to make a rational choice in a democratic vote. The Children Act of 1989 first recognized the rights and capacity of children to have a say in their care.

> ### Box 6.7
>
> The rights of young people with severe learning disabilities to determine their sexual health is a contested area:
> - Should young people with a severe learning disability have sexual relationships?
> - Should they decide whether or not to use contraception?
> - Should they decide if they wish to have children?

In recent years, the courts have ruled that a young woman with a learning disability should be sterilized to avoid the possible trauma of pregnancy and childbirth or abortion, for which it was considered she would not be prepared. It was also deemed in the best interests of a possible child who would not be able to be brought up by the young woman.

In these situations, what do we mean by autonomy? In part, we must mean respecting our clients as persons and helping them to cope with the consequences of their choices. Seedhouse (1988) makes a distinction between creating autonomy and respecting autonomy, which he regards as the central conditions when working for health.

Creating autonomy is making an effort to improve the quality of a person's autonomy by trying to enhance what that person is able to do. In health promotion work, this is often called empowerment. It may involve information to enable clients to make choices or developing the clients' skills in analysing situations and making decisions through increasing self-awareness and assertiveness. As we have stated elsewhere in this book, it is of prime importance in health promotion practice to recognize the limits to individual autonomy, and that social and economic circumstances can constrain individual health choices. Health promoters may claim they are creating autonomy by explaining the health hazards of smoking and thereby enabling individuals to make an informed choice to quit. Yet the autonomy of smokers may be compromised by addiction; their social circumstances in which cigarettes may serve as a 'drug of solace'; as well as advertising, peer pressure and so on.

Respecting autonomy is respecting a person's chosen direction, whether or not it is approved – for example, respecting a pregnant woman's autonomy to smoke. Creating and respecting autonomy are closely related. People cannot express a free wish if they are not aware of the possibilities open to them and thus it may, in some circumstances, be ethically justifiable not to respond to a client's expressed wishes but to attempt to open up other options.

Box 6.8

Is self-determination compatible with the health promoter's goal of seeking health improvement?

Respecting clients' autonomy can be difficult for health promoters. There is often a tendency to give advice, to exert pressure on them to make the 'right' decision or to persuade clients to change their behaviour. The challenge is to accept a role of partner and enabler rather than expert and controller. Ewles & Simnett (2003) identify three common ways in which health promoters hinder rather than respect their clients' autonomy:

1. By imposing their own solutions to the clients' problems

2. By instructing clients on what to do because they take too long to work it out for themselves

3. By dismissing clients' ideas without providing an adequate explanation or the opportunity to try them out.

Box 6.9

Think of some examples from your work when you have attempted to *create* autonomy in your clients so that they are able to express their wishes and wants.

At what point did you decide that the client is autonomous and to *respect* his or her wishes?

Chapter 10 explores a community development way of working which aims to empower people with regard to their own health agenda. It explores this dilemma of control and autonomy, and to what extent community development workers impose, collaborate with or genuinely facilitate local or community health needs. Chapter 9 looks at ways practitioners support individuals to change and whether such approaches are intent on empowering individuals or merely getting them to change.

Perhaps the starkest example of the ethical problems associated with respecting autonomy is that which confronts the health worker when a patient or client chooses not to follow advice or treatment which is known to be beneficial. It would seem straightforward that this is the client's right and the health worker should respect the client's autonomy in choosing such a decision, if the client is properly informed and understands any risks involved. However, the health worker is committed to 'doing good' and may feel it is his or her duty to persuade the client. This is particularly so if the client's decision has implications for other people. Certainly this is paternalistic and putting the health worker's need to do good above the client's wish for autonomy. Yet, by not seeking to persuade or motivate the client, the practitioner may, by omission, be doing harm.

Respecting autonomy involves respecting another person's rights and dignity such that a person reaches a maximum level of fulfilment as a human being. In the context of health promotion and health care this means that the relationship with patients or clients is based on a respect for them as people, and with individual rights. It follows that we must then see them as 'whole people' – with physical, social, emotional and spiritual needs – as fundamentally equal and also as unique individuals.

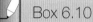

Box 6.10

A patient who has undergone heart bypass surgery continues to smoke after the operation.
- Is it justifiable to refuse further treatment?
- What factors do you take into account in making your judgement?

This extract suggests the following:

> *a doctor who takes seriously his self-imposed and professional obligation to benefit his patient ought to treat the patient if that is what the patient on reflection wants him to do, if some treatment is available which will provide net benefit to the patient ... Of course that in no way prevents the doctor from advising that the most effective way of regaining and maintaining health is to alter one's lifestyle in the relevant way. But coercion will generally be contraindicated by the requirement to respect people's autonomy, and withdrawal of care from those who reject one's advice will generally be contraindicated by a doctor's personally and professionally undertaken duty of care, or obligation of beneficence (Gillon 1990, p. 34).*

Rights in relation to health care are usually taken to include:
- The right to information
- The right to privacy and confidentiality
- The right to appropriate care and treatment.

Health workers are often placed in the position of deciding whether to inform patients or relatives of an adverse prognosis. Although the patient's right to information is usually considered paramount, there are occasions when the health worker's duty of beneficence – to do good and avoid harm – may outweigh this right.

Beneficence and non-maleficence

Frankena (1963) suggests that beneficence means doing or promoting good as well as preventing, removing and avoiding evil or harm. The common good is often put before individual good. Wearing a seat belt may halve the risk of death to the driver but the odds that a particular individual will ever benefit are not great, as few people will be killed on the roads. Rose (1981) termed this the 'prevention paradox', according to which a measure that brings large benefits to the community offers little to each participating individual. The alternative to a mass approach is to focus on risk groups but this may stigmatize certain groups (Naidoo & Wills 2005).

Box 6.11

In the UK the safety of the measles, mumps and rubella vaccine was questioned due to a putative link with autism and Crohn's disease. It was followed by reports of a rise in measles cases because of the large numbers dissenting from the mass immunization programme.

This raises numerous issues central to the ethics of immunization:
- Is getting vaccinated an individual choice?
- Is it right to require individuals to participate in an immunization programme for the sake of the communal benefit of herd immunity?
- Should people be able to refuse a vaccination if they believe it to be dangerous?
- Should the state be able to make immunization compulsory?

Although it could be argued that people have a duty not to infect others and not to simply reap benefits of herd immunity, the risks of vaccination are contestable. Coercion therefore seems unjustified (Holland 2007).

In such circumstances the duty to care has to be extended to include the concept of informed consent. The individual must be informed, and understand the information and implications of any action which is taken to be beneficial. In this way the health worker can be said to be avoiding harm.

In the field of drug education, harm reduction has been adopted as a way of working. This is perhaps more realistic than the encompassing principle of doing no harm. The health care worker recognizes that clients may not wish to change their behaviour, and therefore seeks to encourage a safer way of life and reduce its harm. Drug workers may give clients clean needles and condoms, and provide information about emergency first aid to reduce the risks of HIV infection or accidents.

Box 6.12

Should condoms be provided in prisons?
In England and Wales condoms can be prescribed by the prison medical officer where there is risk of HIV transmission. Condoms are not available in the prisons of Northern Island.

The example of screening illustrates the complexities of ethical decision-making and how attempting to follow the key ethical principles of doing good and avoiding harm is not a simple process. Most preventive services are offered with an explicit promise that they will do some good and an implicit understanding that they will do no harm. Yet what is the nature of that good? Screening, for example, only tells people that they are healthy at the present time. A negative result does not mean that illness will not develop the following year. Screening cannot promise a good outcome. Early detection can mean more effective or less radical treatment in some cases, but there may be no medical benefit and no treatment available. This used to be the case

with HIV infection. However, anti retroviral drug therapies may prevent or delay illness in some people with HIV.

Box 6.13

Consider these points in relation to a screening process with which you are familiar. Do you conclude that screening is of benefit, avoids harm and respects all persons equally?

1. Screening is never wholly routine and inclusive. It is targeted to identified risk groups and therefore excludes certain categories of people, usually on the grounds of age.
2. Screening is spaced because of economic considerations and therefore people may develop the disease in the intervening period.
3. The screening process may foster anxieties.
4. The screening process may be uncomfortable or painful.
5. The call and recall procedures may be poorly handled and the informing of results may take some time.
6. Laboratory protocols may not be rigorous enough, leading to the need for repeat tests.
7. Screening uses high-sensitivity methods which can result in a high number of false-positive results. These people will be subjected to unnecessary worry and distress, and in some cases treatment.
8. Screening uses methods which are less than 100% specific, therefore some people will go away falsely reassured.

Ethically, screening represents the tension between beneficence and non-maleficence. Poorly conducted screening can cause psychological harm from, for example, receiving false-positive results. Unfortunately, the pressure to ensure adequate take-up and to demonstrate success of a service means screening is often 'sold' to the public and consent is often presumed, making refusal seem possible.

Justice

Philosophers suggest three versions of justice:

1. The fair distribution of scarce resources
2. Respect for individual and group rights
3. Following morally acceptable laws.

Thus, justice requires that people are treated equally. But what is meant by equal? Does it mean according to equal need? Or according to merit? Or according to equal contribution? Or ensuring non-discriminatory practices?

For example, the equal distribution of resources can mean different things. It could mean that resources should be distributed equally in mathematical terms. Or should they be distributed according to how much was contributed – thus those that have and can put in most get out most? Or should we apply the Marxist adage 'From each according to his ability, to each according to his needs'?

The National Health Service was established on the basis of free medical care to all those who need it. In an era of scarce resources, demand far exceeds supply. Need is an obvious criterion for distributing care but it is not sufficient. Tudor Hart, whose inverse-care law was described in Chapter 2, observed that those who needed health care most received least (Tudor Hart 1971). As we shall see in Chapter 18, although we may use some objective measurement for the assessment of individual health needs, such as the ability to self-care or to perform certain tasks, this does not overcome the subjective value judgement that is involved in making these decisions. In recent years, health economists have tried to establish some other sort of objective and measurable criteria to compare competing claims – possibly the relative financial costs of treatment or an assessment made on quality-adjusted life years (QALYs), which are described in Chapter 3.

Issues of social justice are glaringly evident in health promotion. We read earlier the evidence of wide differences in health status between different groups in society. Whilst health promoters may be unable to alter society's inequities they may, nevertheless, be able to work on programmes which acknowledge that people's abilities to achieve health differ, which avoid victim-blaming and which tackle discriminatory practices.

Being fair to everyone might seem to suggest adopting public health measures which iron out differences in resources, health care or environmental quality. Yet any kind of state intervention means addressing the issue of individual rights versus the common good. For instance, would it be just that top wage earners should pay 50% income tax to finance public spending on health and welfare? Chapter 7 examines different political perspectives on health promotion, and the fundamental differences between right and left of the political spectrum towards health and welfare.

Telling the truth

The process of health education and information-giving in health promotion also involves complex ethical decisions. Seedhouse (1988) identifies truth-telling and promise-keeping as principles which the health promoter should hold on to when deliberating a course of action. As we saw earlier, the individual's right to information and the health promoter's duty to tell the truth may conflict with the duty of beneficence.

Practitioners want people to make healthy choices. When convinced of the 'good' of an action, practitioners may seek to persuade, perhaps through raising clients' anxiety or selecting the information or evidence. Yet ethical health promotion also includes a commitment to enhancing autonomy. As we saw in Chapter 4, the essential nature of health promotion is that it is based on a principle of voluntarism. It should not seek to coerce or persuade, but rather to facilitate an informed choice.

Box 6.14

Is it ethical to carry out opportunistic health education in primary health care? Consider the example of a patient who goes to her GP with back pain. The doctor takes the opportunity for some health education, and takes the patient's blood pressure and family history. The patient had neither sought this nor was she made aware beforehand of the implications if her blood pressure is found to be raised. The patient has not freely chosen to have her blood pressure checked in this way. Although she gave her consent, it might not be regarded as fully informed.

Campbell (1990) suggests that persuasion is acceptable only if a true picture of various aspects is presented. All education, he argues, involves some persuasion, and it is too simplistic to suggest that a desire to empower and create autonomy rules out persuasion. This means, however, that the health promoter must ensure that clients *seek* advice and help, and are not persuaded against their will. Yet many health promoters would argue that the only way to balance this need to empower people *and* facilitate healthier choices is to make this easier through policy decisions and frameworks (see Chapter 11). This takes us back to the argument that developing healthy public policy prioritizes the public good over individual freedom of choice and may not even be mandated by public opinion.

There may also be debate about the point at which enough information has been collected to justify legislative or coercive means of health promotion. Government bans on beef on the bone and unpasteurized green-top milk are examples where government action has been criticized for removing choice and leading to negative effects on employment and economic activity. Yet government inaction in the field of regulation and labelling of food has also been criticized for removing people's right to make decisions based on information.

In the following chapter we will explore how information about what is deemed 'healthy' is often influenced by political decisions and vested interests.

There is also an increasing trend towards sponsorship for health promotion activities. This ranges from health research sponsored by a tobacco company trust to the sponsorship of health information by drug companies, sanitary wear manufacturers or a local health food shop.

Box 6.15

Is sponsorship compatible with health promotion?

Sponsorship may be acceptable when it comes from enterprises compatible with health promotion principles and practices, and when the acceptance of income does not divert the practitioners from meeting more demonstrable health needs.

Box 6.16

Which of the following would you find acceptable?
- A curriculum pack for schools on puberty, sponsored by a sanitary-wear manufacturer
- A leaflet on safer sex sponsored by Durex, manufacturers of condoms
- A research project on healthy lifestyles supported by a tobacco company trust
- An education project for convicted drink-drivers sponsored by a brewery group
- An information handbook on local support services which includes advertisements for local businesses
- Baby baths and lotions given to maternity workers in low-income countries by baby food manufacturers.

Because the knowledge base of health promotion is changing, there are few areas where recommendations can be made on a factual basis. It is possible to think of numerous examples in recent years where information on the risks or benefits of certain behaviours has changed:

- The advice to exercise for 30 minutes each day and that this may be built up over the course of the day is likely to be disputed by new US physical activity guidelines.
- The importance of reducing saturated fat for those with normal cholesterol levels is disputed.
- Potatoes are no longer thought to be fattening but rather are a good bulk food and source of fibre.
- Moderate amounts of alcohol are now thought to have a beneficial effect on the heart.

Box 6.17

Should the public be made aware of debates over the evidence for health promotion advice? Should interventions be employed when the evidence for their effectiveness is in doubt?

Conclusion

Do practitioners whose work involves decisions affecting the lives of others engage in a moral deliberation about the best course of action? In general, most combine features of utility and deontology. They respect autonomy, try to be honest and fair and avoid victim-blaming. At the same time they try to achieve the best overall solution to any given situation. Yet situations can involve complex layers of decision-making generating many ethical dilemmas. Screening, for example, a frequently unchallenged linchpin of preventive health promotion, raises key issues about its benefits for an individual versus the increase of the social good, as well as questions about the extent to which screening is honestly presented. Before we can make any sort of ethical

judgement we need to be clear about the values and principles which underpin our actions. If we return to the questions asked earlier in this chapter, what do we mean by doing good and avoiding harm? At what point should we switch from creating autonomy to respecting autonomy? What do justice and equity mean in health promotion practice?

Tools to enable clear thinking around ethical issues, such as codes of practice or Seedhouse's (1988) ethical grid, provide a way to clarify decision-making and make the process more transparent. But dilemmas remain, and following different principles (each of which is sound and desirable) may lead to contradictory courses of action. Whilst there may never be absolute answers in ethical decision-making, a way forward is to be clear about which principles and duties you value most, and to encourage an open debate about ethical principles and how these translate into health promotion practice.

Questions for further discussion

- Should we 'sell' health?
- Should there be more legislation to promote health?

Summary

Health promoters need to be clear that what they do involves certain values and principles about what is 'good' health and health promotion. Beneficence, justice and respect for persons and their autonomy are fundamental ethical principles in health promotion. Their application in practice, however, is often problematic. Every situation or potential intervention involves a judgement not only of its possible effectiveness but also of its morality – whether it is 'right' or 'wrong'. In this chapter we have defined these key ethical principles and considered how they are manifested in common dilemmas for the health promotion practitioner.

Further reading

Cribb A, Duncan P 2002 Health promotion and professional ethics. Blackwell, Oxford. *An exploration of ethical issues and their impact on practice. Case studies explore value conflicts and issues such as codes of practice.*

Duncan P 2008 Ethics and law. In: Naidoo J, Wills J (eds) Health studies: an introduction, 2nd edn. Palgrave Macmillan, Basingstoke. *An introduction to the key principles of ethics and law as applied to health.*

The chapter includes a detailed analysis of the ethics of banning junk food advertising.

Hollan S 2001 Public health ethics. Polity, Cambridge. *An interesting and useful introduction to the ethical dilemmas involved in protecting and promoting public health. The book introduces aspects of moral and political philosophies and debates key issues such as screening and immunisation.*

References

Beauchamp T L, Childress J F 1995 Principles of biomedical ethics. Oxford University Press, Oxford.

Campbell A V 1990 Education or indoctrination? The issue of autonomy in health education. In: Doxiadis S (ed) Ethics in health promotion. Wiley, Chichester, pp. 15–27.

Duncan P 2008 Ethics and law. In: Naidoo J, Wills J (eds) Health studies: an introduction, 2nd edn. Palgrave Macmillan, Basingstoke.

Ewles L, Simnett I 2003 Promoting health: a practical guide, 5th edn. Baillière Tindall, Edinburgh.

Frankena W K 1963 Ethics. Prentice Hall, Englewood Cliffs, NJ.

Gillon R 1990 Health education: the ambiguity of the medical role. In: Doxiadis S (ed.) Ethics in health promotion. Wiley, Chichester, pp. 29–41.

Holland S 2007 Public health ethics. Polity, Cambridge.

Kant I 1909 On the supposed right to tell lies from benevolent motives. Cited in: Rumbold G 1991 Ethics in nursing and midwifery practice. Distance Learning Centre, South Bank University, London.

Naidoo J, Wills J 2005 Public health and health promotion: developing practice. Baillière Tindall, London.

Nursing and Midwifery Council 2004 The NMC code of professional conduct: standards of conduct, performance and ethics. NMC, London.

Rose G 1981 Strategy of prevention: lessons from cardiovascular disease. British Medical Journal 282: 1847–1851.

Seedhouse D 1988 Ethics: the heart of health care. Wiley, Chichester.

Sindall C 2002 Does health promotion need a code of ethics? Health Promotion International 17: 201–203.

Society of Health Education and Promotion Specialists 1997 Principles of practice and code of professional conduct for health education and promotion specialists. SHEPS, London.

Tudor Hart J 1971 The inverse care law. Lancet 1: 405.

Chapter Seven

The politics of health promotion

Key points

- Political ideologies
- Politics and globalization
- Politics of health promotion structures
- Politics of health promotion methods
- Politics of health promotion content
- Radical health promotion

OVERVIEW

Politics and health promotion are often thought of as separate activities. However, different approaches to health promotion reflect different political positions. This chapter outlines the diversity of social and political philosophies, which helps us to understand how health promotion has developed in the social and political context of the late 20th and early 21st centuries. Understanding our own values helps us to see the logical consequences for health promotion. The political dimensions of health promotion in relation to its organization, its methods and the content of health promotion activity are then explored.

What is politics?

Heywood (2000) identifies a fourfold classification of politics:

1. Politics as government – party politics and state activities

2. Politics as public life – the management of community affairs

3. Politics as conflict resolution – negotiation, compromise and conciliation strategies

4. Politics as power – the production, distribution and use of scarce resources.

Although these are separate concepts, they are arguably united by the fourth definition – politics as power – that is the main focus of this chapter. In democratic countries, people use their vote to give power to the political party of their choice. The elected party then governs public life and thus wields power on behalf of the populace. Power includes not only material or physical resources, but also psychological and cultural aspects, which may be equally effective in limiting or channelling people.

Power is distributed unequally worldwide, and globalization has contributed to increasing the divide between high-income regions, e.g. Europe, the USA and Canada, and low-income regions e.g. in sub-Saharan Africa. More than 10 million children under the age of 5 die each year, almost all in poor countries or poor areas of middle-income countries (Jones et al 2003). Over half of these deaths are caused by under-nutrition and lack of access to safe water and sanitation (Labonte & Schrecker 2007).

Political ideologies

One of the arenas in which power relationships are manifest is social policy, which may be defined as planned government activities designed to maintain, integrate and regulate society. This includes both welfare and economic policies, ranging from national legislation to local policy developments within local authorities. (See Chapter 11 for a discussion of Developing Healthy public policy.)

Government policies are determined according to its beliefs and ideas – its ideological position. Different political positions give rise to certain types of policy interventions. Analysts have identified many different frameworks and have pointed to the shift in ideologies since the 1960s (Bambra et al 2008). The old mid 20th-century spectrum of political belief from the hard-line left (Marxism) via Socialism and Liberalism to the right wing (Conservatism) no longer describes accurately the political beliefs and ideologies of nations and parties. Globalization, the demise of Soviet rule over Eastern Europe, and the permeation of nation boundaries

through international trade and the forces of nature have given rise to new political beliefs, in particular, the rise of neoliberalism and neoconservatism. These changes are summarized in Table 7.1.

Views on health and health promotion reflect a complex mix of values and beliefs which, in turn, reflect different political ideologies. The central proposition of this chapter is that health, and therefore health promotion, is political. Health promotion takes place in the policy area and embodies ideological values. Ideology is 'a system of interrelated ideas and concepts that reflect and promote the political economic and cultural values and interests of a particular societal group' (Bambra et al 2003, p. 18). The ideological viewpoints of different political parties vary widely. Key beliefs in relation to promoting health on which people differ concern:

- The extent of personal responsibility
- The role of government legislation and intervention
- The role of the economy and whether or not it should be regulated by governments
- Legitimate means to encourage choices and decisions
- The nature of society and the extent to which people are connected to each other
- The extent to which inequalities should be reduced.

On the right of the political spectrum there is a belief in individual self-determination and an antipathy to government intervention which not only restricts freedom but also inhibits enterprise. Conservatism sees inequality as inevitable and beneficial, in that differences stimulate people to succeed, resulting in innovation and productivity. Neoconservatism stresses the need to restore traditional values and a shared culture.

Neoliberalism has evolved since the 1960s as an attempt to combine the twin goals of social justice and economic growth. Neoliberalism is committed towards reducing state intervention in the economy and advocates market deregulation as the means to economic growth and social welfare. Such views are associated with the rugged individualism of Margaret

Table 7.1 A typology of welfare ideologies

Political party	Marxist	New Left	New Right	Conservatives
Political ideology	Socialism	Social democracy	Neoliberalism	Neoconservatism
Role of state	Collectivist, state control	Collectivist	Anticollectivist	Anticollectivist
View of economy	Mixed economy	Mixed economy	Market deregulation and state decentralization	Free market
View of society	Equality of opportunity, economic and political freedom is safeguarded by the state. The state should enable individual self-fulfilment and social justice through redistribution	The state should provide a safety net, although people should be encouraged to fend for themselves	The individual is central. State intervention into economic affairs should be reduced and market economics resurrected	Society is made up of self-interested individuals. Inequalities in wealth are inevitable and desirable because they stimulate innovation and success. Market forces ensure people's needs are met in a satisfactory manner. State intervention should be minimal
View of health care	Universal and free state provision to promote social cohesion and redistribution plus individual provision if desired	State provision to safeguard the vulnerable alongside individual choice and private provision	Paternalistic state should provide a safety net of health care provision, alongside individual responsibility	Individual responsibility and freedom of choice. Needs are best met through the free-market consumerism
Core values	Equality Collective responsibility Humanitarianism Social harmony	Individualism Social justice Collectivism	Individualism Social justice Freedom Responsibility Authority	Tradition Individualism Freedom Self-discipline Choice Competition

Thatcher who famously asserted: 'there is no such thing as society, only individuals and their families'.

Socialism is based on a belief in equality, fellowship and community, or a sense of responsibility for others. The government has a key role to play in ensuring everyone's basic needs are met, redistributing material resources and promoting a sense of social stability and cohesion. Social democracy, whilst embodying the same core beliefs, also embraces the notion of individual choice within a free market.

Box 7.1

In the modern UK, the Labour government elected in 1997 was committed to a 'third way' distinct from both liberal capitalism and democratic socialism. The third way was described by the then Prime Minister Blair as 'rooted in our enduring values of fairness, justice, the equal worth and dignity of all'.

Consider the social policy interventions referred to in these newspaper headlines about particular government policies. What values are being reflected?

- Choose and book – turning patients into consumers
- Hospital providers tender for business
- Child hooligans and trouble-makers – parents must take responsibility
- Surgery refused for obese patients
- Ban on smoking in enclosed places welcomed by health lobby
- Incapacity benefit claimants to be reviewed regularly to check their entitlement to benefits.

At the same time the 1997 election manifesto rejected values and ideology in favour of pragmatism and 'what works'. It is against this background that recent interventions should be viewed as:

- Reviving community
- Promoting responsibility
- Achieving equality through inclusion
- Accountability of individuals and services.

Globalization

Globalization, defined primarily as the economic processes of free trade supporting a global marketplace, is another reason for the shifting positions of political parties. No political party can ignore the immense power of global capitalism, which reaches across the world, ignoring national or regional boundaries. McDonalds, Microsoft and Philip Morris are known worldwide for promoting junk food, internet communication and tobacco respectively. Proponents of globalization argue it is more efficient and allows poorer countries to benefit from the technological advances of more developed countries. Critics of globalization argue that it destabilizes national economies, reduces everything to a market value and increases inequalities of wealth and health. It has been argued that the socioeconomic determinants of health have become globalized, leading to increased inequalities between rich and poor countries as well as within countries (Labonte & Schrecker 2007). Whatever the stance adopted, health promotion needs to develop and function within an increasingly global economy and world.

Globalization in politics is mirrored by globalization in health. Health risks are now increasingly global in their scope and spread, fuelled by the displacement of people (through war and natural disasters), global trade and movement of people and products. For example, the spread of human immunodeficiency virus (HIV)/acquired immunodeficiency syndrome (AIDS) and severe acute respiratory syndrome (SARS) requires continued vigilance and concerted action by nations and international agencies (Kickbusch & Seck 2007).

There are many important challenges to health and health promotion posed by globalization. Lee (2003) identifies the following:

- The loss of the ability to set national health policies
- A global market place with a shifting balance of power between public and private health sectors
- The low profile of health in global policy arenas, e.g. the World Trade Organization.

Equally, globalization opens up new possibilities – of networking, learning from others' experience and sharing of resources – that could be used positively to promote and protect health. The World Health Organization (WHO) Commission on Macroeconomics and Health in 2001 made the case for a reciprocal relationship between health and development, arguing that not only is development vital for health, but health is vital for development. The political challenge for health promotion is to foreground health as a valued goal and a key component of the global public good.

Health as political

In the WHO Alma Ata declaration (World Health Organization 1978) health was seen as both a human right and a global social issue. The Universal Declaration of Human Rights adopted by the United Nations in 1948 proclaimed that 'everyone has the right to a standard of living adequate for the health and well-being of oneself and one's family, including food, clothing, housing, and medical care.' Economic globalization has threatened these views of health as a human right. The People's Health Movement (www.phmovement.org) is a group of political activists and advocates opposed to globalization. This group argues that it is health, not the economy, that should be prioritized.

Within nation states, the political context affects all areas of government policy that have an impact on health, both directly and indirectly. Bambra et al (2003) argue that health is political because power is exercised over it and its correlates (such as citizenship and organization). A recent WHO report (Wilkinson & Marmot 2003) identified 10 social determinants of health: social class gradient, stress, early life, social exclusion, work, unemployment, social support, addiction, food and transport. Evidence suggests that these social determinants of health are the best predictors of individual and population health, that they structure lifestyle choices and that they interact to produce health (Raphael 2003). This in turn leads to the notion of health as political and the outcome of national and international policy decisions. A strong welfare state that provides people with access to the social determinants of health is arguably the best means to promote health (Raphael & Bryant 2006).

The politics of health promotion structures and organization

Internationally and nationally health promotion has enjoyed varying levels of support throughout the 20th and 21st centuries. The first International Conference on Health Promotion in 1986 led to the adoption of the Ottawa Charter for Health Promotion (WHO 1986) whose five action areas (building a healthy public policy, creating supportive environments, developing personal skills, strengthening communities and reorienting health services) are still used widely. This was followed by conferences in Adelaide (1988), Sundsvall (1991), Jakarta (1997) and Mexico (2000) which identified additional areas for action. More recently, the Bangkok Charter (WHO 2005) outlines four key commitments:

1. Strong intergovernment agreements to improve health

2. Health determinants need to be addressed by government

3. Empowered communities and civil societies

4. Good corporate practice to promote health in the workplace, communities and worldwide.

Example 7.3 gives a brief history of political ideologies and their impact on health promotion developments in the UK.

Box 7.2

Can you take politics out of health? Why might people say this?

Box 7.3

A brief history of health promotion in the UK

1800–1900 Public health movement

Arose out of a conservative tradition of reluctant collectivism, that the state had to intervene to ensure national efficiency, economic advantage and social stability

1900–1940 Health education

A liberal laissez-faire agenda which allowed voluntary organizations to provide preventive health education

1940–1970s Rise of prevention

A broadly conservative ideology with the emphasis on individual responsibility for health with information and advice being provided by health professionals; this was coupled with state intervention to provide a safety net for the most vulnerable

1980s The rise of the individual

Despite calls for a coherent national programme to tackle widespread inequalities in health and the WHO Ottawa Charter, New Right ideology dominates the health service; individual freedom is emphasized

1990s The rise of the market

- Emphasis is on public accountability to the consumer in services and the need to consult lay views
- Collaboration is advocated as means of efficiency and to reduce demands on the health service
- Despite an environmental consciousness this is not seen as an agenda for government action

1997 onwards Community, responsibility and equality

- Acknowledgment of the role of socioeconomic factors on health
- Emphasis on public participation in care and services
- Promotion of community cohesion
- Emphasis on the free market, individual choice and the commodification of health as the means to satisfy needs

Several commentators have argued that health promotion in the UK is currently facing a crisis of identity, and is in danger of being subsumed by the new public health (Orme et al 2007; Scott Samuel & Springett 2007). Health promotion has always struggled to have a visible presence and its position within the National Health Service has led to it being viewed as a 'Cinderella' service subordinated to health care provision and the medical model. Since 1997 and the election of the New Labour government, health promotion has been sinking from view, with the disappearance of both its specialist workforce and its lead organization in England (Scott-Samuel & Wills 2007). Health promotion is now just part of the remit of a range of other agencies and staff, including public health practitioners, the National Institute for Health and Clinical Excellence (NICE), health trainers and community development agencies. In many countries the ascendance of neoliberalism combined with traditional biomedical approaches inhibits the wholescale adoption of the Ottawa Charter principles for health promotion (Raphael 2008; Wills et al 2008). For example, in Canada an epidemiological focus on population health has displaced health promotion.

Box 7.4

The following example shows how 'joined-up policy-making' by different agencies can contribute in a coordinated way to the aim of suicide reduction.

Socioeconomic policies

- Employment policies to reduce joblessness
- Neighbourhood regeneration and renewal schemes to promote social cohesion

Environmental policies

- Public housing to reduce homelessness
- Integrated transport policy to reduce isolation

Lifestyle policies

- Health trainers to provide individually tailored encouragement and support to adopt healthy lifestyles, targeted at disadvantaged and vulnerable people

- Reducing access to means of suicide through, for example, blister packs and catalytic converters

Service provision policies

- Training for primary care staff

Integrated health and social care packages to provide 'seamless' care for individuals

- Funding for voluntary mental health agencies

 Box 7.5

What could joined-up policies contribute to the aims of:

1. Coronary heart disease prevention?

2. Cancer prevention?

Health promotion activities are structured by the prevailing policy framework, which has the effect of legitimizing certain approaches and excluding others. Until 1997 in the UK a combination of free-market economics with authoritarianism favoured medical preventive approaches and those which focus on individual lifestyles. Health promotion was seen as a means to prevent morbidity and mortality from specified diseases. Education and advice were the key strategies. Primary care practitioners would identify individuals at risk from a database of the practice population and carry out lifestyle interventions.

Neoliberal ideology sees a more interventionist role for government, although the free-market economy is also emphasized as the means to meet needs. There is an emphasis on partnership working and consumer choice, attempting to transfer free-market economic relationships into the service sector. However there is also recognition that state support and intervention are required to mitigate the inequalities in health driven by socioeconomic

inequalities (Bambra & Scott-Samuel 2005). This runs parallel to a pervasive life course discourse that locates health in the hands of the individual. (See Chapter 2 for more discussion of socioeconomic inequalities in health.)

The politics of health promotion methods

The methods used in health promotion are often viewed as a technical choice. Health promotion specialists are seen as possessing the expertise to decide what methods will prove most effective given the circumstances. However, we shall argue that methods imply political perspectives, and that the choice of which methods to use is not a politically neutral decision.

Health promotion has at its disposal a large repertoire of methods. These are discussed in greater detail in Part 2 (Figure 7.1).

The individual paternalist approach (Conservative)

This approach is expert-led, by professionals, and is focused on the individual. It has a long history, remaining perennially popular. The virtue of professional training is that it gives patients and clients confidence and a clearly demarcated role. Methods focused on the individual send a clear message about individual responsibility for health. Such methods rely on the belief that individuals can make significant changes in their lifestyle or environment. The focus on the individual also implies that everyone has equal resources and means of complying with health promotion messages. This may be viewed as ineffective, or incorrect, and there has been much criticism of these methods as 'victim-blaming' and misconceived (Naidoo 1986). However, such a viewpoint is also politically inspired, which may go some way to explaining its endurance.

By ignoring structural factors which affect the life chances and perceptions of different groups

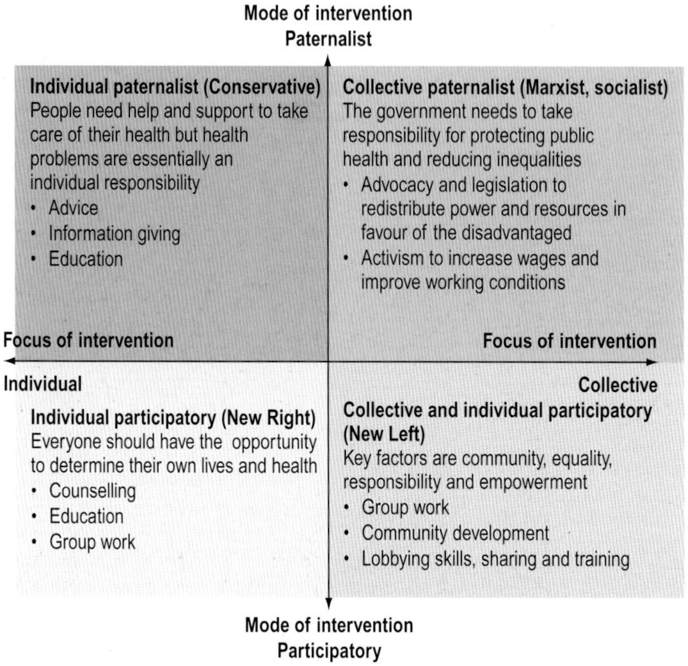

Figure 7.1 • Political philosophies and health promotion methods. Adapted from Beattie (1991, 1993).

of people, the fact that people's personal identity is bound up with their membership of such groups is obscured. Such an approach also ignores the structured inequalities in health status that are linked to socioeconomic status. This approach reinforces professional power by stating that individuals need to comply with expert advice.

The notion of individual free choice is a central tenet of the free-market economy. In economic terms, individualism becomes translated into consumerism, or the right to purchase goods. This approach is linked to the commodification of health, which becomes advertised as a tangible asset that can be bought. For example, sales of organic food and health club memberships have risen sharply in the UK, due in large part to their promotion as routes to health and well-being. This process in turn further exacerbates inequalities in health, as only the richest people can afford these healthier lifestyle choices.

Box 7.6

Do you think there is such a thing as a 'healthy choice'? Is it your role to inform patients and clients about healthy choices?

The individual participatory approach (New Right)

Neoliberalism emphasizes the role of the individual in determining their own choices. The individual participatory approach differs from the paternalistic individual approach by being premised on a different, and more equal, relationship between the health promoter and the client. This approach includes negotiated methods such as counselling, education and group work which take into account people's beliefs, attitudes and knowledge. The client is an active partner in the process and the end goal is enhanced client autonomy. Many professional groups have shifted their practice in recent years and tried to become more client-centred. Many health promoters feel more comfortable using these methods.

Box 7.7

What criticisms can be offered of this approach in terms of promoting the nation's health?

It may be argued that individually negotiated methods are most used and valued by the relatively privileged, healthy and articulate sections of society. Those with the greatest need are least likely to be able to access this kind of health promotion intervention. The focus on the individual maintains the free-market consumerist ethos criticized above.

The collective and individual participatory approach (New Left)

Methods which focus on the collectivity are more likely to be allied to social democratic or socialist political ideologies. The emphasis here is on understanding the processes which shape health outcomes, and assisting people to develop the skills to shape and challenge these processes. The New Left neoliberalist ideology retains a belief in the supremacy of the free market, leading to a focus on individuals and consumerism. The unifying factor is a stress on participation and active involvement, whether of communities or individual consumers. Collective participation, or social capital, is increasingly recognized as an independent source of health as well as self-esteem (Wilkinson 1996). Governments have sought to encourage collective participation through neighbourhood and community initiatives, for example neighbourhood regeneration and renewal interventions.

Individual participation is encouraged through patient choice and shared decision-making in relation to treatment and care. Underlying the commitment to equality is a parallel strand of responsibility.

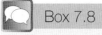

Box 7.8

Choosing Health: Making Healthier Choices Easier Choices (Department of Health 2004) refers to a contract between individuals, communities and the state. Given a goal of increasing physical activity, what might each party be expected to contribute?

Methods of health promotion that encourage participation include individually focused programmes centred on making informed choices and collective approaches that seek to redistribute power by empowering disadvantaged groups through such means as skills-sharing and training and lobbying.

The collective paternalist approach (Marxist, socialist)

The collective paternalist methods of working are associated with Marxist and socialist political beliefs. These beliefs include the primacy of social class, determined by economic status, in predicting social status, culture and life chances. Socialism sees individual identity as shaped by social interaction and membership of social groups. The owners of the means of production (the middle class) and those who only have their labour power to sell (the working class) have conflicting economic goals (to maximize profits or maximize wages accordingly). Class conflict is seen as inevitable according to this perspective.

Karl Marx's (1875) famous phrase 'from each according to his ability, to each according to his need' sums up the socialist goal of equality and social solidarity. Appropriate action uses methods such as the active redistribution of power in favour of the disadvantaged. Such action can be top-down (e.g. advocacy on behalf of lower socioeconomic groups or equity audits to expose inequalities) or bottom-up (e.g. trade union activism to increase wages and improve working conditions). Other methods may include promoting social cohesion through community development (see Chapter 10).

The methods adopted by practitioners in response to particular issues reflect political values about:

- Humanity – the rights of people
- Responsibility – whether health is in the hands of the individual or a result of particular social patterns which are reproduced and maintained by social policies
- The role of the practitioner – whether practitioners should hold power in the form of professional expertise or whether knowledge should be defined and shared by people themselves
- The role of the citizen – whether the citizen has the autonomy and resources to exercise free choices or whether citizens are constrained by social and national norms and the exercise of professional power
- The role of government – whether the state should take an active role in protecting its citizens' health or whether responsibility for health should lie with the individual
- The role of the economy – whether there is a free market and competition or a regulated economy overseen by government.

Box 7.9

Consider the following methods which might be adopted in an HIV and sexually transmitted infection (STI) prevention programme with vulnerable young people:

- Enhancing self-esteem
- Peer education
- Educational media campaign
- Young people's sexual health clinic run by nurses
- Funding for a telephone helpline run by a voluntary self-help group

- Easier and more open access to condoms
- More opportunities for young people to gain work experience and skills
- Creation of hostels and sheltered housing for homeless young people.

What political values are being reflected in each approach?

This discussion has presented the view that the methods chosen to promote health are not politically neutral. Certain methods fit into, maintain and reproduce the ideological assumptions of certain political perspectives. However, it is important not to overstate this view. Methods and ideology are not deterministically linked in a cause-and-effect manner. A variety of methods across all four ideological perspectives may be used by health workers who espouse a particular political viewpoint. There may be convincing reasons for adopting an eclectic methodology to promote health. But it is a fallacy to assume that methods are a technically neutral aspect of the health promoter's activity.

The politics of health promotion content

The previous sections have examined the view that the structure, organization and methods used in health promotion have a political dimension. It is sometimes argued that, although the process of promoting health is a political activity, the content of health promotion is neutral. Our position is that health promotion content is inevitably political. The framing of suitable agendas and the construction of what information is relevant are not value-neutral activities. On the contrary, they imply certain political values.

Box 7.10

What are health promotion priorities for the 21st century?

The Jakarta Conference (WHO 1997) identified the following priorities for worldwide health:

- Urbanization
- Demography (ageing population and population growth)
- Chronic disease
- Sedentary lifestyle
- Resistance to antibiotics
- Substance misuse
- Violence (domestic, civil and international warfare)
- Communicable disease
- Environmental degradation
- Globalization.

Perhaps the clearest example of the political nature of health promotion is the ongoing debate surrounding the social determinants of health. Whilst there is a wealth of research evidence linking poverty and disadvantage with ill health (Davey Smith 2003; Marmot & Wilkinson 2006), different governments have reacted differently. For almost two decades (1979–1997) a Conservative government refused to recognize the evidence on social inequalities and health, referring instead to 'variations in health status between different socio-economic groups within the population' (Department of Health 1992, p. 121). By denying the evidence, a non-interventionist policy could be adopted which argued that the free market is the best means of meeting health needs. By contrast, the Labour government elected in 1997 acknowledges the link between social inequalities and disadvantage and health and has commissioned reports and adopted targets to reduce health inequalities (Department of Health 2003).

Several research studies have confirmed that social democratic countries with strong welfare states, egalitarian ideologies and redistributive policies produce healthier populations, as indicated by lower infant mortality and low-birth-weight rates and increased life expectancy (Navarro & Shi 2001; Chung & Muntaner 2006, 2007; Navarro et al 2006).

 Box 7.11

Should issues such as sustainability and globalization be part of an agenda for health promotion?

Globalization creates new challenges for health promotion to widen its scope of action beyond national boundaries. Creating sustainable healthy environments requires international action. This may appear to be unrealistic for health promoters employed and working in a locality. However international networking, modern forms of communication using the internet and transnational policy-making have increased rapidly in recent years, opening up the possibility for more global health-promoting activity.

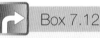 **Box 7.12**

Food labelling in the European Union
The European Union (EU) agreed in 2008 to impose standard nutritional information in food labelling for all prepackaged food across 27 countries. The new labelling scheme was agreed as a means to curb the rise in obesity in the EU. The scheme falls short of the traffic light system advocated by health charities, but went further than self-regulation, which the food industry had lobbied for (*Guardian* 31/1/2008, p. 14).

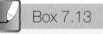 **Box 7.13**

Discuss the claim that evidence-based practice means health promotion is a neutral activity, because scientific methods have been used to determine what works and what doesn't work.

Increasingly, practitioners are called upon to base their work on evidence. The rise of evidence-based practice can be linked to New Right ideas about the accountability of practitioners and services to the 'consumer'. It could also be linked to socialist paternal collectivist ideas, identifying what works best and then requiring practitioners to follow set protocols. Evidence-based practice usually refers to a scientific notion of evidence that prioritizes randomized controlled trials as providing the best evidence (see Chapter 3). However this stance may be criticized for ignoring service users, their values, desires and wants. It may also neglect political and social issues that are too complex to factor into this model of decision-making. Evidence needs to engage with people's views and beliefs rather than pursue abstract notions of health or ill health.

This view of evidence-based practice can also be criticized for adopting a naive view of science as politically neutral. Social scientists (Bauchspies et al 2005, David 2005) point out that science is a social activity like any other, subject to similar constraints. Health-related research does not take place in ivory towers. Researchers have to bid for funds, and provide findings which are acceptable to funders and the academic community. Research indicates that private-sector funding of charitable and non-profit health organizations influences their activities and outputs (Jacobson 2005).

The process of research is therefore not immune to political considerations. What evidence filters through to the general public as the scientific consensus on health topics is also the result of political processes. The very idea of scientific consensus in social science is debatable. There is no issue where there is 100% agreement of the 'scientific facts'. For example, there is an ongoing debate about whether it is social capital or income that is responsible for the better health status of the more advantaged groups.

Being political

We have seen how health promotion arises from and reinforces political values and beliefs and takes place in a political context. Health promoters hold values and beliefs which are underpinned by established sets of ideas or ideologies. Many health promoters are engaged in practice which accords (more or less)

with their personal values. The medical model of health provides a clear role for practitioners because it recognizes their expertise. It also gives a clear role for individuals to act to protect their own health. Some health promoters may find that their professional role at times comes into conflict with their political beliefs and values. A belief in collective health goals and the need to empower people to be involved and take control over factors influencing their health may be at odds with a health promotion role bound by corporate contracts and the need to meet targets.

Box 7.14

Should health promotion have a code of practice that incorporates underpinning political principles? If so, what should be included?

The following activity is designed to help health promotion activists identify where they could make changes in their practice.

Box 7.15

The following are suggestions for developing radical health promotion practice. How many do you think are feasible for you? Be clear and honest about your own political standpoint.
- Develop an equal relationship with clients, where beliefs and values are respected, and information shared
- Try to ensure real community involvement in policies and decision-making
- Try to address health as a collective issue, making explicit the facts about health inequalities and supporting collective action around health issues
- Vet the health education materials you use to ensure they do not reproduce stereotypes or assumptions about gender, class, race, disability, age or sexuality
- Engage in action research in which researchers and researched are partners

- Develop a support network with like-minded health workers, where perspectives can be shared and issues discussed
- Be honest to yourself and others about the limitations of your work role.

Adapted from Adams & Slavin (1985) and O'Neill (1989).

Conclusion

Politics, or the process and study of the distribution of power in society, underpins all human activities, including health promotion. The political scene is in a state of constant flux, with the early 21st century witnessing the rise of neoliberalist ideology and globalization. These processes and values are embedded in the context in which health promoters practise. An understanding and engagement with politics in its widest sense are necessary in order to practise reflectively and in accordance with one's personal values and beliefs.

There is often resistance to the idea that health promotion is a political activity. Accepting the premise that politics is involved in health promotion may be experienced as muddying the waters, for it transforms a situation of relative certainty to one of uncertainty. It is no longer sufficient to rely on professional training to ensure effective health promotion. A whole range of different considerations needs to be taken into account, some of which threaten and call into question the whole notion of professional expertise.

However uncomfortable the process may be, an awareness of the political nature of health promotion is vital to its effectiveness (O'Neill 1989). Accepting the status quo is not an apolitical position but a deeply political one. What exists is not inevitable, but the result of complex forces and historical processes. Things might be otherwise. Health promotion is centrally concerned with a vision of better health for all. This vision may be informed by scientific knowledge and technical know-how, but its overall shape is determined by personal values and beliefs. Part of the task of health promoters is to uncover and hold up to scrutiny their values and beliefs. It is hoped that this and Chapter 6 will help health promoters in this task.

Box 7.16

The following statements reflect particular political philosophies. Can you identify these political philosophies? Which statements do you agree with?

1. There should be a safety net of economic and social support for the needy.
2. Energy and enterprise should be rewarded, not stifled by high taxation.
3. All people in a society have a commitment and responsibility to others.
4. Inequality is inevitable and necessary for development and growth.
5. High levels of benefits make people dependent on support.
6. People today are global citizens and need to focus on global issues like climate change.
7. There is no such thing as class in the modern UK.
8. People should be able to choose the type and level of health care or education they want and can afford.
9. Certain public services are essential and should be run by the state.
10. Macropolitics is of less significance than issues, particularly those affecting local communities.
11. Service users and providers should have an equal say in running public services.
12. People cannot be equal, but everyone should have the same chances.
13. Crime and disorder need to be tackled through the strict enforcement of laws and penalties.
14. Shared values and a common culture are vital to the maintenance of social cohesion.
15. A person's lot in life is determined by luck and accident of birth.

Questions for further discussion

- To what extent may health promotion be said to be a political activity?

- How could an understanding of politics help the health promoter develop more effective practice?

- How have your political values and beliefs affected your practice?

Summary

This chapter has examined the political implications of health promotion structures, organization, methods and content. The central proposition is that health promotion is a political activity, and that to attempt to deny this lessens one's understanding and the possibility of effective action. It has been demonstrated that mainstream health promotion activity is predicated on certain political values. The late 20th and early 21st centuries have witnessed a shift in the political values underpinning health promotion practice, triggered by the new Labour government elected in 1997, the growth of neoliberalist ideologies and the process of globalization. Previous Conservative governments had emphasized a non-interventionist role focused on individual advice and information-giving. The new Labour government has highlighted the social origins of health and given a commitment to act across sectors and boundaries to address the fundamental causes of ill health (Department of Health 2003). This commitment is however limited by New Labour's advocacy of free-market principles and globalization.

The role of the practitioner is still crucial, although it could be argued that the practitioner's function needs to expand to include client advocacy and empowerment with more emphasis on national and international networking and collaborative working across sectors and professions. Whether this shift in practice can occur, given increasing demands on health care services, is problematic. Many practitioners may feel that the broad political framework is now more supportive of health promotion. However, the task of practising in accordance with one's political beliefs remains a challenge.

Further reading

Bambra C, Smith K, Kennedy L 2008 Politics. In: Naidoo J, Wills J (eds) Health studies, 2nd edn. Palgrave, Basingstoke. Chapter 7. *This chapter provides a clear overview of politics as a discipline and applies its methodology and concepts to health issues.*

Harrison S, McDonald R 2008 The politics of healthcare in Britain. Sage, London. *A contemporary review of current provision and explanation of key topics such as rationing, patient and public involvement and interprofessionalism.*

References

Adams L, Slavin H 1985 Checklist for personal action. Radical Health Promotion 2: 47.

Bambra C, Fox D, Scott Samuel A 2003 Towards a new politics of health. Politics of Health Group discussion paper no. 1. University of Liverpool, Liverpool.

Bambra C, Scott-Samuel A 2005 The twin giants: addressing patriarchy and capitalism. Politics of Health Group UK. Available online at: http://www.pohg.org.uk/.

Bambra C, Smith K, Kennedy L 2008 Politics. In: Naidoo J, Wills J (eds) Health studies, 2nd edn. Palgrave, Basingstoke. Chapter 7.

Bauchspies W, Croissant J, Restivo S 2005 Science, technology and society: a sociological approach. Wiley-Blackwell, Oxford.

Beattie A 1991 Knowledge and control in health promotion: a test case for social policy and social theory. In: Gabe J, Calnan M, Bury M (eds) The sociology of the health service. Routledge, London, pp. 162–201.

Beattie A 1993 The changing boundaries of health. In: Beattie A, Gott M, Jones L et al (eds) Health and wellbeing: a reader. Macmillan/Open University, Basingstoke.

Chung H, Muntaner C 2006 Political and welfare determinants of infant and child health indicators: an analysis of wealthy countries. Social Science and Medicine 63: 829–842.

Chung H, Muntaner C 2007 Welfare state matters: a typological multilevel analysis of wealthy countries. Health Policy 80: 328–339.

Davey Smith G (ed) 2003 Health inequalities: lifecourse approaches. The Policy Press, Bristol.

David M 2005 Science in society. Palgrave Macmillan, Houndsmill.

Department of Health 1992 The health of the nation. HMSO, London.

Department of Health 2003 Tackling health inequalities: a programme for action. Stationery Office, London.

Department of Health 2004 Choosing health: making healthy choices easier. Stationery Office, London.

Heywood A 2000 Key concepts in politics. Palgrave, Hampshire.

Jacobson M F 2005 Lifting the veil of secrecy from industry funding of nonprofit health organizations. International Journal of Occupational and Environmental Health 11: 349–355.

Jones G, Steketee R W, Black R E et al 2003 How many child deaths can we prevent this year? Lancet 362: 65–71.

Kickbusch I, Seck B 2007 Global public health. In: Douglas J, Earle S, Handsley S et al (eds) A reader in promoting public health: challenge and controversy. Sage Publications/Open University, London, pp. 159–168.

Labonte R, Schrecker T 2007 Globalization and social determinants of health: introduction and methodological background (part 1 of 3). Globalization and Health 3: 5.

Lee K 2003 Globalization and health: an introduction. Palgrave Macmillan, Basingstoke.

Marmot M, Wilkinson R G (eds) 2006 Social determinants of health, 2nd edn. Oxford University Press.

Naidoo J 1986 Limits to individualism. In: Rodmell S, Watt A (eds) The politics of health education. Routledge and Kegan Paul, London, pp. 17–37.

Navarro V, Shi L 2001 The political context of social inequalities and health. Social Science and Medicine 52: 481–491.

Navarro V, Muntaner C, Borrell C et al 2006 Politics and health outcomes. Lancet 368: 1033–1037.

O'Neill M 1989 The political dimension of health promotion work. In: Martin C J, McQueen D V (eds) Readings for a new public health. Edinburgh University Press, Edinburgh, pp. 222–234.

Orme J, de Viggiani N, Naidoo J et al 2007 Missed opportunities? Locating health promotion within multidisciplinary public health. Public Health 121: 414–419.

Raphael D 2003 Addressing the social determinants of health in Canada: bridging the gap between research findings and public policy. Policy Options March: 35–40.

Raphael D 2008 Grasping at straws: a recent history of health promotion in Canada(in press). Critical Public Health.

Raphael D, Bryant T 2006 Maintaining population health in a period of welfare state decline: political economy as the missing dimension in health promotion theory and practice. Promotion and Education 13: 236–242.

Scott-Samuel A, Springett J 2007 Hegemony or health promotion: prospects for reviving England's lost discipline. Journal of the Royal Society of Health 127: 210–213.

Scott-Samuel A, Wills J 2007 Health promotion in England: sleeping beauty or corpse? Health Education Journal 66: 115–119.

Universal Declaration of Human Rights 1948 UN Department of Public Information, Geneva.

Wilkinson R G 1996 Unhealthy societies: the afflictions of inequality. Routledge, London.

Wilkinson R G, Marmot M 2003 Social determinants of health: the solid facts. WHO Regional Office for Europe, Copenhagen.

Wills J, Evans D, Scott-Samuel A 2008 Hungry for change: politics and prospects for health promotion in England. Critical Public Health (in press).

World Health Organization 1978 Declaration of Alma-Ata. International Conference on Primary Health Care, Alma-Ata, USSR. WHO, Geneva.

World Health Organization 1986 Ottawa charter for health promotion. WHO, Geneva.

World Health Organization 1997 New players for a new era: leading health promotion into the 21st century. 4th International Conference on Health Promotion, Jakarta, Indonesia 21–25 July 1997. Conference report. World Health Organization, Geneva/Ministry of Health, Indonesia.

World Health Organization 2001 Macroeconomics and health: investing in health for economic development. WHO, Geneva.

World Health Organization 2005 The Bangkok charter for health promotion in a globalized world. WHO, Geneva.

Part 2

Strategies and methods

The Ottawa Charter for Health Promotion (World Health Organization 1986) remains one of the most influential policy documents in the history of health promotion. It established the fundamental guiding principles and values of health promotion and described five key action areas:

1. Building healthy public policy
2. Creating supportive environments
3. Strengthening communities
4. Developing personal skills
5. Reorienting health services.

Each of these areas is the focus of a chapter in Part 2 and Part 3 focuses on supportive environments for health. Together these five areas encompass the goals of health promotion: to go 'upstream' and have an impact on the socioeconomic and environmental determinants of health; to focus on population health; to emphasise prevention rather than treatment; and to build capacity in communities and individuals. Whilst social and physical determinants of health were highlighted in the Ottawa Charter, the global, environmental and economic contexts were relatively invisible. This reflects the reality of the 1980s, when such issues were not on the agenda (Hills & McQueen 2007). However many of these issues can be addressed using the strategies outlined in the Ottawa Charter.

Improving the health of the population depends on many factors. Amongst the most important are:

- Tackling socioeconomic inequalities in health
- Making health everybody's business
- Making the healthy choice the easy choice.

These principles, and the values they encompass, underpin the Ottawa strategies. Tackling socioeconomic inequalities in health promotes equity and moves upstream, from a focus on blaming individuals to tackling the policies that shape environments.

The Ottawa Charter called for support for personal and social development through providing information, educating about health and enhancing life skills. By so doing, health promotion increases the options available to people to exercise more control over their own health and over their environments, and to make choices conducive to health. Individual skills therefore include not just knowledge about health issues, but also practical life skills such as negotiation, setting realistic and achievable targets and building self-esteem, all of which have an impact on the ability to make lasting behavioural changes.

Although not specifically flagged up in the Ottawa Charter, using the media is a core health promotion strategy and one that may be put to many different uses. Media coverage may be sought to promote individual lifestyle campaigns, to lobby for policy change or to highlight the importance of socioeconomic determinants of health. Using the media therefore contributes to all the other strategies and is the subject of Chapter 12.

Community development is one of the most fundamental strategies that informed the development of the concept and principles of health promotion, and featured as a strategy in the Ottawa Charter. It was conceived as a process that draws on existing human and material resources in the community to enhance self-help and social support, and to develop flexible systems for strengthening public participation in, and direction of, health matters. A focus on communities provides a route to tackle the social determinants of health through, for example, improving access to education, employment and housing. Strengthening communities is therefore a key strategy in moving upstream. The theoretical and policy base for community action has been informed more recently by research into community capacity building, and concepts such as social capital.

Building healthy public policy remains a key strategy for health promotion, and one that is currently being used in relation to an expanding number of issues, e.g. smoking bans, healthy transport systems and food labelling. It combines diverse but complementary approaches, including legislation, fiscal measures, taxation and organizational change. It requires an interventionist role by government, advocacy by practitioners and co-ordinated and joint action by different sectors. Globalization presents new challenges for international action.

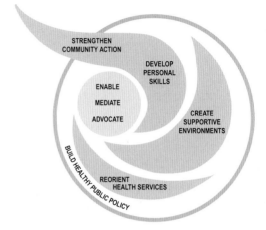

Figure 1 • Key health promotion action areas and strategies. From Ottawa Charter (1986).

Reorienting the health services, from treatment towards prevention, is the subject of Chapter 8. In some respects, this strategy has proved most taxing and impervious to change. There is always a demand that exceeds supply for health services, so trying to shift services away from immediate treatment to long-term prevention is extremely difficult. Treatment is high-profile, media-friendly and politically popular. Prevention is low-profile and its long timescale for effects to be evident makes it politically unpopular.

Creating supportive environments is the subject of Part 3, where different environments are discussed in separate chapters.

The Ottawa Charter stated that all of these actions would be required to promote health and illustrated this in a spiral image (Figure 1). At the heart are the skills of enablement, mediation and advocacy. Increasingly health promotion activities are conducted in combination in a comprehensive approach using a mix of such strategies and at multilevel (national, regional, community) action.

References

Hills M, McQueen D V 2007 At issue: two decades of the Ottawa Charter Promotion and Education(Suppl. 2): 5.

World Health Organization 1986 Ottawa charter for health promotion. WHO, Geneva.

Chapter Eight

8

Reorienting health services

OVERVIEW

Many agencies, services and practitioners contribute to the promotion of health and this chapter outlines the role of these stakeholders and different occupational groups. A reorientation of health services towards prevention was one of the key action areas of the Ottawa Charter (World Health Organization 1986), yet it is the least successfully applied. Health promotion poses several ambitious challenges for the health care sector: to extend the core business of health services from clinical outcomes to quality of life; to extend the focus from patients and relatives to staff and the wider community; and to integrate prevention into care and cure practices. To do so can only be achieved through organizational and funding changes. This chapter discusses these challenges,

the practitioners and agencies involved in promoting health, and how their contribution to health promotion can be mainstreamed and validated. The provision of health and social care services differs widely from country to country, and this chapter focuses on the UK experience.

Introduction

Historically the cure and treatment of illness have taken precedence over the prevention of ill health, or the promotion of positive health in the organization. Most people thinking of health services think of hospitals and family doctors, a focus on treatment, developments in surgery and new techniques and more effective medicines. There is widespread acceptance that prevention is better than cure and it is the only rational way forward for public health. Yet a recent review claims that 1.5 million pounds sterling is spent on prevention and health promotion in the UK each year, which is the sum spent on the National Health Service (NHS) in a day and a half (Wanless et al 2007). Part of the reluctance to invest in prevention is because the benefits accrue over time and so with limited resources and a pressure to demonstrate results, the focus of health services becomes skewed towards care.

Whilst the contribution of health services to longevity is clear, as we saw in Chapter 2 many factors unconnected with health services have a profound impact on health. For many health promotion practitioners, the contribution of health care services in addressing the determinants of health is marginal (Wise & Nutbeam 2007). However health services do have a unique and significant contribution to make towards population health. This chapter argues that health services, defined as 'all the activities whose primary purpose is to promote, restore, or maintain health' (World Health Organization 2000) are critically important in progressing health and human development.

Box 8.1

The Commission on the Social Determinants of Health (World Health Organization 2007, p. viii) has considered the contribution of health systems to equity. In pairs, decide to be A or B and develop some examples and argument to support the statements below:

A. Health systems 'specifically address the circumstances of socially disadvantaged and marginalized populations, including women, the poor and other groups excluded through stigma and discrimination. They also generate wider benefits: a sense of life security, well-being, social cohesion and confident expectation of care in times of illness.'
B. Health systems 'fail to apply their expertise to address the social determinants of health;

fail to contribute to social empowerment in the interests of health equity; institutionalize health care arrangements that create financial and geographic barriers to access for disadvantaged groups; alienate disadvantaged groups through culturally insensitive and sometimes antagonistic health worker and institutional practices; and impoverish the poor whilst allowing the rich to capture greater levels of public health care spending'.

What these statements illustrate is that, whilst health services may be a trusted focal point for any society, they may inadvertently contribute to inequity. In Chapter 4 we outlined the case made for health promotion by the Ottawa Charter of 1986 which stated that health care should encompass traditional education, disease prevention and rehabilitation services but also 'health enhancement by empowering patients, relatives and employees … enabling people to increase control over, and to improve, their health'. Not only would this involve 'open[ing] channels between the health sector and broader social, political, economic and physical environmental components', but it would also demand a 'change of attitude and organization of health services which refocuses on the total needs of the individual as a whole person'.

Box 8.2

Reorienting health services is the least successfully applied of the Ottawa Charter's key action areas (Wise & Nutbeam 2007). What might be the reasons behind this? Is there a case for continued or enhanced action to reorient services?

Resistance to reorienting health services is primarily due to the organizational tradition and culture, particularly within the state-funded NHS, of providing treatment and care. This acute-care paradigm means that all too frequently health practitioners view their role as patching people up and sending them home. Prevention is seen as 'helping people to get better by doing what is good for them', with patient compliance as an important objective. Patients who do not take advice may be seen as demanding and, in some cases, refused treatment if they do not follow recommended behaviour change. In countries funded by social contributions, practitioners who are paid by a fee for service have little incentive for prevention and activities such as managing chronic disease or health education which are time-consuming and bring no financial reward.

Yet there is some evidence of change and a recognition of the need to move towards a national *health* service and away from being a sickness service (Department of Health 2005, p. 119). The focus has shifted from treatment for acute conditions to the management of chronic conditions and the maintenance of optimum health. In recent years, 'self-management', 'collaborative' care, 'shared decision-making' and 'the expert patient' have become integrated into the management of chronic lifestyle conditions such as diabetes. Our companion volume *Public Health and Health Promotion: Developing Practice* (Naidoo & Wills 2005) discusses these moves to involvement and participation by patients and the public in health service planning and delivery in Chapter 6.

A major incentive for the reorientation of health services is economics. Increased longevity and expectations coupled with the rising costs of health services have led to a concern with the cost-effectiveness of services. There is growing evidence of the economic case for shifting focus from treatment to health promotion. A major UK review to examine health care funding needs (Wanless 2002) concluded that the 'fully engaged scenario', in which people self-manage their health and the NHS embraces prevention, is the most cost-effective.

The goals of reorienting health systems are:
- To achieve a better balance between prevention and treatment
- To focus on population health outcomes alongside the focus on individual health
- To achieve better health status for the population as a whole
- To achieve more cost-effective services
- To integrate services maximizing the contribution of the entire workforce.

Promoting health in and through the health sector

In addition to its obvious role of providing health care services, the health sector plays a major role in promoting health through being:
- A major employer – 1.3 million people in the UK (Sustainable Development Commission 2006)
- A purchaser of a wide range of goods and potential support to local economies. Its purchasing power is estimated as 17 billion pounds sterling per year on, amongst other things, food; furniture; medical, cleaning, and office equipment; road vehicles and building materials (Coote 2002)
- A major user of energy and producer of waste and carbon emissions. About 2.4 million tonnes of resources, excluding water and oxygen, is consumed in the NHS, with about 15% being discarded as waste and 1% remaining as stock. The NHS also generates 3.2 million tonnes of emissions, mostly carbon dioxide (Royal Society for Nature Conservation 2004)
- A direct provider of health promotion services
- A means of communicating with large numbers of people, whether as patients, family members, carers, employees, policy-makers, suppliers or health professionals
- A highly valued social institution providing social cohesion in all countries.

The NHS is a social setting just like a school or workplace. It has its own organizational procedures, values and ethos and cultural norms. For it to embrace health (rather than the treatment of disease) as its goal requires a change in all these elements.

Box 8.3

Considering the potential for health promotion, in what ways does the health service provide:

- Opportunity?
- Access?
- Credibility?
- Competence?

The health service is an important setting for health promotion because it offers a range of health professionals the opportunity to integrate health promotion into their practice, and thus to fulfil the early promise of a comprehensive and health-promoting health service.

There are several unique characteristics of the health service setting that make it ideal for promoting health. Use of health services is universal, so that everyone at some point in their lives comes into contact with health service providers. For many more vulnerable groups, such as people with long-standing limiting illness, contact is long-term and frequent. In the UK 97% of the population is registered with a general practitioner (GP) and 70% consult their GP at least once a year. Health practitioners enjoy high levels of trust and credibility amongst the general population and thus have the ability to affect people's knowledge, attitudes and beliefs. The NHS is the country's largest single employer and therefore workplace initiatives may affect a significant percentage of the workforce and their families. All these factors provide good reasons for prioritizing the health services as a setting for health promotion. Chapter 16 discusses the hospital as a health-promoting setting.

Primary health care and health promotion

The 1978 Alma Ata declaration (World Health Organization 1978) defined primary care:

Primary health care seeks to extend the first level of the health system from sick care to the development of health. It seeks to protect and prevent the problems at an early stage. Primary health care services involve continuity of care, health promotion and education, integration of prevention with sick care, a concern for population as well as individual health, community involvement and the use of appropriate technology.

Primary care is often used interchangeably with primary medical care as its focus is on clinical services provided predominantly by GPs, as well as by practice nurses, primary/community health care nurses, early childhood nurses and community pharmacists.

Primary health care (PHC) incorporates primary care, but has a broader focus through providing a comprehensive range of generalist services by multidisciplinary teams that include not only GPs and nurses but also allied health professionals and other health workers. PHC services also operate at the level of communities. The Royal College of General Practitioners (www.rcgp.org.uk) identifies the functions of the PHC team as:

- The diagnosis and management of acute and chronic conditions, treatment in emergencies, when necessary in the patient's home

- Antenatal and postnatal care and access to contraceptive advice and provision

- Prevention of disease and disability

- The follow-up and continuing care of chronic and recurring disease

- Rehabilitation after illness

- Care during terminal illness

- The coordination of services for those at risk, including children, the mentally ill, the bereaved, the elderly, the handicapped and those who care for them

- Helping patients and their relatives to make appropriate use of other agencies for care and support, including hospital-based specialists.

Box 8.4

There are 60 000 primary care physicians in France, about 1.7 per 1000 people, which is double the number in the UK. There are just over two primary care nurses, including health visitors, per doctor in France, which is about half the ratio of the UK.

What effect might this have on the promotion of health?

In many countries, such as France, there has been a move away from PHC in favour of a centralized hospital system. Community care is delivered by medical practitioners with much less involvement in providing a broad PHC with health promotion at its core.

Primary health care principles

The PHC approach is characterized by the following principles:

- A holistic understanding of health as well-being, rather than the absence of disease
- Recognition that the presence of good health is dependent upon multiple determinants; health services are important but so too are housing, education, agriculture and other services
- Health services reflect local needs and involve communities and individuals at all levels of planning and provision of services
- Services and technology are affordable, accessible and acceptable to communities
- Health services strive to address inequity and prioritize services to the most needy.

Primary health care: strategies

PHC strategies need to be consistent with the underlying philosophy of health promotion. In Chapter 5 we discussed various approaches to promoting health, of which education is one approach. Through education, communities and individuals

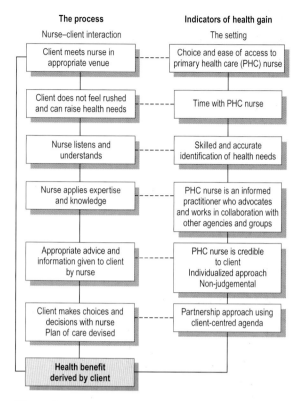

Figure 8.1 • Health-promoting nurse–client contacts. Adapted from Health Education Authority (1998).

gain understanding of the factors influencing their health and can work to gain control over health problems. The term empowerment is often used to describe patient education or any communication with a patient that is client-centred in its orientation. Yet empowering approaches necessitate organizational and environmental change. Figure 8.1 shows how empowerment and health gain can be built into nurse–client contacts.

Box 8.5

What factors might make it difficult for primary care nurses to act in ways which empower their clients?

Much of the health promotion practised in PHC settings is carried out by nurses. Much of this is opportunistic. A client has a consultation or is referred to a member of the PHC team and is identified as 'at risk'. The practitioner takes the opportunity to offer advice, information or a further referral on a health-related issue. In some cases, the practitioner may start a series of brief interventions using motivational interviewing to identify the client's readiness to change (see Chapter 9).

Box 8.6

How many advantages and disadvantages of opportunistic health promotion can you identify? You may have included some of the following:

- Opportunistic health promotion relies on the decisions of individual practitioners. This leads to patchy and uneven implementation, on a basis of chance rather than proven need
- Health promotion remains a marginalized luxury, to be tacked on at the end of a consultation if there is time. Lack of time is an important factor limiting the amount of health promotion undertaken by both GPs and nurses
- Doubts as to the ethics of opportunistic health promotion have been expressed, e.g. raising the subject of smoking with patients consulting for unrelated problems.

The advantages of opportunistic health promotion include:

- Immediate relevance of information
- Highly motivated patients
- The ability to adapt and modify the input to suit individual needs.

The emphasis of recent policy has been on developing more planned and proactive health promotion activities. The need for a risk assessment becomes a key skill enabling PHC practitioners to target health promotion better. For example, only a minority of those at risk of a sexually transmitted infection (STI) attend genitourinary medicine (GUM) clinics, whereas the great majority of adults will access primary care in any one year. Matthews & Fletcher (2001) suggest therefore that GPs are likely to encounter patients from across the risk spectrum for STIs and should develop planned ways of raising the issue of sexual health risks with all patients.

Primary health care: service provision

PHC is the first level of health care which is directly accessible to individuals and communities. This means that effective PHC must be locally based, in proximity to the places where people live and work, easy to access and free at the point of delivery. As the first level of health care services, PHC services need to be well integrated with the secondary and tertiary health care sectors, in order to provide prompt assessment, response, referral and continuity of care for people throughout all levels of the health care system. There is an increasing burden of chronic and complex health conditions, including the frail aged, that will demand care in the community.

The following examples of PHC services describe the Peckham experiment of the 1930s and the recent proposals to reorganize London's health care around polyclinics.

Box 8.7

Do you see any similarities in the following description of two forms of PHC?

The Peckham experiment

The Pioneer Health Centre was started in the 1930s by two doctors concerned about the health of poor people living in south London. The Health Centre tried to address health in a holistic way and incorporated a fitness club, theatre, gym, swimming pool, billiards table, children's nursery, a cafeteria serving healthy, cheap food, a library and medical consulting rooms. For one shilling (5p) a week per family, all of the Centre's facilities could be used. In 1938, 600 families belonged.

It closed during the Second World War, reopening in 1946 when it added a nursery school, youth club, marriage advisory service, Citizen's Advice Bureau and child guidance. It closed in 1950 because it did not fit into the structure of the emerging NHS. The Centre has been revived as Pulse Health and Leisure – a partnership between Southwark Council and Lambeth, Lewisham and Southwark health authorities funded by £3.2 million of lottery money. Its aim is 'to provide a unique leisure, health and fitness resource that encourages local people to invest in their own health and well-being'. The new partnership thus puts the responsibility for health squarely with the individual.

Polyclinics

Polyclinics will offer not just GP services, but also 'antenatal and postnatal care, healthy living information and services, community mental health services, community care, social care and specialist advice all in one place. They will provide the infrastructure (such as diagnostics and consulting rooms for outpatients) to allow a shift of services out of hospital settings. They will be where the majority of urgent care centres will be located. And they will provide the integrated, one-stop-shop care that we want for people with long-term conditions' (Darzi 2007, p. 11, para. 22). The staff in each centre will include GPs, consultant specialists, nurses, dentists, opticians, therapists, emergency care practitioners, mental health workers, midwives, health visitors and social workers (Darzi 2007, p. 92, main table). The shift of much health care out of hospital settings means that in the future 'the bulk of healthcare activity will take place in polyclinics' (Darzi 2007, p. 107, para. 71).

Behind both forms of provision is the notion that health care needs to be closer to home and include the wide range of services that promote health. Whilst the Peckham experiment had a holistic view of individual and community health needs, the polyclinic is firmly rooted in a medical model of care. Whereas the Peckham centre was rooted within its community, inevitably a polyclinic provides centralized services further away and more difficult to access from the disadvantaged communities who use and need PHC the most.

One common argument is that adequate provision of PHC services will mean that more specialized hospital-based services are unnecessary. For example, proper management and monitoring of chronic conditions such as diabetes and asthma should help prevent the development of crises which require hospitalization. As stays in hospital become shorter, the role of the primary health team becomes more important.

Traditional models of PHC that assumed the family doctor would build up a detailed knowledge of patients over time and visit in their own homes are changing, however, and may not be relevant for transient and culturally diverse populations. Consultations in general practice in the UK tend to be short (8–9 minutes) compared to other countries and unable to address adequately the wide range of psychosocial problems experienced by disadvantaged population groups. GP's awareness of possible referral options in the locality is also limited (Popay et al 2007), although innovative 'social prescribing' projects exist such as the one in Stockport, in which a GP may refer to arts, gardening schemes, learning or a self-help library.

Box 8.8

Participation, collaboration, empowerment and equity are core health promotion principles.
- How can people be enabled to increase control over and improve their health?
- How can participation be increased in the planning and implementation of health care?
- How can the contribution of each member of the PHC team be enhanced?
- How can health and social care contribute to sustainable development?
- How can PHC work towards addressing inequalities in health and ensure an equitable distribution of resources?

Participation

It is now accepted that the public have the right to be consulted and to have a say in the policy-making process (the drivers towards patient and public involvement are discussed in our companion volume in Chapter 6 (Naidoo & Wills 2005)). However, the means of public consultation range from formal to informal; one-off events to ongoing contact; and reactive to proactive. Any of the following activities undertaken to increase public participation and involvement could be said to be public health work:

- Supporting patient participation groups in general practice, including lay views in community health profiles
- Seeking feedback from the community on service provision and using this to change practice
- Supporting self-help groups in the community
- Working with community groups on health issues.

Equity

As we saw in Chapter 2, there is a strong argument for advocating greater social and economic equity as a means of promoting health. This refers to equity of both material resources and power (the ability to achieve desired goals). Equity, or being fair and just, is not the same as equality, which is the state of being equal. Whilst equality may be impossible to achieve, providing equal services for people with equal needs and working to reduce known inequalities in health are realistic goals.

 Box 8.9

What can you do in your health promotion role to promote equity?

Most practitioners see the promotion of equity as a political task beyond their role or competence. However, even small steps contribute to greater equity. For example, ensuring clients know their benefit entitlement and claim it, helping clients to fill out the necessary forms or supporting the case for a welfare benefits advisory service to receive health authority funding are all aspects of working for equity to improve material circumstances. Identifying inequities in local services, such as people not registered with general practices, and supporting such groups to gain access to services, is also working for equity. Targeting areas of deprivation for more intensive interventions is another example which is frequently found. The arguments and evidence in favour of targeting small areas or population groups are discussed in more detail in our companion volume (Naidoo & Wills 2005).

Collaboration

Collaboration or partnership working is the third health promotion principle. Collaboration means working together with others on shared projects. Collaboration is necessary because of the many different factors affecting public health, which means that any one agency or organization can have only a limited impact on health. By working together, more fundamental changes can be put into place, with a greater potential to promote health. Government has stressed the need for local authorities to consult widely with their local communities and to work alongside the NHS to promote health. Coterminous boundaries, joint appointments for Directors of Public Health, statutory requirements for joint strategic plans such as local area agreements, and a framework for commissioning services for health and well-being are ways in which this collaboration has moved forward. (Information about current government strategy for health services and local authorities can be found on the websites of the Department of Health at www.dh.gov.uk; the local government authorities at www.idea.gov.uk; or the NHS confederation at www. nhsconfed.org.)

Our companion volume *Public Health and Health Promotion: Developing Practice* (Naidoo & Wills 2005) discusses some of the challenges associated with partnership working across organizational boundaries, such as differences in priorities, organizational ethos, funding arrangements, competition for contracts and geographical boundaries. Enabling factors identified include committed individuals, joint funding and pooling of resources, shared education and training opportunities and existing projects which span different agencies.

of organizational commitment to improving health. The branches describe key areas for health promotion activity and those elements of the setting that contribute to health, e.g. organizational policy and the physical environment.

Box 8.11

To reduce the financial burden on health services there are a number of possible initiatives which aim to prevent ill-health. What are the advantages and disadvantages of each?

- Developing campaigns which focus on top public health priorities, seeking to educate the population to behave differently
- Banning smoking in public places
- Including health education as part of the core remit of community nurses, to be documented and monitored
- Paying primary care doctors an incentive fee to call in 'at-risk' patients such as 25–40-year-old men
- Paying primary care doctors to screen all 'high-risk' patients for specific diseases such as diabetes, kidney disease, stroke
- Creating financial incentives for individuals if they can show they are leading healthy lives by subsidizing insurance schemes
- Working with primary care doctors to discourage overprescribing and scrutinizing diagnoses and resultant interventions
- Developing quality indicators for primary care services.

Box 8.10

Think of an intervention in your health promotion practice concerning the health promotion of a service user.

Reflect on why you did what you did.

Could you have done something different?

Would other health promoters have done the same as you?

If you adopted a public health approach to your work, what aspects of this intervention would change?

How could you:

- Increase participation?
- Promote equity?
- Increase collaboration and partnership working?

NHS Health Scotland has developed a framework to support the development of a health-promoting service, as shown in Figure 8.2.

The roots of the tree suggest the necessity of understanding the underlying conditions that determine health and ill health:

- Biological inheritance
- Physical environment
- Cultural, social, political and economic circumstances.

This understanding of who, when and where is affected enables possible interventions to be identified. The trunk of the tree illustrates the importance

All the above suggestions have been adopted. Most reflect the view that there needs to be incentivization through financing mechanisms or performance management in order for health care organizations to adopt health promotion strategies. As the requirement standard for public health simply requires

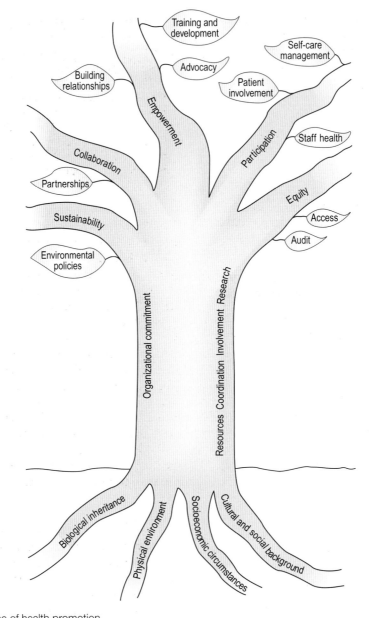

Figure 8.2 • The tree of health promotion.

plans to be in place for disease prevention and health promotion with regard to obesity, smoking, substance misuse and STIs (Department of Health 2004), actions may be interpreted very differently

from routine health education to rehabilitation therapy.

Obesity, for example, is a public health priority. Although primary care may offer potential for health promotion, there are numerous barriers to effective health promotion in primary care. Maryon-Davis (2005, p. 97) describes obesity as a frequently intransigent problem for primary care. He cites:

- Pressure of time in the consultation
- A lack of appropriately trained primary care staff
- A shortage of community dietitians or nutritionists
- The potentially enormous caseload
- Language or cultural barriers
- The intractability of patients' eating habits, exercise behaviour and their clinical condition.

Box 8.12

What might help to improve the management of lifestyle problems in the primary care setting?

Maryon-Davis (2005) suggests the following as ways of overcoming these difficulties in the case of obesity. However these strategies may also be applied to other problems:

- Improved clinical guidelines
- Better training of primary care staff
- At-risk patient registers
- Smarter database search tools
- New quality incentives
- Closer working with other practitioners, e.g. dietitians, counsellors and pharmacists
- More hospital outreach clinics
- Designated GP specialists and practice clustering
- Expanded exercise referral schemes and links with leisure providers
- Subsidized referral to commercial slimming groups
- Better use of patient groups and voluntary and community workers.

Who promotes health?

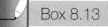

Box 8.13

'Health is a state of complete physical, social and mental well-being, not merely the absence of disease or infirmity' (World Health Organization 1946). Using this well-known definition of health, make a list of who is involved in promoting and protecting the nation's health.

Identifying who promotes health depends on how it is defined. If you adopt a fairly narrow medical model of health, you may have included a range of health sector professionals such as GPs and health visitors. If, however, your definition is wider and health is seen as socially and economically determined, then a much wider range of partners can be seen to promote health. Figure 8.3 illustrates the sectors and range of agencies that can be involved in promoting health. These span international and global interests, national, regional and local levels. Many of these agencies would not regard health as their core business but their activities can make a significant contribution to the promotion of good health in society. Reorienting the work of such agencies and organizations would mean making explicit their health goals and impact.

International

Numerous international organizations such as the World Health Organization have health promotion as a core function. Other organizations, such as the World Trade Organization, responsible for free trade and investment agreements between nations, can have an impact on resource consumption and environmental stress, and on wage rates and thereby the efforts of countries to reduce inequities. The World Bank provides financial assistance to low-income countries and is a major funder of health projects, including mass immunization campaigns and antimalaria projects.

Box 8.14

War and public health

Increasing global interdependence has meant that wars are more likely to affect countries geographically far removed from the conflict, through economic repercussions, emigration patterns and even by direct forms of action such as terrorism. Almost all wars since the Second World War have been fought in developing countries, which has allowed the west to consider war as an exceptional event rather than a mainstream concern for public health. This is despite the fact that in 1990 war was the 16th cause of global burden of disease (Murray & Lopez 1997) and predictions were that by 2020 it would take eighth place, putting it ahead of human immunodeficiency virus (HIV)/acquired immunodeficiency syndrome (AIDS). Wars have also dramatically shaped the spending of the countries of the developing world, which buys approximately 85% of world arms and weaponry. Many of these countries spend more on arms and weapons than on education or health (Levy & Sidel 2002). The five major developed powers (China, France, Russia, the USA and the UK) produce 90% of the world's arms and the arms trade has a role in the perpetuation of conflict (Bunton & Wills 2005).

National

A range of government departments have an influence on health and the government is committed to 'joined-up' policy. The appointment of a Minister for Public Health in England in 1997 was intended to ensure coordination of health policy across government. Health impact assessments are intended to ensure that the health consequences of a range of policies will be considered during their development stage.

 Box 8.15

What is the public health role of the following departments:
- Treasury?
- Department for Transport?
- Department for Children, Schools and Families?

    Could/should that role be developed and made more explicit?

A range of agencies within government have a remit for aspects of health, e.g.:
- Food Standards Agency – regulation of food labelling, food safety
- National Institute for Health and Clinical Excellence – gathering of evidence of effective interventions
- Health Protection Agency – management of health threats, including infectious disease; radiation, chemical and environmental hazards; and emergency response.

In England, following the disbandment of the Health Development Agency, there is no lead agency for health promotion. Health Scotland, the Welsh Assembly and the Health Promotion Agency for Northern Ireland take on this role in the other UK countries. In other countries there are national centres which may coordinate research and knowledge, contribute to policy advocacy and provide a voice for public health and health promotion practitioners, e.g. Public Health Agency for Canada.

Increasingly the corporate sector is recognizing the potential of health as a commodity. In recent years, there has been a huge expansion in gym membership, exercise equipment, organic foods and farmers' markets. Supermarkets promote foodstuffs on the basis of their health-giving potential. The impact of the corporate sector on health through labour market policies and environmental degradation is increasingly recognized (see Chapter 11 on how public policy is being oriented to health).

Local

Authorities and trusts are the different types of organizations that run the NHS at a local level. The whole of England is currently split into 10 strategic

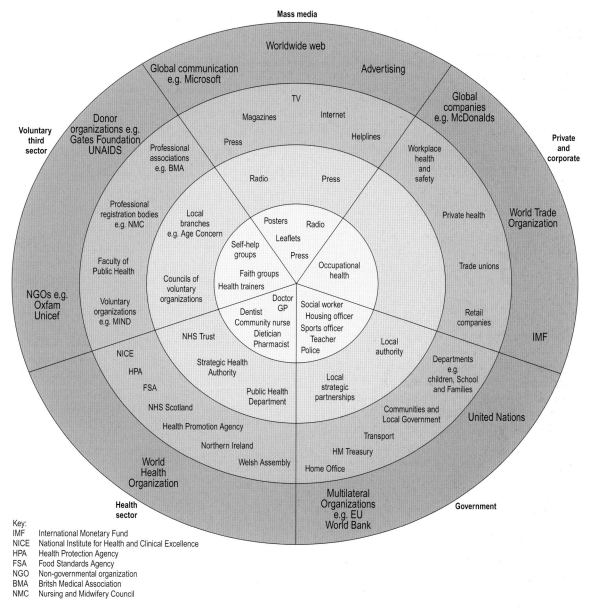

Figure 8.3 • Agencies of health promotion in the UK.

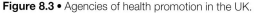

health authorities (SHAs). These organizations were set up in 2002 to develop plans for improving health services in their local area and to make sure their local NHS organizations were performing well. The NHS website (http://www.nhs.uk/aboutnhs/HowtheNHSworks/) provides details on the current structure of the NHS which includes acute trusts that provide hospital-based care; ambulance trusts providing emergency care; mental health trusts and primary care trusts (PCTs).

PCTs are now at the centre of the NHS and control 80% of the NHS budget. They are local organizations with a remit to identify local needs and any problems of equity and commission for the provision of corresponding services. The role of a PCT is to:

- Support and develop the services of GPs and their practice teams
- Provide a range of community health services, such as health visiting and district nursing
- Commission hospital treatment and specialist care for patients
- Directly provide some services.

All NHS bodies have a legal duty to involve and consult the public. Patient and public involvement (PPI) forums were set up in every NHS trust and PCT area to gather views about local health services and provide dialogue with the NHS. Local involvement networks (LINks) will be established for every local authority (LA) area that has social services provision. They will support local people in taking part in planning, developing and making decisions about local services, including monitoring and making their views known about how services are delivered. A health overview and scrutiny committee may review and scrutinize any matter relating to the planning, provision and operation of health services within a local area.

Key functions that have an impact on health, such as housing, transport and sport and leisure, are all LA responsibilities. Prior to the 1970s the public health function was located in LAs but was transferred to the NHS in 1974. Increasingly, LAs and PCTs are now required to work together in planning and providing services. In some areas the Director of Public Health may be jointly appointed by the PCT and the LA. The Local Government and Public Involvement in Health Bill (2006) requires the production of a joint 'strategic assessment' of the health and social care needs of the local population. LAs must produce a community plan to improve well-being in the area informed by a local strategic partnership (LSP) which brings together organizations from public, private, community and the voluntary sector. A local area agreement (LAA) is a 3-year agreement – informed by the community strategy – setting out the priorities for a local area. LAAs cover four basic themes:

1. Children and young people
2. Safer and stronger communities
3. Healthier communities and older people
4. Economic development and enterprise.

Public health and health promotion workforce

PHC services require balance between health promotion, preventive care and illness treatment. This is best achieved through the use of a team drawn from a variety of disciplines, including not only medical and nursing health professionals but also community workers, public health information workers and educators.

The Report of the Chief Medical Officer's Project to Strengthen the Public Health Function (Department of Health 2001) provided a framework for assessing the contribution of the broader public health workforce to the public health function. In particular the document referred to three main categories of employees:

1. Wider contributors
2. Practitioners
3. Specialists.

Reorienting the workforce means identifying health promotion opportunities and also encouraging a way of working which is empowering and enables people to take control over health issues.

Wider contributors

Wider contributors are professionals who have an impact on public health as part of their work, but who may not recognize this, e.g. teachers and social services employees. This part of the workforce is important because they can reach people who are not in contact with the health service and refer them on to sources of advice and support. In order to maximize their contribution, the public health aspects of their work need to be recognized and foregrounded. Teachers provide an example of this failure to recognize the importance of public health and health promotion – although schools are seen as key settings for health promotion in many countries with national standards and with key roles to strengthen the social and emotional well-being of both pupils and staff, health promotion is not part of initial teacher education in many countries (Chapter 13).

There is also a huge informal workforce that contributes to health. Voluntary organizations or non-governmental organizations (NGOs) act as service providers, self-help groups, pressure groups and as sources of education and information. They are involved in statutory structures such as local strategic partnerships and in planning and consultation exercises, such as the community plans. Voluntary organizations are important in providing specialized information, and being close to the community and isolated and vulnerable groups. They can reflect people's experience of a service and give an indication of other needs, acting as a catalyst for change. The precarious funding of many voluntary organizations means they have to expend a great deal of time and effort securing grants and funding, which can make long-term planning difficult and lead to low morale.

Practitioners

Practitioners are a smaller group of professionals who spend most, or all, of their time in public health practice. Changing contracts and more specific definitions of roles and competencies mean that job remits in primary and social care are in a state of constant flux. Any account of working practice is in danger of being both context-specific and out of date in the near future. Increasingly roles are becoming generic such as those within 'the children's workforce' where the skills, competence and knowledge required are similar regardless of professional background or role and apply to a very wide range of workers, including personal advisers, health visitors, midwives, youth workers, family workers, substance misuse workers,

nursery nurses, educational welfare officers, community children's nurses, school nurses and support staff such as learning mentors working in schools.

A brief description of some key roles follows. It illustrates the importance of health promotion in many job remits but also the challenges faced and why, for many individual practitioners, health promotion often slips to the bottom of a busy workload.

Specialist community public health nurses

Health promotion is a priority in the role of specialist community public health nurses such as health visitors and school nurses:

Specialist community public health nursing aims to reduce health inequalities by working with individuals, families, and communities promoting health, preventing ill health and in the protection of health. The emphasis is on partnership working that cuts across disciplinary, professional and organisational boundaries that impact on organised social and political policy to influence the determinants of health and promote the health of whole populations (www.nmc-uk.org).

Increasingly, community nurses are expected to adopt a population focus, adopting community development methods (see Chapter 10), identifying local needs and supporting community and voluntary groups. Community nurses are part of the PHC team and should work closely with other community nurses, GPs and social workers. However health promotion may not always be coordinated or prioritized because health and social care workers tend to concentrate on their own case load.

Because community nurses visit people in their own homes, they are able to build a strong relationship with their clients over a period of time. This enables them to carry out much one-to-one education, counselling and opportunistic health education. District nurses, for example, visit people with chronic sickness or disability at home. Much of their work is with older people (1:4 people over 75 are on a district nurse caseload) and they carry out opportunistic health education as well as liaising between people living in the community and other relevant health and welfare workers. The individualized basis of patient care offers opportunities for health promotion but is also a constraint both in limiting time and also separating district nursing from a population perspective. One study reports a district nurse commenting: 'Public health … it's like anything isn't it … we just don't realise we are doing it … I think maybe we need to be more aware of just what skills we've got' (Arnold et al 2004).

 Box 8.16

The key role of the district nurse

1. Building community intelligence:
   - Sharing information about older patients and their needs
   - Broad public health approach to health needs assessment, e.g. transport to shops; street safety
   - Access to private accounts of health (Scottish Office Department of Health 2001)
2. User participation strategies:
   - Access to the most vulnerable and least heard
   - Access to a large population, both well and ill
3. Working in partnership with individual patients:
   - The expert patient and the contribution of district nurses to patients managing their own condition and educating others.

Mental health nurses

Promoting mental health requires a collaborative approach from a diverse and wide-ranging group of stakeholders. Mental health promotion is often associated with psychiatry and the health and social care services involved in delivering care and treatment to people experiencing mental ill health. Whilst treating mental illness is an important component, mental health promotion is concerned with the mental health and well-being of the whole population throughout the life course. Mental health promotion is delivered in a variety of settings, including schools, the workplace, the community at large and within specific communities such as care homes or prisons (see the Wales Mental Health Promotion Network at www.wales.nhs.uk).

School nurses

School nurses are part of the community nursing service but their role varies enormously. Originally, it was to focus on the detection and treatment of poor hygiene, infestations and malnutrition, but it has since evolved to become routine health surveillance and screening. In common with health-visiting practice, the current role for school nurses is to move away from routine surveillance towards identifying needs and targeting support, e.g. support for children with chronic diseases or the provision of education and counselling on specialized topics such as sexual health. Some areas adopt a life course approach, with the school nurse acting as a navigator for children throughout their school journey.

 Box 8.17

Consider the list of activities below. What challenges and barriers might there be to school nursing extending its role in these ways?
- Health promotion
- Drop-in clinics
- Collaboration with education and social work
- School nurse-led immunization
- School health profiling
- School nurse-led health interviews, e.g. in first year primary.

Midwives

Hospital midwives are involved in antenatal education and the delivery of babies. Community midwives visit all new mothers in their area, and provide support and education as well as monitoring the health of mothers and babies.

Midwives are in an ideal position to extend support to expectant and new families and to provide a service which helps parents to access information and use it effectively to nurture the health of their family. However, they also have an important role in bringing public attention to those issues which are beyond the scope of individuals to change, such as social and environmental obstacles (Crafter 1997, p. 3).

General practitioners

General practice has traditionally been a private and personal consultation between doctor and patient. Health promotion consisted of opportunistic advice or information, often limited by time or a concern not to be 'intrusive'. The contracting of GP services provides additional payments to GPs to carry out preventive work such as immunizations, health checks to identify risk and the giving of advice. Opportunities for planned interventions have increased and there are numerous examples of exercise referral schemes and lifestyle management programmes.

Practice nurses

Practice nurses are directly employed by GPs. Practice nursing is a relatively new profession, although there are now over 25 000 practice nurses in the UK. Their health promotion role has been largely confined to immunization, taking bloods, cytology, lifestyle advice, travel health and health checks, but increasingly they are staffing minor illness centres.

Dentists

There is an increasing emphasis on prevention in dentistry, particularly with children. Dentists receive a capitation fee per child and so have an interest in keeping that child's teeth healthy. Many practices employ a hygienist who gives advice on dental health. Health authorities also have a community dental service which may offer dental health promotion to schools and residential homes.

Pharmacists

The potential of community pharmacies to promote health has been recognized in a national strategy (Department of Health 2005b). Pharmacy staff advise the public on the safe use of medicines, minor ailments and healthy lifestyles. They may also provide specific public health interventions as part of a broader NHS service, for example, weight loss clinics, specialist smoking cessation advice or drug misuse services. In order to maximize their potential, all pharmacies should have areas set aside where members of the public can consult in private with the pharmacist.

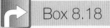 Box 8.18

The role of community pharmacists

Examples of health promotion provided in community pharmacies includes education and advice on:
- Healthy lifestyle (e.g. family planning, smoking cessation)
- Asthma/respiratory diseases (chronic bronchitis, allergies, inhaler devices, medicines and asthma)
- Healthy heart (healthy eating, exercise, high blood pressure, angina, use of aspirin)
- Sexual health (HIV/AIDS, safer sex, infertility, emergency contraception, emotional support, STIs, contraception)
- Safety/prevention (safe use of medicines, dump campaigns, foreign travel, first aid, accident prevention, sports injuries)
- Substance abuse (solvents, alcohol, drugs (illicit or prescription drugs), needle exchange)
- Elderly (advice for carers, compliance devices, mobility aids, incontinence, stoma care, influenza, foot care)
- Parents and babies (breast-feeding, milk substitutes, folic acid, immunization, nappy rash, teething)

- Children (head lice, parasites, meningitis, immunization, vitamins, sugar and salt in food)
- Women's health (breast cancer, cervical cancer, migraine, stress incontinence, thrush, cystitis, menopause, osteoporosis)
- Men's health (prostate problems, heart attacks, lung cancer, stress, indigestion/heartburn)
- Oral health (cancer of the mouth, mouth ulcers, babies' teeth, dentures, dental care, cold sores, sugar-free medicines)
- Skin care (cancer, eczema, psoriasis, acne, sunscreens, scabies) (http://www.rpsgb.org.uk/pdfs/pubhlthguidcommph.pdf).

Box 8.19

Environmental health

The role of environmental health is particularly wide-ranging, encompassing statutory powers relating to food hygiene and pollution (of noise and air), specialist work on safety in the workplace and places of entertainment, and work on sustainability and recycling. Because environmental health officers have wide-ranging statutory powers, their work in health promotion is mainly advice on legislation and enabling people to fulfil those regulations. Their work may thus involve offering training courses or one-to-one advice in establishments.

Allied health workers

Many other professions allied to medicine, such as speech and language therapists, chiropodists, physiotherapists, radiographers and dietitians, have a part to play in health promotion, especially patient education.

Care workers

Population projections indicate a more rapid ageing of the population. People aged 85 and over will comprise 3.8% of the UK population by 2031 and the majority of these will need residential care. Care workers have a key health promotion role to improve fitness and nutrition and thereby minimize illness and dependence. Care workers also have a role in positive mental health promotion and empowering older people to have a degree of control over their lives. Preventing ill health in the frail aged is also important, e.g. the prevention of falls and pressure sores. Residential care workers liaise with GPs, social workers, physiotherapists, chiropodists and catering staff.

Specialists

Specialist advisers in public health are usually public health consultants and specialists working at a strategic or senior management level. They play a role in developing public health programmes and often have specific scientific expertise and accreditation.

Health promotion departments are part of the health authority and are usually accountable to the Director of Public Health. They vary widely in size, from a handful to 50 staff, and consist of health promotion specialists and several support and clerical staff. They have the lead role in initiating, coordinating and supporting health education and health promotion activity within their areas. Health promotion units may have commissioning or providing functions, or both. Commissioning activities include:

- Assessing local health needs
- Contributing to the operational and strategic plans of the health authority
- Reviewing service agreements to ensure that they seek to *promote* health
- Coordinating the plans and services of different agencies.
  Provider activities include:
- Managing health promotion programmes on specific issues such as HIV/AIDS, smoking cessation or coronary heart disease
- Providing advice and consultancy to the public and policy-makers
- Providing training, support and advice to all health promoters and agencies that provide health promotion.

Conclusion

Reorienting health services is a challenging task in which little progress has been made. There are many reasons for the intransigence of the health services to change. PHC is a social system with its own structure and culture which determine the way in which it tackles health and ill health. Its partnerships tend to be client- rather than population-focused, and though based *in* communities, there may be little work *with* communities. It is driven by a medical model of health rather than a social model, and evaluation is still often seen in terms of reduced morbidity and mortality, rather than in terms of health gain processes and outcomes. The priority in primary care is treatment, which means that often patient compliance is valued above patient autonomy and participation. Although progress has been made in prioritizing health promotion, it is still 'bolted on' to core tasks instead of being integral to everyone's work and service delivery. Key health promotion activities, such as addressing health inequalities, are replaced by the need to respond to client demands, which may paradoxically have the effect of reinforcing inequalities by providing more services for more educated and articulate patients. Perhaps the biggest barrier is inertia, or the duplication of ways of working that have served in the past.

On the plus side, there is a large pool of potential health promoters, including many practitioners in primary, secondary and tertiary care services. The effective delivery of health promotion would, in the long run, ease the workload of most practitioners, as well as enabling people to enjoy better health and increased longevity. Health promotion underpins many of the activities already being undertaken by practitioners, e.g. collaboration and partnership working. The economic argument for reorienting health services is robust, and provides a compelling case for action. Pulling all these positive factors together is a long-term and daunting task, but many small steps have already been taken. The ongoing challenge is to keep the reorienting health services agenda foregrounded and to identify ongoing strategies to progress this goal.

Questions for further discussion

- What can be done to reorient the health care sector to take greater responsibility for health promotion? What are the prospects and problems of collaboration with others to promote health in your work?

- How can public health and health promotion professionals engage with the wider workforce in order to build their capacity and promote health?

Summary

This chapter has discussed the potential of the health care sector to promote health and the challenges posed by the medical paradigm. It has outlined the contribution of different agencies and practitioners to health promotion.

Further reading

Scriven A, Orme J (eds), 2001. Health promotion: professional perspectives, 2nd edn. Palgrave Macmillan/Open University, Basingstoke. *A useful insight into what health promotion means in different settings. Interesting accounts of practice will help to increase understanding for collaborative partnerships.*

Scriven A (ed), 2005. Health promoting practice: the contribution of nurses and allied health professionals.

Palgrave Macmillan, Basingstoke. *Discussion of how different roles conceptualize health promotion and examples of practice.*

Naidoo J et al 2007 Who promotes health? In: Earle S, Lloyd CE, Sidell M (eds) Theory and research in promoting public health. Sage/Open University, London, pp. 101–129. *A thorough overview of a range of agencies that promote health.*

References

Arnold P, Topping A, Honey S et al 2004 Exploring the contribution of district nurses to public health. British Journal of Community Nursing 9: 216–223.

Bunton R, Wills J 2005 War and public health. Critical Public Health 15: 79–81.

Coote A 2002 Claiming the health dividend: unlocking the benefits of NHS spending. Kings Fund, London.

Crafter H 1997 Health promotion in midwifery. Arnold, London.

Darzi A 2007 Healthcare for London: a framework for action. NHS London, London.

Department of Health 2001 The report of the Chief Medical Officer's project to strengthen the public health function. Department of Health, London.

Department of Health 2004 Standards for better health. Department of Health, London.

Department of Health 2005a Our health, our care, our say. Department of Health, London.

Department of Health 2005b Choosing health through pharmacy. A programme for pharmaceutical public health 2005–2015. Department of Health, London.

Health Education Authority 1998 Promoting health through primary health care nursing. HEA, London.

Levy S B, Sidel W 2002 The health and social consequences of diversion of economic resources to war and preparation for war. In: Taipale I (ed) War or health? A reader. Zed Books, London.

Maryon-Davis A 2005 Weight management in primary care: how can it be made more effective?. Proceedings of the Nutrition Society 64: 97–103.

Matthews P, Fletcher J 2001 Sexually transmitted infections in primary care: a need for education. British Journal of General Practice 51: 52–56.

Murray C J, Lopez A D 1997 Mortality by cause for eight regions of the world: Global Burden of Disease study. Lancet 349: 1269–1276.

Naidoo J, Wills J 2005 Public health and health promotion: developing practice. Baillière Tindall, London.

Popay J, Kowarzik U, Mallinson S et al 2007 Social problems, primary care and pathways to help and support: addressing health inequalities at the individual level: the GP perspective. Journal of Epidemiology and Community Health 61: 966–971.

Royal Society for Nature Conservation 2004 Material health: a mass balance and ecological footprint analysis of the NHS in England and Wales. Available online at: www.materialhealth.com/download.htm

Scottish Office Department of Health 2001 Nursing for health. A review of the contribution of nurses, midwives and health visitors to improving the public's health. Stationery Office, Edinburgh.

Sustainable Development Commission 2006 NHS good corporate citizenship assessment model. Available online at: www.corporatecitizen.nhs.uk

Wanless D 2002 Securing our future health. Taking a long term view. HM Treasury, London.

Wanless D, Appleby J, Harrison A et al 2007 Our future health secured? Kings Fund, London.

Wise M, Nutbeam D 2007 Enabling health systems transformation: what progress has been made to re-orienting health services? Promotion and Education 2(suppl): 23–28.

World Health Organization 1946 Constitution. WHO, Geneva.

World Health Organization 1978 Declaration of Alma Ata, international conference on primary health care, Alma Ata, 6–12 September. World Health Organization, Geneva.

World Health Organization 1986 Ottawa charter for health promotion. Journal of Health Promotion 1: 1–4.

World Health Organization 2000 The world health report 2000 health systems: improving performance. WHO, Geneva.

World Health Organization 2007 Challenging inequity through health systems. Final report. Knowledge network on health systems. WHO, Geneva.

9

Developing personal skills

Key points

- The role of beliefs, attitudes and values in health-related decisions
- The influence of social norms on health behaviour
- The concept of locus of control
- Health promotion strategies to change attitudes or behaviour

OVERVIEW

People's health behaviour or lifestyles have been regarded as the cause of many modern diseases. Therefore a main focus of health promotion has been on modifying those aspects of behaviour which are known to have an impact on health.

In previous chapters we have argued that such an approach is unlikely to be effective unless it acknowledges how people's behaviour may be a response to, and maintained by, the environment in which they live. Many health promoters, however, see their role as helping people to live their lives to its best potential, which may involve some change in their health behaviour.

This chapter is concerned with those aspects of health behaviour that people can control. Understanding why people behave in certain ways and how they can be helped to maintain chosen behaviours is central to self-empowerment. This chapter explores the usefulness of social psychology which offers several theoretical models that identify the determinants of behaviour change. This can contribute to, if not the prediction, then at least an understanding of how people make decisions about their health. This can be a useful tool in planning health promotion interventions. The influence of specific factors such as individual self-esteem or people's perceptions of control over their lives needs to be taken into account by the health promoter in order to offer practical support and positive experiences in making choices.

Empowerment is a term much used in health promotion. It is a complex concept that encompasses various levels of working for change:

- Individual, working *with* people to develop confidence and control
- Community (see Chapter 10)
- Organizational (see Part 3) to create supportive environments.

Enabling people to change is often assumed by health promoters simply to mean health education. Such programmes are described by Keleher (2007, p. 145) as typically delivered as brief interventions or in a series of sessions covering those things the clinician or health promoter regard as important with compliance as the goal.

Client-centred health education is concerned with a person's agency in decision-making. Such an approach acknowledges that people can take some control over their lives through knowledge, skills and confidence and it may enable people to identify structural barriers and facilitators to their health. This kind of empowering education was described by Paolo Freire (see Chapter 10) in his description of radical adult literacy pedagogy. Frequently however developing personal skills is equated with helping people to change, drawing on psychological theories of behaviour change, motivation and self-efficacy.

Several theories have attempted to explain the influence of different variables on an individual's health-related behaviour:

- The Health Belief model (Becker 1974)
- The Theory of Reasoned Action (Ajzen & Fishbein 1980)
- The Stages of Change model (Prochaska & DiClemente 1984).

This chapter explores the application of these models of behaviour change to health, and considers how an understanding of cognition and decision-making can be incorporated into empowerment and education strategies.

Definitions

According to social psychology theories of behaviour change, people's behaviour is partly determined by their attitude to that behaviour. An individual's *attitude* to a specific action and the intention to adopt it are influenced by *beliefs*, motivation which comes from the person's *values*, *attitudes* and *drives* or instincts, and the influences from social norms.

Beliefs

A belief is based on the information a person has about an object or action. It links the object to some attribute. For example, a person believes that potatoes (object) are fattening (an attribute). Theories of health-related behaviour change are based on the idea that an individual's behaviour will be based on his or her beliefs. In this example, the person will cut down on potatoes if they wish to lose weight. If this person is encouraged to believe that potatoes are not fattening but a useful bulk food, then he or she may include them in the diet. In other words, that information can influence beliefs which will then, in turn, influence behaviour. This simple model is sometimes referred to as the knowledge–attitudes–behaviour (KAB) model. Of course, behaviour change is never quite as simple as that. Information alone is neither necessary nor sufficient for behaviour change. The health risks of smoking are well known and yet 30% of the population continue to smoke.

Values

These are acquired through socialization and are those emotionally charged beliefs which make up what a person thinks is important. A person's values will influence a whole range of feelings about family, friendships, career and so on. For example, values relating to sex and gender give rise to a number of attitudes towards motherhood, employment of women, body image, breast-feeding and sexuality.

Attitudes

These are more specific than values and describe relatively stable feelings towards particular issues. There is no clear association between people's attitudes and their behaviour. Sometimes changing attitudes may stimulate a change in behaviour and sometimes behaviour change may influence attitudes. For example, many people continue to smoke despite a negative attitude to smoking. Yet once the behaviour is stopped, they may develop vehement antismoking views.

People's attitudes are made up of two components:

1. Cognitive – the knowledge and information they possess

2. Affective – their feelings and emotions and evaluation of what is important.

Attitudes are very hard to change. They may be changed by providing more or different information, or by increasing a person's skills. For example, a person's attitude towards the benefits of exercise might be influenced by providing information about different types of physical activity and their effects on the body. It might also be influenced by improved performance which motivates the person and encourages him or her to think of exercise as enjoyable.

Festinger (1957) used the term cognitive dissonance to describe a person's mental state when new information is given which is counter to that already held. This prompts the person either to reject the new information (as unreliable or inappropriate) or to adopt attitudes and behaviour which would fit with it.

Box 9.1

How do people respond to information about the risks to their health from particular behaviours?

Some people may become concerned and change when presented with information about health risks. Others may make some change such as switching to a lower-risk substitute (e.g. low-fat spread). Others may deny their risk, perhaps by underestimating the frequency or amount of their current behaviour.

Drives

The term 'drive' is used in the Health Action model (Tones & Tilford 2001) to describe strong motivating factors such as hunger, thirst, sex and pain. It is also used to describe motivations which can become drives, such as addiction. Some studies suggest that addiction is the consequence of frequently repeated acts which become a habit and its base is a psychological fear of withdrawal (Davies 1997). Social learning theory (Bandura 1977) uses the term instinct to describe behaviours which are not learned but are present at birth. Instincts can override attitudes and beliefs. Hunger, for example, can easily override a person's favourable attitude and intention to diet.

Understanding the impact of people's beliefs in their behaviour is key to addressing those issues. Take the example of smoking:

- If you regard smoking as an addiction (50% of smokers have a cigarette within 30 minutes of waking) then the aim is to help the individual gain control.

- If you regard smoking as a learned behaviour which smokers associate with specific actions and rewards (confidence, less stress) then the aim is to restructure thinking and activities to avoid potentially stressful situations.

- If you regard smoking as having a social meaning (e.g. young women see smoking as providing status) then the aim is to clarify such associations.

Box 9.2

What personal skills are needed to take greater control over one's health? Consider this in relation to a change of behaviour you have made.

Practitioners often prioritize knowledge and information over self-confidence and a belief that change is possible as well as a willingness and motivation to make a change.

The practitioner needs to understand what contributes to people's decision-making about health and what makes some people more amenable to change than others. The social cognition models which we shall now consider highlight the following as important:

- People's views about the cause and prevention of ill health

- The extent to which people feel they can control their life and make changes

- Whether they believe change is necessary

• Whether change is perceived to be beneficial in the long term, outweighing any difficulties and problems which may be involved.

 Box 9.3

How do you explain consistent findings in many studies that show a gap between knowledge and behaviour change, e.g. 70% of the population know about the importance of 5 a day but only 35% of the population act on it (Scottish Executive 2005)?

Such findings illustrate that knowledge of health benefits is only loosely associated with behaviour change. Although opportunities to change are greatest in most affluent areas, little action is taken. Self-reported motivation is unrelated to propensity to change. Understanding the wider cultural frameworks such as pleasure, comfort and convenience underpinning decision-making is essential to motivating individuals and groups.

The following theoretical models try to unpack the relative importance of these factors, recognizing that what people say is not necessarily a guide to what they will do, and that there are numerous antecedent and situational variables.

The Health Belief model

The Health Belief model is probably the best-known theoretical model highlighting the function of beliefs in decision-making (Figure 9.1). This model,

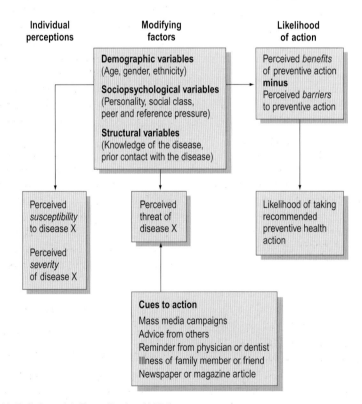

Figure 9.1 • The Health Belief model. From Becker (1974).

originally proposed by Rosenstock (1966) and modified by Becker (1974), has been used to predict protective health behaviour, such as screening or vaccination uptake and compliance with medical advice (e.g. Gillam 1991). The model suggests that whether or not people change their behaviour will be influenced by an evaluation of its feasibility and its benefits weighed against its costs. In other words, people considering changing their behaviour engage in a cost–benefit or utility analysis. This may include their beliefs concerning the likelihood of the illness or injury happening to them (their susceptibility); the severity of the illness or injury; and the efficacy of the action and whether it will have some personal benefit, or how likely it is to protect the person from the illness or injury.

For a behaviour change to take place, individuals:

- Must have an incentive to change
- Feel threatened by their current behaviour
- Feel a change would be beneficial in some way and have few adverse consequences
- Must feel competent to carry out the change.

Box 9.4

Consider the following situation and then try to apply the Health Belief model to see if you can predict how the woman might respond.

A mother of three children under 5 receives a card from her GP informing her that her youngest child should receive a Hib injection to protect him from meningitis. The woman works at a local factory as an hourly paid packer. Her mother cares for the children whilst she is at work, but has no transport.

If we are to use the Health Belief model as a model for predicting health behaviour, we would see the mother as a rational problem-solver who would not only be aware of the causes of Hib meningitis but also the risks of contracting it (the child's susceptibility and severity). We would assume that the

mother would have been made aware of the efficacy of the vaccine and be aware of its protection against one type of meningitis only (*Haemophilus influenzae* B). She would also be aware of any possible side-effects or contraindications. If the mother has had previous children vaccinated with no adverse effects or had this child or other children immunized against other diseases, she is more likely to view this vaccination favourably and have confidence in its effectiveness. In using this model as a predictor of behaviour, we need to take into account the perceived barriers and costs to taking this action. The mother would need to ask her own mother to take the child to the doctor. The child's grandmother may be unwilling or unable to take three children on public transport. Or the mother would have to take time off work with consequent loss of earnings.

Most learning theories are based on the premise that people's behaviour is guided by consequences. If these are positive or deemed to be positive, then the person is more likely to engage in that behaviour. These explanations, which see behaviour as a simple response to positive or negative rewards, do not seem to account for the persistence of health behaviours which have apparently negative consequences, such as smoking or drinking and driving. Short-term gratification is a greater incentive than possible long-term harm.

Becker suggests that individuals are influenced by how vulnerable they perceive themselves to be to an illness, injury or danger (their *susceptibility*) and how serious they consider it to be (*severity*). People's perception and assessment of risk are central to the application of this model. Most people make a rough assessment about whether they are at risk. This seems to be influenced by four factors:

1. Personal experience
2. Ability to control the situation
3. A feeling that the illness or danger is rare
4. Any outcomes are in the distant future.

Where a situation is not well known however, people have an unrealistic optimism that 'it won't happen to me' (Weinstein 1984).

Box 9.5

There are over 250 000 traffic accidents each year with 30 000 casualties, of which 3400 are fatalities. Excess speed is a contributory factor in a significant number of road accidents. In one survey (Scottish Office 1998) 88% of drivers admitted to driving at 40 mph in a 30 mph zone at least sometimes. The current response to speeding is:
- Traffic calming
- Police enforcement
- Media campaigns, e.g. 'speed kills'.

How might an understanding of social cognitions help to target a strategy for safer driving?
  You may have considered people's beliefs about:
- The consequences of accidents
- Likelihood of being stopped by police
- Likelihood of putting people at risk
- Social disapproval
- Perceived control over driving.

Since beliefs may be affected by experience, direct contact with those who have a condition can powerfully affect attitudes exposing stereotypes and prejudice. For example, contact with a person who is human immunodeficiency virus (HIV)-positive or who is living with acquired immunodeficiency syndrome (AIDS) can change beliefs about the fatality of the disease, and about who is affected and how.

Those who work with young people find perceptions of risk are very different. Risk-taking is an important task of adolescence and part of separation from family. It is hard for young people to appreciate the long-term effects of, for example, smoking when 25 can seem old.

Many health education campaigns have attempted to motivate people to change their behaviour through fear or guilt. Drink–drive campaigns at Christmas show the devastating effects on families of road accident fatalities; smoking prevention posters urge parents not to 'teach your children how to smoke'. Increasingly hard-hitting campaigns are used amongst others to raise awareness of the consequences of binge drinking, smoking and drug use. Whether such campaigns do succeed in shocking people to change their behaviour is the subject of ongoing debate (see, for example, Hill et al 1998). Although fear can encourage a negative attitude and even an intention to change, such feelings tend to disappear over time and when faced with a real decision-making situation. Being very frightened can also lead to denial and an avoidance of the message. Protection Motivation theory (Rogers 1975) suggests that fear only works if the threat is perceived as serious and likely to occur if the person does not follow the recommended advice.

Box 9.6

Questioner: 'How do you think you'll be in say 10 years' time, in terms of health?'
K (age 16): 'Dead!'
  T (age 15): 'I don't want to think about tomorrow, let alone 10 bloody years.'
(Health Education Authority 1993)

The Health Belief model suggests that people need to have some kind of cue to take action to change a behaviour or make a health-related decision. The issue needs to become salient or relevant. The cue could be noticing a change in one's internal state or appearance. For example, a pregnant woman stops smoking when she feels the baby move. It could be an external trigger, such as a change in circumstance like change in job or income, or the death or illness of someone close. It could be a comment from a 'significant other' or a newspaper article. Health care workers can be significant others. For example, GPs' advice is taken seriously. The GP has expertise, is trustworthy and has authority, leading the patient to desire to comply. The effects of persuasive communications on attitudes are discussed more fully in Chapter 12 on mass media.

Box 9.7

According to the 2005 Gay Men's Sex Survey (Sigma Research 2005), 50% of sexually active gay men had unprotected anal sex in the previous year. A total of 40% of gay men were unaware of their own HIV status.

Consider how the Health Belief model could be used to explain this health behaviour.

What reasons could you offer for individuals not carrying out their intentions to act in ways that are perceived as beneficial?

Factors associated with HIV-positive men having unprotected sex were.

• Being in a serodiscordant (one partner only HIV-positive) or unknown-status relationship.

• Having 30 or more sexual partners

• Having a high self-rating for attractiveness

• Drug use.

The Health Belief model has been widely criticized. Some of these criticisms relate to its lack of weighting for different factors – all cues to preventive action, for example, are seen as equally salient. It may appear that complex behaviour and actions are informed and chosen via analysis of a set of conceptual components that are isolated from one another. What we have seen so far is that behaviour is far more nuanced with many different interwoven arguments and scripts. The model may not be particularly helpful in predicting behaviour or identifying those elements that are important in influencing people to change, but it does highlight the range and complexity of factors involved.

Theory of Reasoned Action and Theory of Planned Behaviour

According to the Theory of Reasoned Action (Ajzen & Fishbein 1980), behaviour is dependent on two variables:

1. Attitudes – beliefs about the consequences of the behaviour and an appraisal of the positive and negative aspects of making a change

2. Subjective norms – what 'significant others' do and expect and the degree to which the person wants to conform and be like others.

These two influences combine to form an intention.

Ajzen & Fishbein (1980) acknowledge that people do not necessarily behave consistently with their intentions. The ability to predict behaviour will be influenced by the stability of a person's belief. Stability is determined by strength of belief, how long it has been held, whether it is reinforced by other groups to which the individual belongs, whether it is related to and integrated with other attitudes and beliefs and how clear or structured it is.

The Theory of Reasoned Action differs from the Health Belief model in that it places importance on social norms as a major influence on behaviour. Figure 9.2

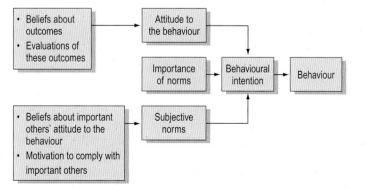

Figure 9.2 • The Theory of Reasoned Action. From Ajzen & Fishbein (1980).

shows the significance of this factor in the Theory of Reasoned Action. Social pressure may be exerted through societal norms (such as those relating to weight and body image), community norms, the peer group and the beliefs of 'significant others' (such as parents or partners).

The motivation to comply with perceived social pressure from 'significant others' could cause individuals to behave in a way that they believe these other people or groups would think is right. The influence of so-called peer group pressure (even if it does not amount to pressure) can be very powerful within a small group if the individual values membership of that group or wants to belong to it. Young people have many potential social pressures and increased social competition due to internet websites such as MySpace and Facebook, and are exposed to marketing and advertising that may encourage early adoption of a teen lifestyle.

Box 9.8

Think of an occasion where social norms have influenced a health-related decision on your part. What was the most powerful aspect of this influence? Consider the following example of conformity with social norms.

'Bill works in a predominantly male office. At the end of the day, five or six people adjourn to a local bar. The men are eager to establish themselves by buying a round of drinks. Bill waits until everyone has finished before offering to buy a round, by which time someone else has got to the bar. Bill usually only drinks one pint of beer but he stays until everyone has bought a round – six pints.'

The role of modelling has been particularly important in health promotion. Concern has been expressed that indirect modelling of behaviour may come from the media. For example, people on television are able to drink heavily without any apparent ill effects (Hansen 2003). Direct modelling is sometimes assumed to be less influential, but models who have status and credibility, such as musicians and people in sport, have been used to present health promotion messages. If people are influenced by role models, then health promoters may themselves be taken as exemplars.

Box 9.9

Should health promoters 'practise what they preach'?
    Think of some examples where practitioners' behaviour may be at odds with the health improvement they wish to promote.

Some health promotion programmes use the influence of the peer group to promote positive health. The rationale is that peers may be seen as having more credibility, are able to communicate in appropriate ways and are models to follow, although doubts may be expressed about the skills and information that peer educators possess (Wilton et al 1995; Harden et al 1999).

Social norms include peer group or family beliefs, but also what are perceived to be 'general' norms as conveyed by, for example, the mass media. What is important is what the individual believes other people do, not the actual extent of the activity. The World Health Organization has identified the importance of formal and informal social networks to support individuals and give people assistance in the pursuit of health (Wilkinson & Marmot 2003). Group techniques, such as those used by Alcoholics Anonymous, appear to have some success by getting clients to identify with the group through personal testimony and a public commitment, which encourages the group to provide support for each other.

Bandura's (1977) social learning theory suggests that the health choices people make are related to:

- Outcome expectancies (whether an action will lead to a particular outcome)
- Self-efficacy (whether people believe they can change).

Perceptions of self-efficacy are based on people's assessment of themselves – whether they have the knowledge and skills to make changes in their behaviour and whether external factors such as time and money will allow that change.

Box 9.10

How might observing others' behaviour influence our own? To what extent does believing we can do something enable us to do it? How does thinking influence our behaviour?

Self-efficacy is determined by:

- Our previous experiences of success and failure (e.g. having lost weight before)
- Relevant vicarious experiences (e.g. seeing someone else lose weight)
- Verbal/social persuasion (e.g. being told you can do it)
- Emotional arousal (e.g. being scared).

Personal judgement of worth expressed in the attitudes people hold towards themselves is also part of a sense of self-efficacy. We talk of high or low self-esteem in the sense of feeling more or less worthwhile and valued. Self-concept is a global term which refers to all those beliefs which people have about themselves – about their abilities and their attributes. It includes ideas about appearance, intelligence and physical skills. It is built and modified through our perceptions of the way other people behave towards us, how we are accepted and affirmed, or rejected and criticized. It will thus also derive from having a network of social support.

The development of self-concept and self-esteem has been at the centre of work in health education and promotion. It is assumed that people with high self-esteem are likely to feel confident about themselves and have social and life skills which will enhance their feelings of personal efficacy. Because of these feelings of personal effectiveness, the person's self-esteem is enhanced.

Box 9.11

The Expert Patient Programme

The Expert Patient Programme is a National Health Service-based training programme which provides opportunities for people with long-term conditions to develop new skills to:

- Manage their condition better on a day-to-day basis.
- Become key decision-makers in their own care.
- Take more control over their lives.

Many health education programmes, particularly those targeted at young people, have been based on the premise that there is a relationship between low self-esteem and health behaviour. However a survey by the Joseph Rowntree Foundation (Perri et al 1997) found that those who had ever tried drugs had similar levels of sociability as young people in general but were more at ease and had a more relaxed attitude to the future. Programmes such as Drug Abuse Resistance Education (DARE) which aim to boost self-esteem by equipping young people with better skills to resist peer pressure and make independent decisions are thus unlikely to prevent drug experimentation.

Box 9.12

Intention and behaviour in sexual decision-making

Personal or 'micro' factors are played out in many issues of choice and real-life decision-making is often not a rational process.

A study of HIV-positive people and sex (Ridge et al 2007) found that, although they may have the intention to use a condom, 'irrational feelings' such as intimacy, trust and desire could all influence perceptions of risk.

Ajzen further developed the Theory of Reasoned Action and recast it as the Theory of Planned Behaviour (Ajzen 1991) (Figure 9.3). This model incorporated another variable – that people's behaviour is a consequence of their perceived control. People differ in the extent to which they think they can make changes in their lives. Social learning theory suggests that the ways in which people explain the things that happen to them are a product of their childhood experiences. Those who are rewarded for their successes and punished consistently and fairly will come to believe that they are in control of their lives. Those who have inconsistent rewards or punishments irrespective of their behaviour are more likely to see events as a consequence of chance and their own role as irrelevant (Rotter 1954).

Control in the context of health can be understood in terms of:

- Internal locus of control (the extent to which individuals believe that they are responsible for their own health)
- External locus of control (people who believe that their actions are influenced by powerful others, chance, fate or luck).

Box 9.13

What strategies can practitioners use to help build their clients' confidence so that they feel more able to make changes in their health behaviour?

Research has focused on categorizing attitudes to health by using a locus of control measure such as a multiple-choice inventory. It has been assumed that those who have a strong internal locus of control will see themselves as more coping, and more able to act decisively and capably and will be those people who undertake preventive health actions or change to more healthy behaviours. So far it has generally been found that there is only a weak relationship between feelings of control and specific behaviours, although associations have been found with smoking cessation and weight loss and the propensity to use preventive medical services (Wallston et al 1978). Indeed, a lifestyle survey of 9000 adults found that 'unhealthy' kinds of behaviour are more likely to be associated with an internal locus of control (Blaxter 1990). At the same time, those who recorded positive or responsible attitudes to health were also more likely to have a high locus of control. This confirms the argument earlier in this chapter that specific behaviour cannot necessarily be predicted from attitudes.

People who register as 'externals' on the multidimensional health locus of control scale are those with lower levels of education, and of lower socioeconomic class – in other words, people who have every reason to believe that they do not have much control over their lives or health status. Figure 9.4 is a diagrammatic representation of some of the influences

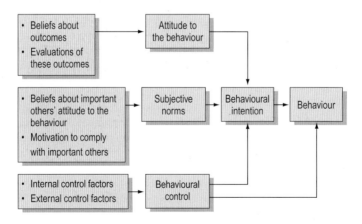

Figure 9.3 ● The Theory of Planned Behaviour. From Ajzen (1991).

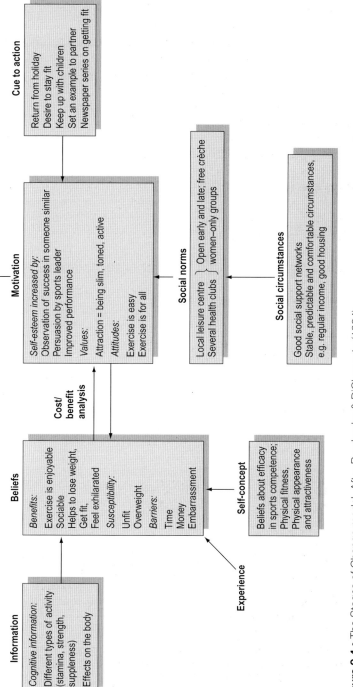

Cue to action

Return from holiday
Desire to stay fit
Keep up with children
Set an example to partner
Newspaper series on getting fit

Motivation

Self-esteem increased by:
Observation of success in someone similar
Persuasion by sports leader
Improved performance

Values:
Attraction = being slim, toned, active

Attitudes:
Exercise is easy
Exercise is for all

Social norms

Local leisure centre } Open early and late; free crèche
Several health clubs } women-only groups

Social circumstances

Good social support networks
Stable, predictable and comfortable circumstances,
e.g. regular income, good housing

**Cost/
benefit
analysis**

Beliefs

Benefits:
Exercise is enjoyable
Sociable
Helps to lose weight,
Get fit,
Feel exhilarated

Susceptibility:
Unfit
Overweight

Barriers:
Time
Money
Embarrassment

Self-concept

Beliefs about efficacy
in sports competence;
Physical fitness,
Physical appearance
and attractiveness

Experience

Information

Cognitive information:
Different types of activity
(stamina, strength,
suppleness)
Effects on the body

Figure 9.4 • The Stages of Change model. After Prochaska & DiClemente (1984).

on a person's decision to take up an exercise programme. It shows how confidence to participate in physical activity could be built through positive attributions such as fitness and weight loss and through successful performance. Social support networks will also be crucial in maintaining commitment.

The Stages of Change model

So far in this chapter we have discussed the factors influencing the decisions people make in relation to their health.

Prochaska & DiClemente's transtheoretical model (1984, 1986; Prochaska et al 1992) is important in describing the process of change. The model derived from their work on encouraging change in addictive behaviours, although it can be used to show that most people go through stages when trying to change or acquire behaviours.

Box 9.14

Many people have had experiences of knowing what they ought to do and not doing it. Most people have tried and failed at some point in their lives to make a change in their health behaviour, such as giving up smoking or losing weight. Think about one of your experiences of failing to make a change. Why do you think the change did not last:

• Lack of motivation?
• Lack of support?
• Lack of knowledge?
• Lack of time or other resource?

Now think about a change you have managed to make. Why do you think you were able to stick to this decision?

Figure 9.5 illustrates this process and identifies the following stages.

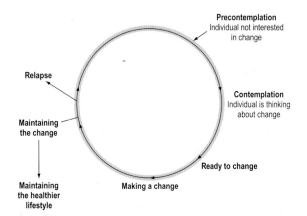

Figure 9.5 ● Health-related behaviour change: the example of exercise in women.

Precontemplation

Those in the precontemplation stage have not considered changing their lifestyle or become aware of any potential risks in their health behaviour. When they become aware of a problem, they may progress to the next stage. Assessing a client's readiness to change is a key first step.

Contemplation

Although individuals are aware of the benefits of change, they are not yet ready and may be seeking information or help to make that decision. This stage may last a short while or several years. Some people never progress beyond this stage.

Preparing to change

When the perceived benefits seem to outweigh the costs and when the change seems possible as well as worthwhile, the individual may be ready to change, perhaps seeking some extra support.

Making the change

The early days of change require positive decisions by the individual to do things differently. A clear goal, a realistic plan, support and rewards are features of this stage.

Maintenance

The new behaviour is sustained and the person moves into a healthier lifestyle. For some people maintaining the new behaviour is difficult and the person may revert or relapse back to any of the previous stages.

Change is not a smooth process. Whilst few people go through each stage in an orderly way, they will go through each stage. This has proved helpful for many health care workers who find it reassuring that a relapse on the part of their clients is not a failure, but that the individual can go both backwards and forwards through a series of cycles of change – like a revolving door. Thus a smoker may stop smoking many times before finally giving up completely. Nevertheless the client is still aware of the benefits of giving up smoking and health care workers may be able to focus on such small changes, which can provide themselves and their clients with a sense of achievement and identifiable progress.

Whilst individuals may not have an awareness of contemplating, actioning and maintaining change, the intention will be based on individuals deciding that it is in their best interests to change. The key to successful interventions then is for a client to be motivated. Health promoters must bear in mind that their clients may not share their perceptions about the worth of a particular behaviour.

Motivational interviewing is a non-directive client patient-centred counselling style that aims to help clients explore their ambivalence about changing their behaviour. It starts with an exploration of the clients' readiness to change (in keeping with the transtheoretical model of change) and how important change or the behaviour is to them (Miller & Rollnick 2002). Central to this technique is the view that motivation is enhanced if the client articulates the costs and benefits of change. The client's confidence that change can happen is bolstered by support, discussion of barriers and negotiated action plans.

Box 9.15

How might you help someone to decide to make a change in her health behaviour?
- What questions might you use to help the client explore her situation?
- How would you identify her readiness to change?
- How would you help someone to weigh up the pros and cons of making a change?
- What support would you offer to help someone to stick to the change she makes?
- How would you help her to cope with difficult situations or setbacks?

These techniques are widely adopted. Some have much in common with counselling techniques, as summarized in Table 9.1. One of the principles of motivational interviewing is that people feel some ambivalence about their health behaviour. One way of helping a person to become clearer is to use a decision balance matrix in which clients work out the costs and benefits of changing or not changing their behaviour, as illustrated in Figure 9.6 with a person exploring cannabis use.

Box 9.16

Health trainers
The White Paper *Choosing Health: Making Healthy Choices Easier* (Department of Health 2004) proposed the development of a new role for improving health – health trainers. These are people drawn from local communities and trained to reach those who want to adopt healthier lifestyles but don't necessarily use local services.

Table 9.1 Using client-directed counseling techniques

Do	Don't
Summarize your understanding of the client's thoughts and feelings	Interrupt or finish sentences
Look and sound interested	Advise or tell the client what to do
Keep eye contact and use positive body language	Disagree or contradict (raise alternatives)
See things from the client's point of view	Project your own beliefs or feelings on to the client
Ask open questions to get more information	Assume your experiences are the same as the client's
Be curious rather than intrusive	Constantly repeat the same paraphrases, e.g. 'it sounds like' or 'you feel like'
Give the client time to think as well as talk	Pretend you understand if you don't. Ask for more explanation
Respond to what the client is saying rather than trying to lead the conversation	

From Michie et al (2006).

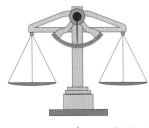

	Advantages	Disadvantages
Changing my behaviour	Might lose weight
Feel healthier
Save a bit of money	Friends might think I'm boring
Might get bored
Not changing my behaviour	Feel relaxed
Something to do
Be with my friends
Sleep well	Put on weight
Feel paranoid sometimes
Argue with friends and family
Smoker's cough

Figure 9.6 • Exploring ambivalence about cannabis use.

Self-empowerment approaches have at their centre the principle of participation. These techniques allow people to examine their own values and beliefs; explore the factors which affect the choices they make; and develop the skills to act upon their intentions. In addition to techniques such as motivational interviewing and client-centred counselling, educational drama, story-telling, assertiveness and negotiation skills training, and problem-solving may be used.

The prerequisites of change

All the models of behaviour change discussed in this chapter suggest that people are involved in a rational processing of information when they make a decision. People are not usually so consciously rational, as this study of the health beliefs of working-class mothers in south Wales illustrates:

> In the subjects we studied there was little evidence of a rational approach to the personal decision-making process, i.e. a weighing up of the advantages and disadvantages of a particular change followed by a decision to act. Instead any change was a consequence not just of thought but also a mix of emotion, habit, impulse, social influences and bolshie lack of forethought, which is so typically human (Pill & Stott 1990).

Pill & Stott's study of self-initiated change shows the importance of precipitating life events and the minor part played by health concerns. For example, women who gave up smoking did so to save money and those who took up exercise did so to join in with their children.

The importance of considering the social context and everyday life is brought out clearly by this study, which showed that eventually most women reverted to their original behaviours because of the influence of partners or children, or because it was too difficult to juggle personal and family priorities.

The evidence from people who have changed their health behaviour suggests that there are certain minimum conditions required for that change to take place.

The change must be self-initiated

Some people react adversely or wish to contain any attempt to look at their 'unhealthy behaviour'. To some people, their behaviour may not seem unhealthy at all but may constitute a clear source of well-being, its benefits far outweighing its risks. There is a clear message here for those health promoters who work with individual clients and who are sometimes accused of 'telling people what to do' – people will only change if they want to.

The behaviour must become salient

Most health-related behaviours, including smoking, alcohol use, eating and exercise (or lack of it), are habitual, and built into the flow of everyday life such that the individual does not give them much thought. For a change to occur, that behaviour or habit must be called into question by some other activity or event so that the behaviour becomes salient. For example, a smoker going to live with a non-smoker causes the smoking behaviour to be reappraised. The death of a relative from breast cancer may similarly prompt a woman to go for screening.

The salience of the behaviour must appear over a period of time

The habitual behaviour needs to become difficult to maintain. The new behaviour must, in turn, become part of everyday life. For example, one reason why people on diets often resume their previous eating pattern is because they are made constantly aware of the diet and it is never allowed to become a habit. Similarly, exercise is often not maintained because it requires effort; hence the advice to reluctant 'couch potatoes' to build physical activity into their daily life by walking to work or running up stairs rather than going out to exercise at a pool or gym.

The behaviour is not part of the individual's coping strategies

People have various sources of comfort and solace, and will resist change to these behaviours. It is sometimes possible to enable clients to identify alternative coping strategies. For example, a person who eats chocolate when depressed may be encouraged to become physiologically aroused by taking up jogging.

The individual's life should not be problematic or uncertain

There is a limit to a person's capacity to adapt and change. For example, those living on low incomes will be stretched by coping with poverty and its uncertainties. Having to make changes in their health behaviour may be too much to expect for people whose lives are already problematic.

Social support is available

The presence and interest of other people provides reinforcement and keeps the behaviour salient. Changing one's behaviour can be stressful and individuals need support. The influence of peer group pressure and support is not given sufficient weight in the various psychological theories of change.

 Box 9.17

Think about an attempt you have made to enhance your health, e.g. giving up smoking, losing weight.
• Were you successful in the change?
• What influenced you to make the change?
• Can you identify any specific triggers that prompted you to make the change?
• How do your family and friends regard the behaviour?
• What were the costs and benefits of making the change?
Look at the list of minimum conditions above. Do any of these factors help to explain your success or failure in making the health-related behaviour change?

Conclusion

What is clear from this outline of psychological theories of behaviour change is that none provides a full explanation. However, the variables identified by these models do appear in people's accounts of their health behaviour:

• Perceptions of risk and vulnerability
• Perceptions of the severity of the disease
• Perceived effectiveness of the behaviour in contributing to better health
• Perception of own ability to make a change
• Perception of how significant others evaluate the behaviour.

Whilst these models may not help to predict who will adopt preventive or protective health practices, they can help to plan programmes of education by making clear those factors which influence decisions.

Elsewhere in this book we argue that a focus on people's health lifestyles can minimize the structural barriers such as poverty or discrimination that may make choices more difficult for some groups. The client-centred approaches described reflect a shift away from traditional didactic and persuasive methods. Their aim is to enable clients to have the understanding and skills to translate intention into practice. Those most likely to benefit, however, are people with good education and literacy, social support and personal and economic resources. For this reason such approaches must be accompanied by broader programmes that make the healthier choice the easier choice.

Questions for further discussion

• Do social psychology theories help you to understand the reasons why people may or may not change their health behaviour?

• What factors should health promoters take into account when helping clients to change their health behaviour?

Summary

This chapter has reviewed the role of psychosocial factors in health behaviour and discussed three theoretical models. These models have been used to explain and predict health-related decisions, such as screening or compliance to a medical regimen. All the models identify some common variables which influence the likelihood of a person adopting 'healthy' behaviours: beliefs about the efficacy of the new behaviour; motivation and whether they value their health enough to change; normative pressures and the influence of significant people around them. The limitations of the role of social psychology in health promotion are outlined but it is concluded that an understanding of those factors influencing individual behaviour can help in planning appropriate health promotion interventions.

Further reading

Bennett P, Murphy S 1997 Psychology and health promotion. Open University, Buckingham. *A very useful textbook which examines how behaviour and the social environment contribute to health status.*

Ogden J 2007 Health psychology: a textbook 4th edn. Open University, Buckingham. *An accessible textbook on psychological theory integrating case studies and examples of research studies.*

Payne S, Walker J 1996 Psychology for nurses and the caring professions. Open University, Buckingham.

A clear and comprehensive introduction to social psychology.

Pitts M, Phillips I K 1998 The psychology of health 2nd edn. Routledge, London. *A useful textbook with a topic focus including exercise, nutrition and drugs.*

Rollnick S, Mason P, Butler C 1999 Health behaviour change: a guide for practitioners. Churchill Livingstone, Edinburgh. *A really useful guide for practitioners using brief interventions with clients. It describes techniques and includes case study material.*

References

Ajzen I 1991 The theory of planned behaviour. Organisational Behaviour and Human Decision Processes 50: 179–211.

Ajzen I, Fishbein M 1980 Understanding attitudes and predicting social behaviour. Prentice Hall, Englewood Cliffs, New Jersey.

Bandura A 1977 Social learning theory. Prentice Hall, Englewood Cliffs, New Jersey.

Becker M H (ed). 1974 The Health Belief Model and personal health behaviour. Slack, Thorofare, New Jersey.

Blaxter M 1990 Health and lifestyles. Tavistock/Routledge, London.

Davies J B 1997 The myth of addiction, 2nd edn. Harwood, Reading.

Department of Health 2004 Choosing health: making healthy choices easier. Stationery Office, London.

Festinger L 1957 A theory of cognitive dissonance. University Press, Stanford.

Gillam S 1991 Understanding the uptake of cervical cancer screening: the contribution of Health Belief Model. British Journal of General Practice 41: 510–513.

Hansen A 2003 The portrayal of alcohol and alcohol consumption in television news and drama programmes. Alcohol Concern, London.

Harden A, Weston R, Oakley A 1999 A review of the appropriateness of peer delivered health promotion interventions for young people. EPPI Centre Social Science Research Unit, Institute of Education, University of London, London.

Health Education Authority 1993 The health action pack. HEA, London.

Hill D, Chapman S, Donavan R 1998 The return of scare tactics. Tobacco Control 7: 5–8.

Keleher H 2007 Empowerment and health education. In: Keleher H, MacDougall C, Murphy B (eds) Understanding health promotion. Oxford University Press, Melbourne, pp. 141–152.

Michie S, Rumsey N, Fussell A et al 2006 Improving health: changing behaviour. NHS Health Trainer Handbook. Available online at: www.nsms.org.uk/public/CSDDownload.aspx?casestudy = 53&document + 29.

Miller W, Rollnick S 2002 Motivational interviewing: preparing people to change, 2nd edn. Guildford Press, London.

Perri S, Jupp B, Perry H et al 1997 The substance of youth: the role of drugs in young people's lives today. Joseph Rowntree Foundation, London.

Pill R M, Stott N C H 1990 Making changes: a study of working class mothers and the changes made in their health related behaviour over five years. University of Wales College of Medicine, Cardiff.

Prochaska J O, DiClemente C 1984 The transtheoretical approach: crossing traditional foundations of change. Don Jones/Irwin, Harnewood, IL.

Prochaska J O, DiClemente C C 1986 Towards a comprehensive model of change. In: Miller W R, Heather N (eds) Treating addictive behaviours: processes of change. Plenum, New York.

Prochaska J O, DiClemente C, Norcross J C 1992 In search of how people change. American Psychologist 47: 1102–1114.

Ridge D, Ziebland S, Williams J et al 2007 Positive prevention: contemporary issues facing HIV positive people negotiating sex in the UK. Social Science and Medicine 65: 755–770.

Rogers R W 1975 A protection motivation theory of fear appeals and attitude change. Journal of Psychology 91: 93–114.

Rosenstock I 1966 Why people use health services. Millbank Memorial Fund Quarterly 44: 94–121.

Rotter J B 1954 Social learning and clinical psychology. Prentice Hall, Englewood Cliffs.

Scottish Executive 2005 The Scottish Health Survey 2003. Blackwells, London.

Scottish Office 1998 The speeding driver. Scottish Office, Edinburgh.

Sigma Research 2005 Consuming passions. Sigma, London.

Tones K, Tilford S 2001 Health education; effectiveness, efficiency and equity, 3rd edn. Nelson Thornes, London.

Wallston K A, Wallston B S, DeVellis R F 1978 Locus of control and health: a review of the literature. Health Education Monographs 6: 107–117.

Weinstein N 1984 Why it won't happen to me; perceptions of risk factors and susceptibility. Health Psychology 3: 431–457.

Wilton T, Keeble S, Doyal L et al 1995 The effectiveness of peer education in health promotion: theory and practice. HEA, London.

Wilkinson R, Marmot R 2003 The social determinants of health: the solid facts, 2nd edn. WHO Europe, Copenhagen.

Chapter Ten

Strengthening community action

- Defining community development
- Community development in health promotion
- Working with a community development approach
- Community development activities
- Dilemmas for practice

OVERVIEW

We have seen in previous chapters how there are many different ways of working for health. Strengthening community action is one of the key action areas identified in the Ottawa Charter (World Health Organization (WHO) 1986). This chapter focuses on community development – a strategy which aims to empower people to gain control over the factors influencing their health. Working with communities to increase their participation in decisions affecting health is an essential aspect of health promotion. This chapter begins by defining what is meant by a community and goes on to explore different ways in which health promoters can work with communities. Some of the dilemmas that confront the health promoter who wants to work in this way are discussed and illustrated using examples of community development projects.

Defining community

The concept of community is frequently used in discussions about health and health care. In general, the context of the community is taken to be desirable; thus we have care in the community, community policing and community education, all of which are seen as preferable to alternative (non-community) practice. In contrast to the state or the bureaucratic organization, services provided by and in the community are viewed as being more appropriate and sensitive. But what is the community which is referred to in these ways?

There are different ways of defining a community, but the most commonly cited factors are geography, culture and social stratification. These factors are viewed as being linked to the subjective feeling of belonging or identity which characterizes the concept of 'community'. Other characteristics of communities are social networks or systems of contact, and the existence of potential resources such as people's skills or knowledge.

Box 10.1

- Which communities do you belong to?
- Are these the same communities which your parents belonged to?
- What are the key characteristics of these communities?

Geography

A community may be defined on a geographical or neighbourhood basis (see Chapter 15). A well-known example is the East End of London, but this use of community is not restricted to working-class or urban areas. It is this notion of community which gives rise to 'patch'-based work, where people such as social workers, police officers or health visitors are assigned a geographically bounded area. The assumption is that people living in the same area have the same concerns, owing to their geographical proximity. This in turn rests on an assumption that the physical environment is a key factor in influencing health and social identity.

Culture

Community may be defined in cultural terms, as in 'the Chinese community' or 'the Jewish community'. Here the assumption is that common cultural traditions may transcend geographical or other barriers, and unite otherwise scattered and disparate groups of people. There is an expectation that members of a cultural community will assist each other and share resources. The most commonly cited elements of a common cultural heritage are ethnic origin, language, religion and customs.

Social stratification

A community may be based on interests held to be common, which are usually the product of social stratification. Thus we have 'the working-class community' and 'the gay community'. This definition implies that members of a community share networks of support, knowledge and resources which may transcend other boundaries, even national ones.

Box 10.2

Which definitions of community are being used in the following quotations?
- 'A number of individuals with something in common who may or may not acknowledge that connection' (Health Education Authority 1987)
- 'A specific group of people who share a common culture, values and norms, and who are arranged in a social structure according to the relationships the community has developed over a period of time' (Nutbeam 1998)
- 'A locality which comprises networks of formal and informal relationships, which have a capacity to mobilise individual and collective responses to common adversity' (Barclay Report on Social Work 1982)
- 'People with a basis of common interest and network of personal interaction, grouped either on the basis of locality or on a specific shared concern or both' (Smithies & Adams 1990, p. 9).

Most definitions of community tend to suggest that it is a homogeneous entity. However, it is obvious that any geographical community will include people whose primary identity is based on different factors, e.g. class, race, gender or sexual orientation. People who feel united by a shared interest, e.g. pensioners, or the unemployed, will also be members of other communities, geographical and otherwise. People may belong to several different communities, some of which may have more salience for the individual than others. In practice, people may find their allegiance to different communities shifting at different points in their life span.

The meaning and significance of community vary enormously. How one defines community is important because it influences how practitioners understand the dynamics within communities and the potential challenges that may present when working with them. Some communities may be easier to work with than others and practitioners may feel more comfortable working with some communities than others.

Defining community development

Community development has been defined as:

Building active and sustainable communities based on social justice and mutual respect. It is about changing power structures to remove the barriers that prevent people from participating in the issues that affect their lives. Community workers support individuals, groups and organisations in this process (Standing Conference for Community Development 2001).

Community development is both a philosophy and a method. As a philosophy its key features are:

- A commitment to equality and the challenging of attitudes and practices which discriminate against and marginalize people
- An emphasis on participation and enabling all communities to be heard
- An emphasis on lay knowledge and the valuing of people's own experience
- The collectivizing of experience and seeing problems as shared, and working together to identify and implement action
- Recognizing the skills, knowledge and expertise that people contribute
- The empowerment of individuals and communities through education, skills development and sharing and joint action.

There is a difference between community-based work and community development. Many practitioners may work in the community, organizing projects to meet people's health needs or doing outreach work where a professional service such as screening is extended into the community to make it more accessible. The Sure Start programme is an example of a community project providing early educational interventions in specific areas. Table 10.1 illustrates some of the differences between community-based work and community development work.

The community development approach has been influenced by the work of Paulo Freire, a Brazilian educationalist who worked on literacy programmes with poor peasants in Peru and Brazil during the

Table 10.1 Characteristics of community-based versus community development models

Community-based	Community development
Problem, targets and action defined by sponsoring body	Problem, targets and action defined by community
Community seen as medium, venue or setting for intervention	Community itself the target of intervention in respect to capacity-building and empowerment
Notion of 'community' relatively unproblematic	Community recognized as complex, changing, subject to power imbalances and conflict
Target is largely individuals within either geographic area or specific subgroup in geographic area defined by sponsoring body	Target may be community structures or services and policies that impact on the health of the community
Activities largely health-oriented	Activities may be quite broad-based, targeting wider factors with an impact on health, but with indirect health outcomes (empowerment, social capital)

After Labonte (1998).

1970s. Freire saw education as a way to liberate people from cycles of oppression. He aimed to engage the people in critical consciousness-raising or 'conscientization', helping people to understand their circumstances and why they have been oppressed. The process of 'conscientization' begins with problem-posing groups which seek to break down barriers and establish a dialogue between individuals and between individuals and the facilitator. Eventually a state of praxis is reached in which there is a common understanding and development of action and practice, whereby people collectively can transform their circumstances. The process is summarized as:

- Reflection on aspects of reality
- Search and collective identification of the root causes of that reality
- An examination of their implications
- Development of a plan of action to change reality (Freire 1972).

Community development is a recognized way of working which has given rise to a specific profession – community development workers, who are generally employed by local authorities to support, facilitate and empower communities. Community development workers have their own training courses, qualifications and professional associations.

Community development and health promotion

Community development is a recurring theme in health promotion. In the 1960s the Women's Movement emphasized the need to reclaim knowledge about our bodies and control over our lives. Shared personal experience led to a new understanding of health issues as well as providing positive effects and social cohesion for participants. Black and ethnic-minority groups also addressed health issues, particularly the effect of racism within the health services (Jones 1991).

In the 1970s and early 1980s numerous community development projects were set up, mostly funded and located outside the National Health Service (NHS). Inner-city decline prompted youth work, neighbourhood centres and planning groups which drew attention to the relationship between poverty, health and inequalities in service provision (Rosenthal 1983). Within the health services, community development approaches remained marginalized.

In the latter part of the 1980s there was widespread lip service to the notion of community development, stimulated in part by WHO.

Box 10.3

Consider the following statements from WHO on the importance of participation, involvement and community development. What do you think contributed to this emphasis on working with 'the community'?

'The people have a right and a duty to participate individually and collectively in the planning and implementation of their health care' (WHO 1978).

'Health for all will be achieved by people themselves. A well-informed, well-motivated and actively *participating community* is a key element for the attainment of the common goal' (WHO 1985, p. 5, original emphasis).

'Health promotion works through concrete and effective community action in setting priorities, making decisions, planning strategies and implementing them to achieve better health. At the heart of this process is the empowerment of communities, their ownership and control of their own endeavours and destinies' (WHO 1986).

'Community action is central to the fostering of health public policy' (WHO 1988).

'Health promotion is carried out by and with people, not on or to people. It improves the ability of individuals to take action, and the capacity of groups, organisations or communities to influence the determinants of health. Improving the capacity of communities for health promotion requires practical education, leadership training and access to resources' (WHO 1997).

Community development has been seen as the central defining strategy for health promotion (Green & Raeburn 1990). By the mid-1980s the Community Health Initiatives Resource Unit estimated that there were 10 000 local projects in existence. By the 1990s the lead health promotion agencies for developing strategies were under pressure as community development was seen as too radical. Its focus on structural causes of inequality, such as class, race and gender, was not acceptable to New Right political ideology (see Chapter 7 for more discussion of this). The Community and Professional Development Division of the Health Education Authority (HEA) was disbanded. The National Community Health Resource (NCHR) lost its funding from the HEA and Community Health UK (CHUK) lost its funding from the Department of Health.

Yet the 1990s also saw an emphasis on the concept of 'community'. Strategies for service delivery were linked to the notion of community, and care in the community, community policing and community education emerged as key policies. The focus on the community needs to be seen in relation to the developing crisis in the role of welfare state provision and broader debates around accountability. Chapter 7 has shown how neoliberal concerns to retreat from welfare have been linked to a focus on individuals as consumers of services. Devolved services and an emphasis on participation and 'consumer involvement' were all strategies designed to achieve these aims.

'Third-way' politics in the UK draws upon ideas of communitarianism – that we are all linked together as citizens. Communal relations such as trust and reciprocity are to be valued and government action aims to bolster social capital (see Chapter 15 for a discussion of how neighbourhoods and the community became a focus for policy and analysis). A new government department of communities and local government, a public service agreement to build more cohesive, empowered and active communities, and Chapter 4 of the public health White Paper *Choosing Health: Making Healthy Choices Easier* (Department of Health 2004) all

show a commitment to working through communities to create a stable, inclusive society.

The tradition of community development has radical roots and is closely associated with work to challenge the status quo, redistribute resources and address power imbalances across society. Although many have welcomed the adoption of once-radical terms such as empowerment and participation into mainstream policy language, there are those who suggest this mainstreaming of community development has diluted its aims and processes and resulted in a gulf between theory and practice (Berner & Philips 2005). There have been warnings that such 'state-commissioned' community development results in 'not government by communities but government through communities' (Shaw 2005). The policy focus on communities to bring about change (e.g. in neighbourhood renewal or antisocial behaviour) leads to communities, rather than society, being seen as responsible for the problems they face. This may be viewed as an extension, from individuals to communities, of the 'victim-blaming' principle.

Working with a community development approach

The ways in which community development is carried out vary enormously. However there are a number of core principles underpinning community development work, which overlap and link together. These principles are:

- Participation
- Community empowerment
- Community-led
- Social justice.

Participation

Participation, engagement and involvement are terms that are frequently used in the health sector. While these terms have different meanings they all relate to a central aspect of community development, that of

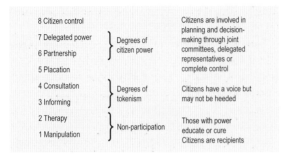

Figure 10.1 • Arnstein's ladder of participation. Adapted from Arnstein (1971).

increasing people's involvement in decisions, service design and delivery. The emphasis in community development on increasing people's power and control means increasing their participation in decision-making. Participation may be thought of as a ladder which includes many different activities (Figure 10.1). At the low or weak end, it may mean consultation to 'rubber-stamp' plans already drawn up by official agencies. At the high or strong end of the spectrum, it may mean control over the setting of priorities and implementation of programmes.

Box 10.4

Consider the following examples of participation. Where would you place them on Arnstein's ladder?
How could they be moved up the ladder?
- A public forum to discuss the provision of mental health services
- The attendance of a mother at a court hearing about the care of her child
- The use of care plans for elderly people living in residential homes
- An inner-city locality project funded by local and health authorities: a health visitor is given a 0.5 secondment to lead the project; the focus is on providing appropriate preventive services.

Community empowerment

Empowerment as a health promotion approach is discussed in Chapter 5 and the distinction is made between empowerment of individuals and empowerment of communities. Empowering communities is a core principle of community development and has been defined as:

> *a process by which communities gain more control over the decisions and resources that influence their lives, including the determinants of health. Community empowerment builds from the individual to the group to the wider collective and embodies the intention to bring about social and political change (Laverack 2007, p. 29).*

Community empowerment begins through a process of critical consciousness-raising whereby individuals and communities begin to question and challenge the social justice of their situation (Ledwith 2005) (see the section on defining community development earlier in this chapter for a more detailed discussion of critical consciousness-raising).

Laverack (2007) identifies nine domains or areas of influence of community empowerment as a way of further clarifying how we understand this term:

1. Improves participation
2. Develops local leadership
3. Builds empowering organizational structures
4. Increases problem assessment capacities
5. Enhances the ability of the community to 'ask why'
6. Improves resource mobilization
7. Strengthens links to other organizations and people
8. Creates an equitable relationship with outside agencies
9. Increases control over programme management.

Community-led

In contrast to professionally determined priorities, community development starts with priorities identified by and common to communities. The term community-led requires us to make a commitment to learning from communities, being accountable to communities and working in partnership. This is not without its tensions, for example when needs and priorities identified by communities are not compatible with those identified by statutory and funding bodies. An important aspect of community development work is legitimizing people's knowledge about health and illness and giving this a voice. Not only does this pose a challenge to medical dominance; it is also very different from the systematic research into needs which we describe in Chapter 18. Establishing the needs of the community also means a shift towards more participatory and locality-based involvement.

Box 10.5

- How important do you think community development is as a health promotion strategy?
- How does it compare with other approaches such as the medical preventive, individual empowerment, educational, behaviour change or social change approaches?

Social justice

Community development recognizes that inequalities exist within society and that some communities are more privileged and better resourced – and consequently more healthy – than others. Community development sees these inequalities as having been created by society and therefore amenable to change by society. Community development seeks to strengthen civil society in a democratic and participatory way by giving a voice to communities that are disadvantaged or oppressed (Craig et al 2004). In so doing, it focuses on the determinants of

health rather than on individual lifestyles. This may mean:

- Working to promote the health of disadvantaged groups
- Increasing the accessibility of services
- Influencing the commissioning of services
- Acting as an advocate and representing the interests of disadvantaged groups
- Building a social profile of the community, highlighting the relationship to health status.

The community development approach is challenging. It offers the prospect of change for health but there are many practical difficulties to overcome (Table 10.2).

Types of activities involved in community development

A large number of activities may be included as part of a community development approach:

- Profiling
- Capacity-building
- Organizing
- Networking
- Negotiating.

Profiling

Undertaking a community profile is much broader than a needs assessment. Community profiling involves the community, statutory and voluntary organizations in identifying the community's needs, particular issues and resources. It is an important and early stage of the community development process. Profiling creates a better understanding of both the strengths and challenges within a community whilst simultaneously developing the skills and capacity of community members (Hawtin & Percy-Smith 2007). The key task of a community development worker is to build a picture of the community, identifying key individuals, groups and resources, and get to know the community formally and informally.

Table 10.2 Advantages and disadvantages of the community development approach

Advantages	Disadvantages
Starts with people's concerns, so it is more likely to gain support	Time-consuming
Focuses on root causes of ill health, not symptoms	Results are often not tangible or quantifiable
Creates awareness of the social causes of ill health	Evaluation is difficult
The process of involvement is enabling and leads to greater confidence	Without evaluation, gaining funding is difficult
The process includes acquiring skills which are transferable, for example communication skills, lobbying skills	Health promoters may find their role contradictory. To whom are they ultimately accountable – employer or community?
If health promoter and people meet as equals, it extends principle of democratic accountability	Work is usually with small groups of people
	Draws attention away from macro issues and may focus on local neighbourhoods

Building networks and identifying communities takes time. The role of the community worker is to build on initial research and contact with people living and working in the community, so that the needs identified can be expanded upon and solutions developed (see Chapter 18).

Box 10.6

Many community nurses compile community profiles. How could these be used to facilitate community development?

Capacity-building

Capacity-building is working with individuals and groups within communities to recognize and develop the skills and resources they have (their assets) in order to identify and meet their own needs. The Charity Commission sees it as being concerned with two key areas of work:

1.   Providing opportunities for people to learn through experience – opportunities that would not otherwise be available to them

2.   Involving people in collective effort so that they gain confidence in their own abilities and their ability to influence decisions that affect them (Charity Commission 2000).

Box 10.7

Community capacity-building: untangling the web in Prestonpans
The Scottish Executive provided three free public internet access points in Prestonpans as part of its initiative to get more people in Scotland online. Staff at these access points noticed that they were very underused and did not seem an effective way to introduce new users to computing or the internet. During an open day to launch the community website participants were able to get hands-on experience, sign up to a short course and get a personal follow-up from staff. This increased the community's use of the internet.

Organizing

An important area of work that community development workers are engaged in is the process of helping to organize the community to work together effectively. This may include helping to establish small self-help groups or organizing community events such as health forums.

 Box 10.8

Refugee action
A refugee advocate describes their role:

Community development can be quite an invisible job, but the relationships you build with groups over the months or years is vital. By getting to know different groups, you can identify the issues they face and where they can work together. We have strategic bodies at one level, and the communities and grassroots activity at another level, and community development somewhere in the middle. If you take that out, the structures will collapse; the issues which need to be addressed by policy makers just won't reach them ... one of the things I have done is to help set up a Refugee Forum. The refugee community organisations now come together in a group and talk about their issues, what action they want to take and how to make a strong voice (Mani Thapa, Community Development Officer Refugee Action, quoted in Community Development Exchange, undated).

Networking

Networks are the ties that link people together within a community. Gilchrist (2004, 2007) identifies two different types of networks: those linked by strong ties and those linked by weak ties. Networks linked by strong ties are based on bonds of friendship or family relations and are those we are most likely to turn to for daily support and companionship. Networks based on weak ties link different clusters of networks together. They have been described as the links that operate over the whole network forming bridges between sections of the community or between organizations. Both types of network are an important

asset within a community and are an indicator of levels of social capital. Strong networks create opportunities for skills, information and learning to be shared across the community, to create synergy and lead to more effective community action. Building such networks by making the links between individuals, groups and local organizations is therefore an important part of the community development worker's role.

Negotiating

Community development work recognizes the diversity and division that exist within communities. Communities are not homogeneous entities but include hierarchies, imbalances in power and differences. Such diversity must be negotiated and managed in order to achieve a consensus, particularly in relation to prioritizing needs and agreeing actions to meet needs. As well as negotiating and managing conflict within communities, the community development worker must negotiate and advocate on behalf of the community. This may involve negotiating with funding or statutory bodies to ensure that the needs and views of the community are heard and considered.

 Box 10.9

Community development in practice
Carol Osgerby, Community Health Development Worker for West Hull Primary Care Trust describes community development work:
Question: Please explain your job as simply as possible.
Answer: When people want their community to get more healthy and prevent illness, I help them to set up groups and keep them going, by encouraging them and helping sort out problems.
Question: Please describe a typical week.
Answer: *Monday*: Work on an evaluation of the health impact of community groups. Later, I join a local walking group to talk to them about raising funds and developing the group.
Tuesday: Prepare display materials for Thursday's event. Attend a committee meeting of a local Community Orchard. Discuss insurance,

tenancy agreement and annual budget. Agree to work with the secretary to draft a funding application and help them make contacts with other similar groups so they can share information.

Wednesday: Catch up with paperwork and e-mails. Team meeting in the afternoon. We are a team of four community health development workers, trying to cover a city of 250 000 people.

Thursday: More paperwork, and reading the latest on the reorganization of public health in Hull. Later I attend a health event at a community centre where I run a quiz about food labelling and offer tasters of fruit smoothies. Get into discussion with many of the residents and workers there about nutrition, exercise, slimming and assorted queries about health care and illness. My real aim is to publicise community groups, and maybe make some links that could lead to new projects. In the evening I attend a neighbourhood management meeting. Good turnout of residents, as well as council staff, Community Empowerment Network, youth workers, etc. I help to get residents' ideas on to paper.

Friday: Meet with the Community Orchard secretary to help draft a budget and fill in grant application form. We discuss how we can encourage local residents to get involved in winter, when there is less physical work to do. Later, I work on our community groups newsletter.

Question: Please describe what you feel makes your work specifically 'community development'.

Answer: Community development develops and leaves behind structures that were not there before, and those structures are managed by members of the community. A vital part of community development is to support individuals to develop skills which they can use to develop community groups, organizations and networks. When I'm asked to take on a new piece of work, I ask myself: 'Is there potential to produce a project which is truly led by the community it's meant to serve?' If not, to me it's not community development. You have to respect the ability of the communities you work with to make their own decisions (Community Development Exchange (CDX) information sheet).

Box 10.10

Read the excerpt in Example 10.9 and then discuss the following questions:
- What positive outcomes have been attributed to community development health promotion projects?
- Are these outcomes unique to community development?

Dilemmas in community development practice

The question of whether the community development worker is engaged in radical practice or supporting the status quo is at the root of much of the ambiguity surrounding practice. Common dilemmas facing the community development worker relate to funding, accountability, acceptability, the role of the professional and evaluation.

Funding

Most community development projects are funded by statutory agencies, such as health and education authorities, sometimes in partnership, through joint funding. Other projects which might come under the label 'community development' belong in the voluntary sector, and are funded from a variety of sources, including direct government grants and independent fund-raising. Most community development work is funded in the short term only. Lack of security and the impossibility of guaranteeing an input in the long term increase the problems of planning and evaluating such work. Insecure funding arrangements can also subvert a project's focus, leading workers to spend time fund-raising instead of working around defined issues.

Accountability

All community development workers have a dual accountability: to their employers and to their communities. Funding agencies naturally require projects to be accountable, and this can lead to problems where the priorities of the community and the agency are not the same. Organizational objectives such as service take-up may become incorporated into the community development worker's role.

Community and worker responses to issues may also differ. For example, both may identify safety as a priority, but whereas the worker may respond by advocating structural changes such as better lighting and common responsibility for shared areas, the community might respond by advocating increased vigilance or the exclusion of specific groups, families or individuals.

Community development workers may feel themselves to be trapped in the role of mediator, informing statutory services about community needs and informing the community about how services work so that people can participate.

Acceptability

Employing authorities often view community development as not quite respectable. Community development may be seen as absorbing unacceptably large amounts of time and resources for dubious results. Community development tends to focus on small numbers of people whereas employers tend to be responsible for large populations. The long-term nature and diffuse outcomes of community development are at odds with the organizational need to allocate resources on the basis of demonstrable results.

Issues which are raised through a community development approach (such as discrimination in service provision) may be unacceptable to employing authorities. By allying themselves with dissent, community development workers may be seen as betraying the organization.

Community development workers may also find that they need to establish and negotiate their role before they are accepted by a community. The role of the worker is ambiguous. Their status and employment set them apart from the community in which they are working. Relationships of trust may need to be created before any other work can take place.

Role of the professional

Community development also poses problems for workers whose primary training lies in other areas.

Problems may arise from the different kind of client–worker relationship envisaged in professional training and community development work. Professional workers are taught a particular area of expertise and tend to assume that they know what is best for their clients. They may be sensitive to individual circumstances but the secondary socialization encountered during professional training reinforces the notion of expertise.

Box 10.11

A health visitor wishes to adopt a community development approach in her work. She has identified setting up a postnatal mothers' group as an appropriate project.

- What arguments might she use in favour of this kind of work?
- What arguments might her manager use against it?

The health visitor might argue that such work is important for health because it increases self-esteem, autonomy and confidence, and a sense of belonging. She could argue that such work is effective. For example, postnatal networking amongst mothers could prove effective in reducing mental illness amongst this client group. The health visitor might also argue that time spent on setting up the group will reduce claims on her time in future, and is therefore a cost-effective option.

The health visitor's manager might respond that there is not enough time to carry out such work. Full caseloads and many other priority claims (such as visiting all new mothers and carrying out child development check-ups) mean there is no spare time available for other activities. The manager might also argue that such activities need to be thoroughly evaluated and of proven effectiveness before resources can be committed.

Sociologists argue that professional culture is actually an occupational strategy designed to increase the status and rewards of the professional group (Freidson 1986; Johnson 1972). By acquiring professional jargon, expertise and qualifications, professionals can justify their right to practise and defend their area of work.

By contrast, community development workers see their role as that of catalyst and facilitator rather than expert. Their task is to enable a community to express its needs, and support the community in meeting those needs themselves. This requires a different worker–client relationship, based on egalitarianism and the sharing of knowledge. For professionals, whose identity is bound up in their work role, this can be a difficult switch to make.

The skills involved in community work also tend to be different from those acquired in professional training (unless this includes community development). Key skills concern process rather than content and include:

- Organizational skills, e.g. developing appropriate management structures such as management committees or steering groups
- Communication skills, e.g. consultation and communication with a variety of groups, including community groups, funding agency and coworkers
- Evaluation skills, e.g. monitoring the impact of interventions and self-evaluation.

Box 10.12

- Which of these skills are covered in your professional training?
- How much time is devoted to these areas compared to other areas in the curriculum?
- Do you think your professional training has equipped you to practise community development?

Evaluation

Community development has often been described as difficult to evaluate because it works on so many levels, is a long-term strategy and encompasses so many strands of work. However, many of the principles used for evaluating health promotion work discussed in Chapter 20, particularly around assessing process, impact and outcomes are relevant. Barr (2002) provides a useful checklist of questions to consider when evaluating community development work which reflect the principles and goals of this approach:

- Are we gaining a new understanding of community issues and needs?
- Are we being effective in tackling them?
- Are we being inclusive?
- Are the participants achieving their personal goals?
- Are we building community assets and resources?
- Is our work empowering people?
- Are we building a culture of collaboration, participation and sustainable change?
- Are we learning from our experience?
- Are we contributing to health and well-being?
- Are we making the best possible use of the resources we have?
- Do we have the evidence we need to influence future decisions?

As part of the drive to build an evidence base in community development work as well as to support work of practitioners, a number of evaluation models that provide frameworks for assessing work have been developed. The ABCD model was developed by the Scottish Community Development Centre to support both the planning and evaluation of projects and provides a framework for measuring participation and empowerment (Barr & Hashagen 2000). This model was used as the basis for the Learning Evaluation And Planning (LEAP) model. LEAP provides a strategy through which community representatives and professionals jointly consider:

- What needs to change?
- How will we know it has changed?
- How will we change it?
- How will we monitor what we do?
- How will we learn from our experience?

The answers to these questions are used to devise a framework against which community activity is planned, monitored and evaluated.

Box 10.13

Consider the following statement: Community development is about ...
- Trying to create a 'better' community
- Getting the community to do what the authorities want them to do
- Promoting equal access to resources
- Getting the community to take responsibility for its own problems
- A political process
- Controlling social unrest by providing diversionary activities
- Helping people to see the root causes of problems
- Providing people with opportunities to become involved in decision-making.

Which of these statements would you say were true? What issues or dilemmas were raised when you were thinking about these statements?

Conclusion

Community development does not fit tidily into most health promoters' working lives. In contrast to how most health promotion workers have been trained, community development relies upon a different set of assumptions about the nature of health and a different set of skills. This can make it a problematic activity to undertake. However, practitioners who have espoused community development are enthusiastic about its potential and outcomes. It is claimed to be the most ethical and effective form of health promotion, and one which makes a real impact on people's lives.

What [inner-city community health projects] are doing is creating a climate in which some of the most oppressed and deprived sections of our urban communities can find a voice with which to challenge the forces which both determine their health and control the quantity and quality of health services to which they have access (Rosenthal 1983).

Community development does appear to address many of the problems inherent in more traditional forms of health promotion. It avoids victim-blaming, addresses structural causes of inequalities in health and seeks to empower people. This goes some way to explain its popularity with health promoters.

Community development has been endorsed both at the international level, by various WHO declarations, and at the local level, by project workers. It is not such a popular option at the middle level of large-scale organizations, including the NHS. This is in part due to the practical difficulties of implementation and evaluation. However, there are also ideological conflicts if community development is to be practised within the NHS. It has been stated that community development represents a challenge to the medical model of health, and previous experience in the UK has also demonstrated that it is perceived as an overtly political strategy. The political implications of community development have been attacked from both the right and left wings of the political spectrum. Community development has been viewed as both a subversive left-wing activity and a subtle means of policing and controlling communities.

A global review of community projects has shown that they do tackle broader influences on health and promote health behaviour change in individuals (Gillies 1997).

Box 10.14

Community development in Costa Rica

A comprehensive community development programme in Costa Rica involved links across government departments, health and local authorities working together, local people contributing to decision-making through local social action committees, needs assessments, educational opportunities for women and microenterprise developments to boost income in the poorest groups. The programme led to improved infant mortality rates, improved access to services and improved social, economic and physical environments. The key elements of success were:

- Involvement of local people in identifying needs
- Committed and open partnerships between agencies
- Involvement of local people in planning and decision-making through local action committees
- Training and support for volunteers, peer educators and local networks (Gillies 1997).

Questions for further discussion

- Would you consider adopting a community development approach in your work?
- Do you think community development has advantages over other health promotion strategies?

Summary

This chapter has examined the history and theoretical underpinnings of community development as an approach to health promotion. We have seen that community development is often viewed by workers as the most ethical and effective means of promoting health. At the same time, its practice poses dilemmas for the health promoter and its evaluation is fraught with problems. However, we would argue that the reasons put forward for the privileged position of community development are sound. Practical difficulties should not obstruct the continuing development and spread of this health promotion strategy. On the contrary, what is needed is a more open outlook from statutory organizations, and a willingness to experiment with this kind of strategy.

Further reading

Lloyd C E, Handsley S, Douglas J et al 2007 Policy and practice in promoting public health. Sage/Open University, London. *An accessible textbook which explores the potential for communities to be involved in promoting their own health.*

Henderson P, Thomas D 2001 Skills in neighbourhood work, 3rd edn. Routledge, London. *Describes the skills and techniques for working with communities.*

Laverack G 2007 Health promotion practice; building empowered communities. Open University Press, Buckingham. *Combines theory with practice in discussing how to build community empowerment using experiences from the UK, Asia and Africa.*

Useful websites include:

Community Development Exchange: www.cdx.org.uk

Community Development Foundation: www.cdf.org.uk

People and Participation: www.peopleandparticipation.net

Scottish Community development Centre: www.scdc.org.uk

References

Arnstein S R 1971 Eight rungs on the ladder of citizen participation. In: Cahn S E, Passelt B A (eds) Citizen participation: effecting community change. Praeger, New York.

Barclay Report on Social Work 1982 National Institute for Social Work. Social workers: their role and tasks. Bedford Square Press, London.

Barr A 2002 Learning evaluation and planning. A handbook for partners in community learning. Community Development Foundation, London.

Barr A, Hashagen S 2000 ABCD Handbook. A framework for evaluating community development. Community Development Foundation, London.

Berner E, Philips B 2005 Left to their own devices? Community self help between alternative development and neo-liberalism. Community Development Journal 40: 17–29.

Charity Commission 2000 The promotion of community capacity building. The Charity Commission, London.

Community Development Exchange (undated) CDX information sheet; community development in action. CDX, Sheffield.

Community Development Exchange (CDX) information sheet. Available online: at http://www.cdx.org.uk/files/u1/cd_in_action_07__2_pdf

Community Health Initiatives Resource Unit/London Community Health Resource 1987 Guide to community health projects. NCVO, London.

Craig G, Gorman M, Vercseg I 2004 The Budapest Declaration; building European civil society through community development. Available online at: http://www.iacdglobal.org/documents/general/BudapestDeclaration4683D.pdf#search = %22The%20Budapest%20Declaration%22 on 9/2/08

Department of Health 2004 Choosing health: making healthy choices easier. Stationery Office, London.

Freidson E 1986 Professional power. The institutionalization of knowledge. Chicago University Press, Chicago.

Freire P 1972 Pedagogy of the oppressed. Penguin, Harmondsworth.

Gilchrist A 2004 The well connected community. A networking approach to community. Policy Press, Bristol.

Gilchrist A et al 2007 Community development and networking for health. In: Orme J, Powell J, Taylor P (eds) Public health for the 21st century. Open University/McGraw Hill, Maidenhead.

Gillies P 1997 The effectiveness of alliances or partnerships for health promotion. Conference working paper. 4th International Conference on Health Promotion, Jakarta, Indonesia.

Green L W, Raeburn J 1990 Community wide change: theory and practice. In: Bracht N (ed) Health promotion at the community level. Sage, California.

Hawtin M, Percy-Smith J 2007 Community profiling; a practical guide. Open University Press, Buckingham.

Health Education Authority 1987 Leaflet on community department. HEC, London.

Johnson T J 1972 Professions and power. Macmillan, Basingstoke.

Jones J 1991 Community development and health education: concepts and philosophy. In: Community development and health education, vol. 1. Open University Press, Milton Keynes.

Labonte R 1998 A community development approach to health promotion: a background paper on practice tensions, strategic models and accountability requirements for health authority work in the broad determinants of health. Prepared for Health Education Board of Scotland, Research Unit on Health and Behaviour Change, University of Edinburgh.

Laverack G 2007 Health promotion practice; building empowered communities. Open University Press, Buckingham.

Ledwith M 2005 Community development; a critical approach. Policy Press, Bristol.

Nutbeam D 1998 Health promotion glossary. WHO, Geneva.

Rosenthal H 1983 Neighbourhood health projects – some new approaches to health and community work in some parts of the United Kingdom. Community Development Journal 18: 120–130.

Shaw M 2005 Political, professional, powerful: understanding community development. Transcript of introductory presentation – Community Development Exchange Annual Conference, 23–25 September 2005, Leeds.

Smithies J, Adams L 1990 Community participation in health promotion. HEA, London.

Standing Conference for Community Development 2001 Strategic framework for community development. SCCD, Sheffield.

World Health Organization 1978 Alma Ata 1978: primary health care. WHO, Geneva.

World Health Organization 1985 Targets for health for all. WHO Regional Office for Europe, Copenhagen.

World Health Organization 1986 The Ottawa charter for health promotion. Health Promotion 1: iii–v.

World Health Organization 1988 Adelaide recommendation on health public policy. WHO, Adelaide.

World Health Organization 1997 New players for a new era: leading health promotion into the 21st century.

4th International Conference on Health Promotion, Jakarta, Indonesia 21–25 July 1997. Conference Report World Health Organization, Geneva/Ministry of Health, Indonesia.

Chapter Eleven

Developing healthy public policy

Key points

- Defining healthy public policy (HPP)
- Advantages and drawbacks to using an HPP approach
- The history of HPP
- HPP at different levels – global, national and organizational
- The potential of HPP to promote health
- Resources and skills required for HPP
- The practitioner's role
- Evaluating the effectiveness of HPP

OVERVIEW

Healthy public policy (HPP) was identified in the Ottawa Charter (World Health Organization (WHO) 1986) as one of the five key strategies for promoting health. HPP focuses on changing the environment in order to make the healthy choice easier. Health is affected by many different policy areas:

Everyone has the right to a standard of living adequate for the health and well-being of himself and of his family, including food, clothing, housing and medical care and necessary social services, and the right to security in the event of unemployment, sickness, disability, widowhood, old age or other lack of livelihood in circumstances beyond his control (Universal Declaration of Human Rights Article 25(1)).

HPP therefore includes all the major areas of policy that are the responsibility of democratic governments – employment, welfare, education, transport, food and health and social services. Relevant policies may also be instigated by private commercial organizations or devolved government agencies. Promoting HPP across this range of agencies and issues appears to be a daunting task. How to make inroads into this aspect of health promotion is the subject of this chapter, which examines the infrastructure required to facilitate HPP, the role of the practitioner and the potential of this approach to promote health. Readers are referred to Chapter 4 of our companion volume (Naidoo & Wills 2005) for a more detailed discussion of the policy process.

Defining HPP

Policy is a contested term, with meanings ranging from intentions to decisions and strategies. Milio (2001, p. 622) in a glossary of definitions describes it as 'a guide to action to change what would otherwise occur, a decision about amounts and allocations of resources: the overall amount is a statement of commitment to certain areas of concern; the distribution of the amount shows the priorities of decision makers. Policy sets priorities and guides resource allocation'. We shall adopt a broad definition of policy as a plan of action to guide decisions and actions. Policy can be developed and implemented at many different levels, from organizational to national to international. Whilst policy may be allocated to a specific sphere, such as health, education or transport, in practice its effects are often wide-ranging and extend beyond the sphere originally targeted. Figure 8.3 in Chapter 8 illustrates the many agencies and organizations that promote health in some way. At government level the Treasury, for example, tries to influence individual behaviour through taxation of unhealthy products whilst the Department of Children, Schools and Families tries to do this through school-based health education. Joined-up policy-making is the term used to refer to integrated policy-making across different spheres. The determinants of health are multiple and interconnected, so in order to be effective, policy also needs to be holistic. It is often assumed that policy, once made and adopted by the relevant agency, translates smoothly into the intended action and anticipated outcomes. However this is the exception rather than the rule. Policy is (re)interpreted at all levels and its practical application may diverge from the original intention. It is therefore not enough to make policy; it must be followed through, monitored and supported by appropriate training and resources.

WHO has defined HPP as: 'placing health on the agenda of policy makers in all sectors and at all levels, directing them to be aware of the health consequences of their decisions and to accept their responsibilities for health' (WHO 1986, p. 2). This is a very broad definition, as is the Ottawa Charter's (WHO 1986) definition of HPP as a central plank for health promotion. The Ottawa Charter cited the following fundamental resources for health: peace, shelter, education, food, income, a stable ecosystem, sustainable resources, social justice and equity. This embraces all governmental activities, except, ironically enough, the provision of health services, although they might be counted as part of the social justice and equity resources. The Second International Conference on Health Promotion in Adelaide, Australia in 1988 (WHO 1988) explored HPP. It called for a political commitment to health by all sectors and an explicit accountability for health impacts.

Further international conferences focused on the globalization of health and the need for international cooperation to tackle the determinants of health. The Sundsvall Conference concentrated on the global, interlinked nature of environmental change to promote health (WHO 1991). The Jakarta Declaration (WHO 1997) and the Mexico conference (WHO 2000a) focused on the interlinked nature of social, economic and political development for health. The Bangkok Charter (WHO 2005) sought to make health promotion central to the global development agenda, and called for commitments from governments, communities and the private corporate sector to address health determinants and reduce inequalities.

> ### Box 11.1
>
> Are there any core values that should underpin HPP? If so, what are they?

Some core values underpinning HPP may be inferred from the conferences and charters outlined above and are also discussed in Chapter 4. These include:

- Equity – an active redistribution of the material resources required for healthy living, e.g. income, housing
- Upstream focus – concentrating on the socioeconomic determinants of health rather than individual lifestyles

- Participation – the involvement of all interested partners including governments, practitioners and the public
- Collaboration – working across organizational and national boundaries to meet agreed goals
- Sustainability – meeting existing needs without compromising the ability of future generations to meet their own needs.

What is clear from the above definitions resulting from the WHO international conferences is the broad scope of HPP, encompassing as it does all levels of government from international to national to local.

No policy would claim to have adverse health effects and most would claim to increase well-being in some way, albeit indirectly. Yet many policies may have apparently contradictory effects. For example, it has been argued that the overall economic effect of a reduction in smoking would be negative, due to the loss of tobacco tax revenue to the exchequer, and the extra demand on services due to people living longer. Economic policies that increase the income of the wealthiest have been defended on the grounds that there would be a 'trickle-down' effect, despite evidence that increases in relative inequality are detrimental to health (Wilkinson 1996). The application of stringent animal and environmental welfare regulations in the UK has resulted in an increase in meat imports from other countries where the same regulations do not apply. The consequences of policy programmes therefore need to be thought through in some detail. Health impact assessment (HIA) is an approach that does just this. HIA enables the identification, prediction and evaluation of likely changes to health, both now and in the future, as a consequence of a policy programme or plan. HIA recognizes that health is affected by a broad range of determinants linked in various pathways. For example, a HIA of a policy to extend licensing hours would weigh up the benefits and disadvantages of the proposal's impact on individuals, the local community, the environment and the economy. Whilst the proposal may benefit the local economy, disadvantages to health, law and safety, and community cohesion are likely.

HIA as an approach is likely to become more widespread as various international agreements require an assessment be made of the likely impact of policy. For example, the European Union requires the establishment of mechanisms to ensure a high level of human health protection in the definition and implementation of all Community policies and activities (article 152 of the Treaty of Rome).

Box 11.2

Health impact assessments in London

Congestion charges

Prior to the introduction of congestion charging in London, an HIA concluded that the scheme had the potential to improve health by:

- Promoting other modes of transport, e.g. cycling and walking
- Reducing emissions
- Segregating modes of transport through road reallocation
- Linking transport
- Economic and spatial development to encourage economically and socially sustainable communities (http://www.londonshealth.gov.uk/pdf/transprt.pdf).

Hosting the Olympic Games

Hosting the 2012 Olympic Games in London is anticipated to bring economic benefits to local communities. It might be assumed that the construction of additional sporting facilities will improve the opportunities for physical activity amongst the local population. However this is not necessarily the case. The extent to which members of a community will use facilities and opportunities is almost impossible to quantify in advance. There may also be an adverse health impact (e.g. air and noise pollution) on the community during the construction phase. A rapid HIA concluded that the overall impact will be positive: 'there will be greater benefits to the local communities arising from increased employment and income opportunities, greater physical activity and enhanced community cohesion' (http://www.londonshealth.gov.uk/PDF/Olympic_HIA.pdf).

The history of HPP

HPP has a long and illustrious history. Many would date its origins in the UK to the 19th century and the rise of the Sanitary Reform Movement, prompted by concerns about the spread of disease in overcrowded industrial slums. Edwin Chadwick's *Report from the Poor Law Commissioners on an Inquiry into the Sanitary Conditions of the Labouring Population of Great Britain* (1842) made it clear that the poor did not have the power to change their conditions, and that protecting and promoting their health were tasks of local government. The 19th century saw a plethora of legislation and regulations to protect and promote health – a trend that was carried on into the 20th and 21st centuries (see Example 11.3).

Box 11.3

Landmarks in healthy public policy in the UK during the 19th, 20th and 21st centuries

1842 Edwin Chadwick's *Report from the Poor Law Commissioners on an Inquiry into the Sanitary Conditions of the Labouring Population of Great Britain* is published

1843 The Royal Commission on the Health of Towns is established

1844 The Health of Towns Association is founded

1845 Final report from the Royal Commission on the Health of Towns is published

1848 Public Health Act for England and Wales requires local authorities to provide clean water supplies and hygienic sewage disposal systems, and introduces the appointment of medical officers of health for towns

1854 John Snow controls a cholera outbreak in London by removing a contaminated local water supply

1866 Sanitary Act – local authorities had to inspect their district

1868 Housing Act – local authorities could ensure owners kept their properties in good repair

1871 Local Government Board (which became the Ministry of Health in 1919) was established

1872 Public Health Act makes medical officers of health mandatory for each district

1875 Public Health Act consolidates earlier legislation and the tone changes from allowing to requiring local authorities to take public health measures

1906 Education Act establishes the provision of school dinners

1907 Education Act establishes the school medical service. Notification of Births Act and the development of health visiting is encouraged

1967 Road Safety Act set a legal limit of 80 mg of alcohol per 100 ml of blood and imposed a 70 miles per hour speed limit

1968 Clean Air Act to reduce air pollution and respiratory diseases

1974 National Health Service (NHS) reorganization – community and public health services transferred from local authorities to the NHS

1974 Heath and Safety at Work Act requires all employers to secure the health, safety and welfare at work of all employees

1977 Housing (Homeless Persons) Act places a duty on local authorities to house homeless persons

1983 Seat belt legislation. Wearing of seat belts in rear seats becomes law in 1991. Children to be restrained in car seats becomes law in 2006

1988 Water Bill requires privatized water suppliers to conform to health standards

1989 Tax subsidy on unleaded petrol

2000 The Food Standards Agency, an independent body, is established to protect the public's health and consumer interests in relation to food

2004 Smoking ban in all public places introduced in the Republic of Ireland

2005 Pubs and clubs able to apply for unlimited extension to opening hours

2005 Civil Partnership Act (2005) allows same-sex couples to enter a civil partnership, giving them the same next-of-kin rights in relation to health care as married couples

2006 Smoking ban introduced in all public places in Scotland

2006 Work and Families Act extends maternity and adoption leave from 6 to 9 months' paid leave, to be taken by the father or the mother

2007 Smoking ban in all public places introduced in England, Northern Ireland and Wales

2007 Junk food advertising banned from television programmes aimed at young children (4–9-year-olds)

The 19th-century view of public health was dominated by the effects of the physical environment on health. The 21st-century view of public health is ecological, whereby economic, environmental and social factors interconnect and have an impact on health. Current health concerns include ensuring that everyone has access to green space, a safe environment, mobility and transport, as well as clean, safe land and water. Everyone should be able to use renewable energy, reduce waste products to a minimum and use efficient recycling methods.

Regulation is just one way in which policy can support health. Governments may also use fiscal or monetary means such as taxing unhealthy products or hypothecation (a dedicated tax to support a specific purpose, e.g. funding cycling routes through a congestion charge on motor vehicles). Policy can support health through the provision of services, e.g. recycling facilities.

There is clearly a role for individual champions of public health. The story of John Snow, who stopped the cholera epidemic in Soho in 1854 by removing the handle of the Broad Street water pump, illustrates the importance of the epidemiological (studying the incidence and prevalence of disease) approach in public health (Figure 11.1). Previously, people had believed that bad air (miasma) from the rubbish and waste in the slums was responsible for the spread of disease. Snow's successful action demonstrated that cholera was a waterborne disease which could be prevented by the provision of clean water supplies.

Single-issue pressure groups or non-governmental organizations (e.g. Help the Aged; Friends of the Earth) may also act as champions lobbying and advocating for specific policies. An example is Oxfam's lobbying to change trade-related aspects of intellectual property rights (TRIPS) regulations in relation to patented medicines. Publicity showing how human immunodeficiency virus (HIV)-positive patients in South Africa and Zimbabwe could not afford patented drug therapies set the scene. Oxfam then launched a sustained campaign to ensure that low-income countries have access to medicines at minimal cost, including the right to access non-patented medicines. At the time of writing (2008) the campaign is ongoing.

There is also a role for research to establish the links between determinants and health. Credible research needs to document the severity of the problem and the effectiveness of the proposed solutions. The British Medical Association (2003), for example, has called for more evidence to show that improved housing can improve health. Lobbying to translate research findings into plain English and spell out their implications for health is also important. The gathering of robust evidence for the effectiveness of HPP, given the long timescales and complexity of interrelated factors, has proved to be problematic. The lack of a robust evidence base for HPP has been commented on by

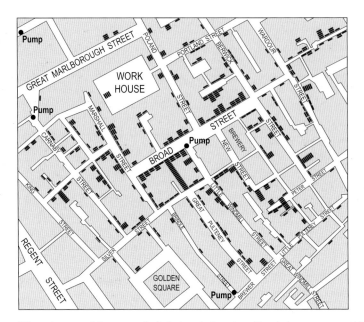

Figure 11.1 • A portion of Snow's map of the spread of cholera in London. Purple bars represent the number of fatal cases in each house. The position of the Broad Street pump from which all the victims had obtained water is also marked.

policy-makers and researchers (Petticrew et al 2004).

Many factors impacting on health operate on a global scale that transcends national boundaries, e.g. infectious diseases, poverty and food shortages, war and civil conflict and climate change. At the global level, international organizations such as the United Nations (UN), WHO, the World Trade Organization, the World Bank and the International Monetary Fund (IMF) are all hugely influential in affecting the socioeconomic determinants of health. An example of global health-promoting policy-making is the WHO's establishment of a Commission on Social Determinants of Health in 2005 and the UN Millennium Development Goals, which include targets to reduce poverty, hunger, child and maternal mortality, and infectious diseases; and to promote universal primary education, gender equality and environmental sustainability (United Nations Development Programme 2006).

The impact of global players is not always beneficial. For example, financial bodies such as the World Trade Organization support free-trade policies which often benefit middle- and high-income countries rather than low-income countries. The IMF has imposed structural adjustment programmes in low-income countries, which has had the effect of reducing their public spending, including spending on health. There is a 'brain drain' of skilled health professionals from low-income countries to middle- and high-income countries, which leads to a spiral of reduced service delivery and further migration of professionals (Sanders et al 2003).

The role of states is usually emphasized in HPP but policy is also made at other levels. In Part 3 we discuss how settings such as schools and hospitals can be supportive environments for health. Organizational policies, such as those relating to cultural competence for example, may have an impact on working practices.

Key characteristics of HPP: advantages and barriers

Box 11.4

Take a topic, e.g. obesity, sexual health or drug use. Identify a range of health promotion interventions including educational, behavioural and policy-making. What might be the advantages of an HPP approach to health promotion? And what might be the disadvantages?

HPP as an approach to health promotion has many strengths. Perhaps most important is its recognition of the multiple socioeconomic environmental determinants of health, and the necessity to change these determinants in order to promote health. Alongside this recognition and 'upstream' focus goes a commitment to reducing inequalities in health and promoting equity. An upstream approach also has economic benefits. A positive impact on determinants of health will prevent much ill health and disease, thus averting the need to spend money on services and treatment. Prevention is typically far more cost-effective than treatment.

HPP has the potential to make clear inroads into the state of the health of the public. McPherson (2001) states that 30% of coronary heart disease and 25% of all cancers are preventable through appropriate public health action. If achieved, this reduction would have economic as well as health benefits. The potential of HPP to achieve dramatic shifts in behaviour and attitudes is another reason for its popularity.

Box 11.5

Smoke-free workplaces in the Republic of Ireland

An evaluation of the legislation introducing smoke-free workplaces in the Republic of Ireland

in 2004 reported very positive results. There were dramatic declines in reported smoking in all venues, including restaurants (from 85% to 3%), bars and pubs (from 98% to 5%). Support for the ban from smokers increased, with 83% of smokers reporting that they thought the smoke-free law was a good or very good thing. Nearly half (46%) of smokers said the law made them consider quitting, and of smokers who had quit following the ban, 80% reported the law had helped them quit and 88% that the law helped them to stay quit (Fong et al 2006).

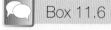

Box 11.6

Why, given the benefits outlined above, has HPP such a low profile?

There are many barriers to achieving HPP. Hunter (2003) identifies several barriers, including the tendency of both the government and the public to focus on health services instead of public health, and the silo mentality of government departments that means cross-departmental working to promote public health remains an aspiration rather than a reality. Public health issues tend to be 'wicked issues' (Rittel & Webber 1973). Wicked issues are complex issues that are not well understood and not amenable to easy manipulation or solution. Public health issues, such as sustainability or reducing health inequalities, are multidisciplinary in nature, and effective action is likely to require a long timescale, well beyond political parties' terms of office. As Hunter (2003, p. 17) puts it: 'Almost by definition public health issues are wicked issues.'

Opponents of an HPP approach might argue that it removes personal responsibility, and supports a 'nanny state' that dictates to its citizens their opportunities and behaviours. Indeed, Beattie (1993) described legislative action in his model of approaches to health promotion as authoritative and 'top-down'. Those who subscribe to conservative and individualistic political beliefs and ideology might be particularly likely to hold this view. This criticism has been met by the proposal that governments should act as stewards, guiding and protecting the health of the public, but not replacing the need for individual responsibility. Stewardship is about collective responsibility, which requires agreement about what needs to be done. The WHO ranks stewardship as more important than health service delivery or funding, because 'the ultimate responsibility for the overall performance of a country's health system must always lie with government' (WHO 2000b).

Joffe & Mindell (2004) argue that the focus should shift from telling people what to do to making healthy choices easier; that the state should shift from being a 'nanny state' to a 'canny state' – one 'that is clever, prudent, capable, and shrewd' (Joffe & Mindell 2004, p. 967). There are therefore several roles that governments may adopt in order to pursue healthy public policies. Some, such as the 'nanny state', appear old-fashioned and deeply unpopular. Others, such as stewardship or the 'canny state', appear more contemporary and in tune with a range of current values and ideologies in which the people in a civic society determine direction and government 'steers' but does not 'row' (Giddens 1998). Any form of legislative action requires agreement by the public. Tones has argued that, without health education, HPP would not be possible. Health education can not only set an agenda, e.g. environmental concern, but can also help 'to create a climate of opinion that will enable government, for example, to institute and claim the credit for change without risking electoral unpopularity' (Tones 2001, p. 14).

Box 11.7

Identify a health issue of concern to you, e.g. obesity, alcohol, smoking, mental health.

Go 'upstream' and try to identify the socioeconomic factors implicated in this health issue. Then try to define what policies might make an impact upstream on this issue. What agency or organization is responsible for this policy? What steps could you take to lobby for such a policy?

Resources and skills required for HPP

Box 11.8

Identify an example of HPP, e.g. smoking ban, food labelling regulations, transport policy to promote walking and cycling, neighbourhood regeneration. What kind of skills and resources are necessary to formulate and implement HPP?

Influencing, planning for, and operationalizing, HPP calls for a variety of skills. The required skills include health education, partnership working, lobbying, advocacy, managing, leadership and public relations. The Ottawa Charter (WHO 1986) described three key skills that would be necessary to act on the five action areas – mediation, advocacy and enablement. The competences for public health practice (www. skillsforhealth.org.uk) currently include a key area in policy and strategy development and implementation which calls for an understanding of the policy-making process, different methods of HIA and interagency working.

The policy-making process is complex and has been described elsewhere (Naidoo & Wills 2005, Chapter 4). The four key stages are (Walt 1994):

1. Problem identification and issue recognition

2. Policy formulation

3. Policy implementation

4. Policy evaluation.

An understanding of the policy-making process is crucial. A variety of different skills are needed at each stage. For example, stage 1, problem identification and issue recognition, may require research, lobbying and advocacy in order to prompt awareness of a particular issue. HIA can raise awareness of health impacts.

Partnership working is an important element within the policy process. The benefits and statutory requirements for collaboration are outlined in Chapter 5 of our companion volume (Naidoo & Wills 2005). Identifying key stakeholders, clarifying their interests in the proposed policy and making links with others to present a united agenda for change is all part of the wider policy process. Chapter 8 outlines the roles of some agencies. An awareness of different organizational cultures and their interests is vital for partnership working. Key skills are how to influence, negotiate, facilitate and manage in a multiagency environment to bring about change.

Public health advocacy has been described as the process of overcoming structural barriers to public health work (Chapman & Lupton 1994). It means influencing and then expressing public opinion to influence policy-makers' judgements about what is politically desirable and acceptable (Kemm 2001). Presenting the case for a policy might mean finding areas of overlap or congruence between the interests of the people you are representing and the key people with influence. Advocacy may also be used to present the case against a policy. The use of the mass media in advocacy is discussed further in Chapter 12.

Box 11.9

Think of a recent policy change in your workplace. How was the policy implemented? Was there resistance to the policy? Was implementation successful?

It cannot be assumed that once a policy has been approved the implementation stage is straightforward. This stage may be particularly problematic for policies that affect organizational working. Implementation involves getting the agreement of those who are affected by it, and their commitment to its operationalization. There is often resistance to the imposition of change from above. Frontline workers or 'street-level bureaucrats' (Lipsky 1979) have been identified as playing a key role in the implementation and delivery of policy changes, with the capacity to progress or impede the policy process.

Although in an ideal world HPP would be a rational process, in reality policy-making is not rational but incremental, or what has been labelled 'muddling through' (Lindblom 1959, Tones & Green 2004). Ideally policy-making would be driven by clarity about the problem, desired goals and outcomes and the best means of achieving these. This in turn would require an objective assessment of all alternatives at each stage of the policy process. The outcome would be the best possible choice, and there would be consensus about this. In reality, policy-making is incremental and typically considers a restricted range of options, blurs the distinction between goals and implementation, and achieves consensus about small changes rather than radical overhauls.

Box 11.10

The Framework Convention on Tobacco Control (WHO 2003)

The Framework Convention on Tobacco Control (FCTC) is an attempt to challenge the powerful economic interests of the tobacco industry and tobacco growers, and protect individual nations and populations from their power. The FCTC was agreed by the member states of the WHO in 2003, following almost 4 years of negotiation. Lobbying from antitobacco pressure groups and the tobacco lobby's persistent manoeuvring from the inside had made the creation of the FCTC a difficult task. By 2004, 131 countries had signed the treaty and 21 had ratified it. The USA was a notable omission to those ratifying the Convention. The FCTC is the first global health treaty and came into force in 2005 (Beaumont et al 2007).

The practitioner's role in HPP

Although many practitioners might not think of HPP as being part of their work remit, there are a number of ways in which practitioners might become involved. Depending on job role and employing organization or service, practitioners may take on a range of roles in relation to HPP. These roles range from leading the process, sharing the vision and promoting the benefits of the HPP approach, to active involvement in the process of lobbying, advocacy and partnership working.

Box 11.11

Your local council is proposing a new transport plan to encourage cycling and walking. The plan includes congestion charging, the introduction of cycling lanes and dedicated lanes for cars carrying more than one person. Proponents argue that this will encourage people to integrate exercise into their personal travel plans. Opponents argue the scheme will lead to more congestion and longer travel times due to reduced road space and more speed restrictions. The council is inviting consultation with all interested parties. What, if anything, would you see as your role as a practitioner? How, if at all, would this differ from your role as a member of the public?

As a practitioner faced with a proposed new policy affecting your clients, you would probably consider it your duty to assess the plan in terms of its likely impact on the health of your clients. This might include initiating discussions and forums with clients to gauge their reaction to the proposal, or a more ad hoc process of sounding things out with individuals as and when you deem it appropriate. Perhaps you would take it upon yourself to translate research findings into plain English, or to spell out the likely effects of the proposed policy. You might propose that a rapid HIA is undertaken which would ensure the views of community groups are heard. You might also take the issue up with your professional association, and get them involved in the issues.

As a member of the public, you might be involved in the same spectrum of activities (apart from working with professional associations). However your role and expertise would be different, and you would engage as an interested member of the public rather than as a practitioner with a duty of care. This might give you more freedom to voice your opinions and make your principles and values known.

Box 11.12

How, if at all, has the policy process been covered in your professional training?
Has your training included skills helpful for those engaging with the policy context and process?

The policy context, process and implementation, as well as specific skills helpful for those engaging with policy, tend to be neglected areas within professional training. This is the current situation despite the fact that practitioners are often crucial in determining whether or not a policy achieves its goals. Policies need to be implemented in order to have an impact. This will usually involve a change in working practices, and there is a tendency to resist change within organizations. Change is often stressful and time-consuming, and unless people are convinced of its merits, there may well be resistance. Inertia or misinterpretation of what is required may also mean policies get no further than the paper they are written on. In order to be effective, practitioners need to be 'on board' and committed partners in implementing policies. This in turn depends on whether and how their organization has engaged them in the policy-making process.

Within the health services there is a long history of continual change and reorganization. This can lead to a degree of cynicism and lack of engagement with the policy-making process. For many, policy implementation in the past has been experienced as increased levels of micromanagement, leading to a negative stance towards policy. However policy-making is a powerful professional tool, and the skills for effective engagement in the policy process need to be embedded in professional training.

Evaluating an HPP approach

 Box 11.13

How would you evaluate the impact of the ban on advertising 'junk food' during television programmes targeted at children?

Evaluating the impact of policies is often difficult, due to the long timescale involved, the lack of controlled comparisons and the complexity of factors and relationships affected by policy changes. Areas that are commonly researched in order to assess the impact of policy changes are:

- Knowledge of the policy change
- Attitudes towards the policy change – for or against
- Self-assessed behaviour change following the policy change
- Independently assessed behaviour change, e.g. monitoring before and after sales of products or use of services
- Media coverage of the policy change – amount; positive or negative
- Economic analysis to demonstrate whether or not the policy change is cost-effective

More details of the evaluation process are given in Chapter 20.

Conclusion

HPP is a vital cornerstone of health promotion. Policy is a complex phenomenon that exists at many different levels. HPP has a sound rationale and some notable successes, but remains rather underused as a strategy. This is probably due to its complexity and the fact that responsibility for HPP often falls between agencies and practitioners. HPP is inevitably affected by politics, values and ideologies, all of which are constantly shifting. This provides another reason for the relatively low profile of HPP. The potential of HPP to be an effective and efficient means of promoting health and preventing ill health suggests that it should be embedded in professional training. The ability to understand and engage effectively in the policy process should be part of every practitioner's professional skills base.

Questions for further discussion

- To what extent do you engage with policy issues as a practitioner? Would you like to increase or decrease your level of engagement?
- Select a controversial new policy, e.g. the smoking ban, and search the newspapers for reporting about this issue. What issues are highlighted in media coverage about this issue?
- Do you think the increase in policies focused around health is a sign of the 'nanny state', or of stewardship in the interests of public health? How would you defend your position?

Summary

This chapter has outlined what HPP is, its history and its potential benefits. Barriers to forming and implementing HPP have also been discussed. The practitioner's role in HPP has been considered.

Further reading

Hunter D J 2003 Public health policy. Polity Press, Cambridge. *A readable, engaging and comprehensive account of public health policy. National, European and international policies affecting health are all discussed.*

Lloyd C E, Handsley S, Douglas J et al (eds) 2007 Policy and practice in promoting public health. Sage and Open University Press, London. *A comprehensive discussion of public health policy at different levels (global, national, local) and within different settings. Policy principles such as partnership working and collaboration are also discussed in depth.*

Naidoo J, Wills J 2005 Public health and health promotion: developing practice 2nd edn. Baillière Tindall, London. *Chapter 4 on the policy context gives a detailed account of the policy process and the realities of engaging with policy.*

Pitt B, Lloyd L 2008 Social policy and health. In: Naidoo J, Wills J (eds) Health studies: an introduction, 2nd edn. Palgrave Macmillan, Hampshire, Chapter 7. *A concise overview of the discipline of social policy with a focus on health. The chapter includes a historical account and a discussion of methodological issues, including policy analysis and the policy process.*

References

Beattie A 1993 The changing boundaries of health. In: Beattie A, Gott M, Jones L et al (eds) Health and wellbeing: a reader. Macmillan/Open University, London, pp. 260–272.

Beaumont K, Douglas J, Heller T 2007 Making and changing healthy public policy. In: Lloyd C E, Handsley S, Douglas J et al (eds) Policy and practice in promoting public health. Sage and Open University Press, London.

British Medical Association 2003 Housing and health: building for the future. BMA, London. http://www.bma.org.uk/ap.nsf/AttachmentsByTitle/PDFhousinghealth/$FILE/housinghealth.pdf

Chadwick E 1842 Report from the poor law commissioners on an inquiry into the sanitary conditions of the labouring population of Great Britain. Poor Law Commission, Home Office, London.

Chapman S, Lupton D 1994 The fight for public health; principles and practice of media advocacy. BMJ Publishing, London.

Fong G T, Hyland A, Borland R et al 2006 Reductions in tobacco smoke pollution and increases in support for smoke-free public places following the implementation of comprehensive smoke-free workplace legislation in the Republic of Ireland: findings from the ITC Ireland/UK survey. Tobacco Control 15(Suppl. 3): iii5–iii58.

Giddens A 1998 The third way. The renewal of social democracy. Polity Press, Cambridge.

Hunter D J 2003 Public health policy. Polity Press, Cambridge.

Joffe M, Mindell J 2004 A tentative step towards healthy public policy. Journal of Epidemiology and Community Health 58: 966–968.

Kemm J 2001 Health Impact Assessment: a tool for healthy public policy. Health Promotion International 16: 79–85.

Lindblom C 1959 The science of muddling through Public Administration Review 19: 79–88

Lipsky M 1979 Street level bureaucracy. Russell Sage, New York.

McPherson K 2001 Are disease prevention initiatives working? Lancet 357: 1790–1792.

Milio N 2001 Glossary: healthy public policy. Journal of Epidemiology and Community Health 55: 622–623.

Naidoo J, Wills J 2005 Public health and health promotion: developing practice, 2nd edn. Baillière Tindall, London.

Petticrew M, Whitehead M, Macintyre S J et al 2004 Evidence for public health policy on inequalities: 1: The reality according to policymakers. Journal of Epidemiology and Community Health 58: 811–816.

Rittel H, Webber M 1973 Dilemmas in a general theory of planning. Policy Science 4: 155–169.

Sanders D, Dovlo D, Wilma M et al 2003 Public health in Africa. In: Beaglehole R (ed) Global public health: a new era. Oxford University Press, Oxford.

Tones K 2001 Health promotion: the empowerment imperative. In: Scriven A, Orme J (eds) Health promotion professional perspectives, 2nd edn. Palgrave Macmillan, Hampshire, pp. 3–18.

Tones K, Green J 2004 Health promotion: planning and strategies. Sage, London.

United Nations Universal declaration of human rights article 25(1). United Nations, Geneva.

United Nations Development Programme 2006 Millennium development goals. Available online at: http://www.undp.org/mdg/goallist.shtml

Walt G 1994 Health policy: an introduction to process and power. Zed Books, London.

Welsh Assembly Government and Directorate of Learning Disability Services, Bro Morgannwg NHS Trust 2006 Health challenge Wales: accessible information on healthy living. Public Health Strategy Division, Welsh Assembly Government, Cardiff.

Wilkinson R 1996 Unhealthy societies: the afflictions of inequality. Routledge, London.

World Health Organization 1986 Ottawa charter for health promotion: an international conference on health promotion. November 17–21. WHO, Copenhagen.

World Health Organization 1988 Second international conference on health promotion. WHO, Adelaide, Australia.

World Health Organization 1991 Third international conference on health promotion. WHO, Sundsvall, Sweden 9–15 June.

World Health Organization 1997 New players for a new era: leading health promotion into the 21st century. 4th International Conference on Health Promotion, Jakarta, Indonesia 21–25 July 1997. Conference report. World Health Organization, Geneva/Ministry of Health, Indonesia.

World Health Organization 2000a Fifth global health promotion conference. WHO, Mexico City.

World Health Organization 2000b The world health report 2000 – health systems: improving performance. WHO, Geneva.

World Health Organization 2003 Framework convention on tobacco control. WHO, Geneva.

World Health Organization 2005 Bangkok charter for health promotion. WHO, Geneva.

Chapter Twelve

Using media in health promotion

Key points

- Nature of media effects
- Role of mass media
- Using mass media
  - Planned campaigns
  - Unpaid coverage
  - Media advocacy
  - Social marketing
- Effectiveness of mass media
- Communication tools

OVERVIEW

Communication of information and advice is central to health promotion strategies. A knowledge of how communication between the sender and receiver of messages takes place and an understanding of the medium through which communication occurs are therefore important tools for the health promoter. Mass media is a powerful agent of communication, reaching large numbers of people. In addition to the traditional media (radio, television, press) new forms of media, most notably the internet, have changed communication patterns and coverage. The mass media now combines the capacity to reach large numbers of people with the capacity to be accessed individually as and when people choose. Mass media has a long history of persuading people to buy a vast array of products and lifestyles which create ill health, such as tobacco, alcohol and fast cars, through both paid advertising and current affairs coverage. Paid advertising and campaigns, unpaid news coverage, social marketing and media advocacy are all used to promote health. Practitioners also use posters, leaflets and other tools to enhance communication with service users. This chapter looks at the potential and limitations of using various media in these different ways to promote health. Readers can find a more detailed discussion of health communication and social marketing in Chapter 8 of our companion volume (Naidoo & Wills 2005).

Introduction

The term mass media includes any communication which reaches large sections of the population. Examples of mass media are television and radio broadcasting and print media such as newspapers, posters and leaflets. The mass media is a 'broad-spectrum' intervention, as distinct from 'narrow-gauge' personalized interventions tailored to individuals and small groups. The use of public announcements to promote health also has a long history:

Box 12.1

In 1603 James I, King of England, made a public declaration that smoking is:

A custom, lothesome to the eye, hateful to the Nose, harmful to the brain, dangerous to the Lungs and in the black stinking fume thereof, neerest resembling the horrible Stigian smoke of the pit that is bottomelesse ... by the immoderate taking of tobacco, the wealth of a great number of people is impaired and their bodies unfit for labour.

More recently, the powerful effects of propaganda during the Second World War were influential in persuading health promoters to adopt a similar strategy. In 1953 John Burton, the editor of the *Health Education Journal*, stated that:

> *The first 10 years of our existence could well be called the era of propaganda. Health education has been realised mainly in terms of mass publicity on all fronts. Ad hoc exhortations have been directed at the public following closely the patterns of commercial advertising (Burton, cited in Tones 1993, p. 128).*

However, by this time there had already developed a concern that such a strategy was not working and that the role of the mass media in health promotion needed to be redefined:

> *Many [have come] to feel that mass publicity methods were expensive and relatively ineffective in changing people's health habits and beliefs, and that health education would have to be planned on a more personal basis (Burton, cited in Tones 1993, p. 128).*

Box 12.2

What functions or roles do you think the mass media plays in modern life?

The relationship between the media and the public is complex. In addition to its primary function of informing and entertaining, the media plays a pivotal role in social cohesion, defining what is normal and desirable, and what is not. McQuail (2005) identifies several different roles played by the media:

- The main source of essential information
- The arena where public-life affairs are played out
- The source of definitions and images of social reality
- Where values are constructed and expressed
- A benchmark for what is normal.

The mass media is important to health promotion because it is so widely used. Many public health issues, e.g. human immunodeficiency virus (HIV)/acquired immunodeficiency syndrome (AIDS), alcohol misuse and smoking have been the subject of extensive mass-media campaigns. The aim of such campaigns is usually to raise awareness or present a message advocating healthy lifestyles (Figure 12.1). Beattie (1993) describes the use of the media as 'health persuasion', by which he means a top-down conservative method designed to infuse an audience with information.

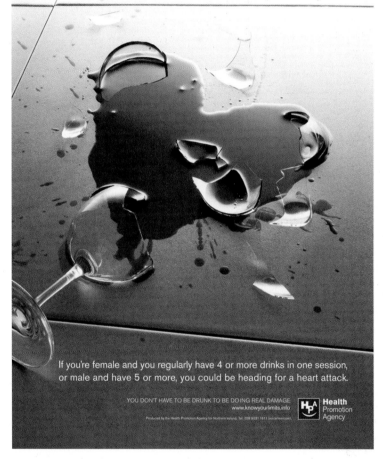

The more you drink, the greater your risk of a heart attack.

If you're female and you regularly have 4 or more drinks in one session, or male and have 5 or more, you could be heading for a heart attack.

YOU DON'T HAVE TO BE DRUNK TO BE DOING REAL DAMAGE
www.knowyourlimits.info

Health Promotion Agency

Figure 12.1 • Alcohol poster from Health Promotion Agency Northern Ireland. Reproduced with permission from the Health Promotion Agency for Northern Ireland: photography, David Gill.

The media may also be an unhealthy influence, advertising unhealthy products, e.g. fast food, or transmitting unhealthy messages, e.g. that drinking excessively is fun and fashionable. The media also plays a major role in constructing society's views on health issues and services. What health issues are covered, and the slant the reporting takes, are powerful forces in public discourse around health.

The nature of media effects

The mass media is a distinctive form of communication with specific properties, including:

- Large scale
- Standardized content
- One-directional flow
- Impersonal
- Based on a market relationship (McQuail 2005).

These characteristics include both strengths and weaknesses when the aim is to promote health. Although a mass audience is guaranteed, with favourable cost implications, 'correct' reading, understanding and recall of the intended message by the target audience is by no means certain. A great deal of research is needed to develop suitable messages that will appeal to the target audience and to evaluate their real-life impact. Chapter 8 in our companion volume (Naidoo & Wills 2005) discusses the nature of health promotion messages.

Views on the effects of the mass media have shifted from an early belief that the mass media could produce dramatic changes in attitudes and behaviour to the opposite view that the media has negligible effects (Gatherer et al 1979). Today there is a more tempered view, which regards the media as influential in certain circumstances and in specific ways. For example, a recent systematic review concluded that the use of mass media in promoting the use of health services was effective (Grilli et al 2002). The West Yorkshire Smoking and Health Trial (McVey & Stapleton 2000) demonstrated that a prolonged, heavy-weight, well-resourced mass media campaign can contribute to a significant reduction in smoking prevalence.

Lasswell (1948) presents the following model of mass communication:

Who says *what* in *which channel* to *whom* with *what effect?*

Lasswell's model is useful in flagging up all the key stages of the process of mass communication:

- *Who?* The credibility of the source of the message
- *What?* Information, entertainment, news, advice
- *Which channel?* Television, radio, poster, internet, mobile phone
- *Whom?* Who is the target audience in terms of, for example, age, gender, socioeconomic class, ethnic group, personality, able-bodied or living with disabilities
- *What effect?* Changes in knowledge, attitudes, beliefs, behavioural intentions, actual behaviour

This model was developed with traditional forms of mass media in mind, and its applicability to newer forms of instant and overlapping communication and technologies has been questioned (Chamberlain 1996). The new technologies, such as text messaging or social network sites, are particularly relevant if young people are the target group. Young people are media-literate, i.e. they can access, understand and create communications using a variety of new technologies, including the internet and mobile phones. These new forms of communication may be used to promote health. Text messaging has been successfully used to improve self-management of diabetes (Franklin et al 2006), and has also been used to engage young people in health messages (Dobkin et al 2007). Atkin (2001) has argued that the new interactive and individually tailored communication technologies empower users. Benefits of these new means of communication include relative anonymity, avoidance of stigmatization and marginalization and immediate access wherever people are.

Four main models of how the media affects audiences have been suggested:

1. Direct effects (linear causal)
2. Two-step or diffusion of innovation model
3. Uses and gratifications
4. Cultural effects.

Direct effects (linear causal)

This model likens the effects of the mass media to a hypodermic syringe that has an immediate and direct effect on its audience. It assumes a passive audience which can be swayed by manipulative mass media. This view prompted the development of political broadcasts intended to shift voting intentions.

Box 12.3

In 1938 Orson Welles broadcast a radio version of H G Wells' classic science fiction story *The War of the Worlds*. Thousands of American listeners assumed that the story of an imminent alien invasion from outer space was real and panic spread as people started to flee (Cantril 1958).

This view has since been replaced by an aerosol spray analogy:

> *Rather than being a hypodermic needle, we now begin to look at mass communication as a sort of aerosol spray. As you spray it on the surface, some of it hits the target: most of it drifts away; and very little of it penetrates (Mendelsohn 1968).*

Box 12.4

Some people argue that representations of people consuming large quantities of alcohol, being violent or engaging in unsafe sexual activities encourages viewers to do the same. They argue for tighter censorship and controls. Others argue that censorship stifles public debate and different views and opinions, and removes personal freedoms. What do you think?

Two-step or diffusion of innovation model

This model suggests that mass communication influences key opinion leaders who are active members

of the mass-media audience. These opinion leaders then spread ideas to other people through interpersonal means of communication (Katz & Lazarsfeld 1955). The process of diffusing innovation or new ideas through a population is based on the finding that the adoption of new behaviours typically follows an S-shaped trajectory (Rogers & Scott 1997). There is usually a slow initial uptake followed by rapid acceptance, as opinion leaders or early adopters (who are usually from higher socioeconomic groups) communicate the benefits, and then a final slowing as a minority (who tend to be from isolated traditional communities) resist acceptance or change. This suggests that the mass media may be important in raising awareness and communicating basic information, but interpersonal sources, such as friends, peers and known 'experts', are most influential in persuading people to make changes.

Uses and gratifications

This model tends to see the audience as more active in selecting and interpreting communications. It suggests that people use the media to meet their own needs, reinforcing existing beliefs or rejecting or reinterpreting communications that do not fit their existing values or beliefs.

Cultural effects

This model sees the media as having a key role in creating beliefs and values about health, medicine, disease and illness. The ways in which these are presented, from the kindly doctor in soap operas, to news bulletins on miracle cures and high-tech interventions, all contribute to people's understanding of health (see, for example, Lupton 1994). Many studies use discourse analysis to reveal the underlying values, concepts and messages implicit in media portrayals of health and ill health. For example, Joffe & Haarhoff (2002) analyse the ways in which diseases such as Ebola are presented as deadly uncontrollable viruses whilst simultaneously giving the message that such diseases pose little threat to the UK. Harrabin et al (2003) argue that public health is neglected in

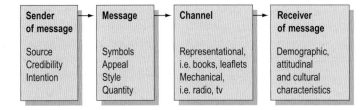

Figure 12.2 • Media messages.

the media. Public health's long timescale and basis in numerical data make it unattractive to the mass media. Instead, 'shock horror' stories of crisis within the National Health Service (NHS) or the appearance of rare diseases tend to dominate the news headlines.

 Box 12.5

Monitor media coverage on television, in magazines, on radio, in broadsheet and tabloid newspapers for items about health over a 1-week period. Use the following categories to allocate coverage by type:
• Medical dominance, e.g. medical breakthroughs, high-technology interventions
• Crisis or scare stories, e.g. failures in services or outbreaks of unusual diseases or illnesses
• Individual consumerism and lifestyles, e.g. stories about how to choose and access healthier lifestyles and health services
• Celebrities illustrating how health or antihealth behaviours can be perceived as attractive
• Social, economic or political health determinants, e.g. policy changes and how these might affect health
• Environmental or global determinants of health, e.g. the loss of agriculture and the ability to grow food due to climate change.
Does the media coverage you monitored fit into these categories?
  Which categories were least/most common? What are the implications of this?

How much of the coverage was in entertainment programmes?
  Think about and find some examples of how the following are represented in popular media culture:
• Doctors
• Hospitals and health care services
• Chronic illnesses, e.g. coronary heart disease, cancer
• Acute illnesses, e.g. flu
• Social and environmental health
• Individual state of positive health and well-being
• Prevention of ill health
• Protection of health.

Communication is concerned with the transmission of messages from a sender to a receiver. Messages are coded into signs and symbols which have meaning within specific codes. The message is encoded by the sender, and decoded by the receiver (Figure 12.2). The intention is that messages should be decoded and understood according to the intentions of the sender, but this can be problematic when using the mass media. This is because the mass media targets large audiences simultaneously, and, unlike direct personal communication, there is typically no feedback loop from the receiver back to the sender of the message. This means messages may be interpreted in ways that were not anticipated or intended by the sender. This is one reason why researching the target audience and piloting messages is an important stage in the planned use of the mass media for health promotion.

The role of mass media

Mass communication has been used in health promotion in the following ways:

- To raise public awareness through:
  - Providing information
  - Reminding the population of the effects of their health-damaging behaviour and the benefits of adopting healthy behaviours and lifestyles
- Media advocacy – creating a climate of opinion conducive to policy change through maintaining the salience of an issue and making sure it is thought about
- Social marketing – using the 'marketing mix' (see Box 12.12) to achieve behaviour change.

There are two main ways in which mass media is used:

1. Planned campaigns and advertising. This has the advantage of reaching large numbers of people from all social classes and population groups quickly. Messages can be developed and targeted to meet specific objectives. A downside is the necessity for adequate funding in order to make an impact.

2. Unpaid publicity and media advocacy. This has the advantage of low cost and a greater credibility, as messages are not seen as being directly promoted by health organizations. A downside is the lack of control over what appears in the media, which means messages may be misinterpreted or refuted.

Planned campaigns

Mass-media campaigns have been used by national health promotion agencies in the UK and worldwide to promote various health messages. Different media, including billboards, press advertisements and radio announcements, have been used, but television is the principal medium because, although it is expensive, it reaches much larger audiences and

recall has been shown to be better. The end goal of most media campaigns is to achieve a specific behaviour change, although their ability to achieve such aims is disputed. Harrabin et al (2003) state that members of the public may alter their health related behaviour due in part to the information and advice they get from the media.

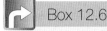 Box 12.6

Evaluation of mass-media campaigns

1. Sun safety – evaluation of repeated campaigns in Australia using the mass media to promote sun protection measures among children concluded that they 'may contribute to short-term increases in some sun protection behaviours; however, as their impact is not sustained they should be repeated and supplemented by educational, policy and environmental strategies' (Smith et al 2002, p. 51).

2. Weight gain – a repeated campaign aimed at preventing weight gain in the Netherlands resulted, after the final campaign wave, in high awareness (88%) and message recall (68%) and positive attitudes and motivation. However the campaign had mixed effects on self-efficacy and negative effects on risk perception (Wammes et al 2007).

3. Physical activity – well-funded, imaginative and consistent mass-media campaigns that promote realistic goals can play a role in contributing to increasing physical activity levels. However other factors also need to be present, e.g. partnership working, supportive cultural norms, funding for local initiatives and participatory strategies (WHO 2004).

These examples suggest that on their own, mass-media campaigns are unreliable in achieving behaviour change. However, used in combination with other strategies, such as personal reinforcement from trusted peers or experts, or policy changes affecting the environment, mass-media campaigns can be effective.

Mass-media campaigns adopt a variety of tactics to communicate their message, including emotional appeals, shock tactics and reassurance. The evidence on whether or not fear is an effective strategy is inconclusive. Early studies showed that people may attend, comprehend and retain information when shocked, but may also become resistant or deny the relevance of the message (Montazeri et al 1998). The use of fear appeals in social marketing has been criticized for its relative ineffectiveness and its unintended negative consequences (e.g. anxiety, complacency and increased social inequity) (Hastings et al 2004). However a review of mass-media antismoking campaigns (Grey et al 2000) concluded that 'threatening' and 'supportive' approaches could complement each other and contribute to overall effectiveness. What was important was an appeal to the emotions, coupled with supportive messages. It is also important to present a clear action which individuals feel confident they can take (Barth & Bengel 2000).

Extensive reviews of media campaigns now conclude that they may be successful if their goals are reasonable and there is no expectation of immediate results. Tones & Tilford (2001) refer to the hierarchy of communication effects which suggests that simple awareness or market penetration is relatively easy to achieve; to inform or reinforce attitudes is more difficult, and to have any effect on behaviour is even more difficult. They identify certain preconditions for success:

- Favourable public opinion, which is most likely when there has been extensive market research at the design stage
- Time available for the presentation of complex information
- Support through interpersonal communication.

Box 12.7

How would you evaluate a mass-media campaign to reduce drink-driving?

Evaluation of a mass-media campaign to reduce drink-driving could take many forms. Evaluation studies often look at coverage (the percentage of the target population who were exposed to the message), recall (the percentage of the population who could accurately recall the message) or the impact of the campaign on behaviour. Behavioural indicators include statistics relating to the incidence of drink-driving, but the evaluation would probably also examine the incidence of alcohol-related car accidents as this is the main cause for concern and is likely to be better monitored than drink-driving. The evaluation might also include examining the cost-effectiveness of such a campaign (see Example 12.8).

Box 12.8

Mass-media campaigns to reduce drink-driving

Two systematic reviews of mass-media campaigns to reduce drink-driving and related car crashes agree that such campaigns are effective. Tay (2005) found that mass-media campaigns significantly reduce drink-driving and alcohol-related crashes and result in large savings. Elder et al (2004) found an average decrease of 13% in alcohol-related crashes following mass-media campaigns, and concluded that the benefits to society outweighed the costs.

Unpaid media coverage

The term 'unplanned' is used to describe media coverage that is not specifically paid for as part of a campaign. Health promotion has become increasingly concerned to generate news stories. Campaigns can extend their reach enormously through unpaid coverage.

The mass media has no responsibility to promote health and so if they address such issues it is because the issues are inherently newsworthy, or have been packaged by health promoters to become newsworthy. The tendency to sensationalize means that it is the emotional, the dramatic or the tragic that gets space. Stories tend to relate to individuals, and issues which concern population groups such as older people or the determinants of health thus are ignored. The emphasis on behavioural journalism means that personalities or real-life case studies are also prominent. Newsworthiness depends less on the importance of an issue than on its immediate impact, which is often heightened by being linked to celebrities in emotive ways. For example, the involvement of celebrity Jamie Oliver led to a dramatic increase in media coverage of children's diets and healthy school meals.

Box 12.9

Newsworthiness of health issues
Chapman & Dominello (2001) found that newspaper coverage of tobacco and health issues could be significantly affected and increased through a strategy of proactive press reports. The key to increased media coverage was to use newsworthy aspects, e.g. the use of celebrities, moral panics or medical scares, to contextualize the story. Giving a local spin to general stories will also ensure coverage in regional media.

Although such tactics may increase coverage of the work of health promoters and put across health messages, the ability of the media to distort and sensationalize should always be remembered. An editorial in *The Observer* newspaper in 1994 commented: 'There is nothing quite so irresponsible as the media in hot pursuit of a health scare and nothing quite so gullible as the public presented with one'. The editorial had been prompted by a concern about necrotizing fasciitis (a tissue-destroying disease caused by a strain of bacteria) which was neither new nor on the increase, but which had prompted headlines such as 'Killer bug eats my body' or 'Flesh-eater on the move'.

Reid (1996) observes that media interest can be generated by the commissioning of surveys or research reports. However, such reports frequently result in health scares because of poor reporting and misunderstanding of statistics and the concept of risk. An example is the research study linking the measles, mumps and rubella (MMR) vaccine to the development of autism and Crohn's disease in young children, which led to a drop in MMR uptake immediately following the press reports.

Box 12.10

Take a current issue which has received a lot of media coverage, e.g. bovine spongiform encephalitis (BSE), young people's alcohol and drug use or the rising incidence of obesity, especially amongst children and young people.
• What is helpful and useful about such coverage?
• What is unhelpful and not useful?
• On balance, would you try to get more or less media coverage?

Although the generation of unpaid publicity can be effective and at minimal cost, it is difficult to sustain a high level of coverage for more than a few days. Health promoters need persistence and creativity to keep issues prominent in the media. There is also a need for media training for health promoters in skills such as writing press releases, networking and design in order to access and use the media to its full potential.

No Smoking Day (NSD) is an example of a successful ongoing event. NSD is a charity with no budget for advertising, yet it succeeds in generating media coverage of the day as well as increasing the use of quit-smoking helplines. Evaluation of this public awareness campaign, which is supported by local activities, demonstrates its effectiveness. In 2004 an estimated 1 in 7 of UK smokers claimed to have quit or reduced their consumption on NSD. Among those who participated, 11% were still non-smokers 3 months after the event (Owen & Youdan 2006).

Media advocacy

Public policy is rarely a consequence of direct approaches to policy-makers and increasingly there is a recognition that public opinion can influence decisions. Media advocacy is a particular strategy of using the media to try to generate public concern about the ways in which the legislative, economic or environmental context affects public health. Examples include promoting the smoking ban in public places and the debate surrounding food-labelling regulations. Media advocacy is therefore a means of applying pressure for policy change to advance public health objectives (Wallack & Dorfman 1996). Often there is major opposition from established economic interests to the proposed policy change. The conflicting interests in many health-related areas can lead to split loyalties, and there have been calls for media advocacy to be undertaken independently of any official health promotion or public health posts (Regidor et al 2007). Media advocacy objectives are:

- To get an issue discussed
- To get an issue discussed differently
- To discredit opponents
- To bring in new voices
- To introduce new facts or perspectives
- To shift risk perceptions.

Chapman (2004) lists 10 questions that can be used to guide careful planning and lead to positive results, including identifying desired public health objectives and media advocacy objectives, and how to frame the issue in a favourable light, including what sound bites, symbols and words to use, and how it might be personalized. Weinreich (1999) identifies five key stages in media advocacy:

1. Planning (including formative research and audience segmentation)
2. Designing messages and materials
3. Pretesting
4. Implementation
5. Evaluation and feedback.

Chapman & Lupton (1994) emphasize the importance of the media in achieving policy change: 'There are few instances in the recent history of public health where advocacy staged through the news media has not played a pivotal role in effecting the changes sought by public health workers.' An example of successful media advocacy involving international cooperation was Infact's Nestlé boycott of the 1970s and 1980s which led to the World Health Organization's International Code of Marketing for Breast Milk Substitutes (McKee et al 2005). Direct action can also be successful, as evidenced by the Billboard Utilising Graffitists Against Unhealthy Promotions (BUGA-UP), an Australian group which targeted tobacco advertising (Figure 12.3) (McKee et al 2005).

> ## Box 12.11
>
> Consider the ways in which mental health issues are reported in the media.
> How could the media be actively used to get mental health issues discussed differently?

Stuart (2006) has shown how entertainment and news media provide images of mental illness that emphasize danger, criminality and unpredictability. This kind of coverage has a negative impact on people with mental health problems, leading to further stigmatization.

Social marketing

Just as commercial companies are able to get the public to buy products (even those they may not really need), so health promoters should be able to get people to choose healthy behaviours. Some of the techniques of marketing are now being widely used in health promotion to influence the acceptability of healthy lifestyles so that they seem desirable and easy to adopt. One of the limitations of mass-media campaigns is that they are a one-way communication process and tend to adopt a uniform population message.

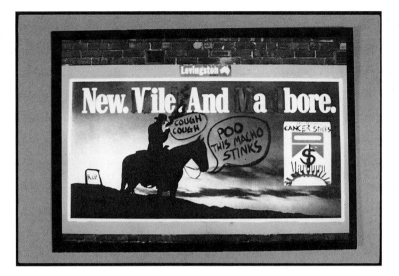

Figure 12.3 • Defaced billboard. Courtesy of Cecilia Farren.

Increasingly, health promoters are making use of social marketing techniques that allow specific groups to be targeted (Naidoo & Wills 2005). Marketing segments the population into different subgroups based on attitudes and behaviour as well as cruder socioeconomic and demographic variables.

Commercial marketing is based on the idea of 'exchange' – that the marketer tries to provide something the consumer wants at an acceptable price. Health promoters are beginning to recognize the importance of formative research, which carefully identifies what people see as the benefits of particular health behaviours, so that these can be incorporated into the campaign message. In a sense this is merely an application of the Health Belief model (see Chapter 9) which suggests that for people to make a change in their health behaviour they need to see the benefits outweighing costs such as time and effort.

Marketing a commercial product is very different from trying to sell health. Advertising typically mobilizes existing predispositions, whereas health promotion typically tries to counter them. For example, advertising associates the product (beer, crisps) with something people desire, such as fun. All too often, health promotion messages are about not indulging, and therefore by implication, not having fun (don't drink and drive, eat less fat). Advertising is selling things in the here and now, to be consumed and enjoyed immediately. By contrast, health promotion messages are often about forgoing present enjoyment for future benefits.

As we have seen, selling a product is a complex and carefully researched process. The needs of the market have to be identified, messages developed which will appeal to the market segment that is being targeted, and a comparison made of different media channels and their relative effectiveness in reaching a general and the targeted population. Together these aspects make up the marketing mix.

Box 12.12

The marketing mix: the four Ps:
- *Product* – the product or behaviour and its key characteristics which can contribute to the product image
- *Price* – the value of the product and how important it is to the audience

- *Place* – where the product is available
- *Promotion* – the means by which the product is promoted (advertising, publicity, personal communication).

Social marketing – the application of marketing principles to 'sell' ideas, attitudes and behaviours to benefit the target audience and society in general – poses additional challenges. Additional Ps have been suggested for social marketing, including:

- *Positioning* – identifying attitudes and beliefs that are congruent with the message and therefore reinforce it
- *Publics* – potential audiences
- *Partnership* – joint working between organizations with similar goals
- *Policy* – supportive policy environment, perhaps achieved through media advocacy
- *Purse strings* – social marketing is often financed through limited public funding sources)

(Lefebvre & Flora 1988; Weinreich 1999).

Box 12.13

Choose an issue which you think could be promoted through social marketing, e.g. sun safety, sensible drinking, safer sex, breast screening.

Use the Ps framework above to plan your social marketing strategy.

What the mass media can and cannot do

Research and evaluation of the use of the mass media in health promotion have led to a reassessment of its potential and limitations (see particularly Tones & Tilford 2001). It is now accepted that the mass media can:

- Raise consciousness about health issues, e.g. drink-driving

- Contextualize an issue within a value framework, e.g. childhood obesity as a result of parental negligence
- Help place health on the public agenda, e.g. nutritional content of fast food
- Convey simple information and single messages, e.g. put babies to sleep on their backs
- Change behaviour if other enabling factors are present, e.g. encourage smokers already committed to giving up.

Factors which enable behaviour change include existing motivation, supportive circumstances and advocating simple one-off behaviour change (e.g. carry a donor card, install a smoke alarm).

Using the media is more effective if:

- It is part of an integrated campaign, including other elements such as one-to-one advice.
- The information is new and presented in an emotional context.
- The message resonates with popular values or is linked to celebrities.
- The information is seen as being relevant for 'people like me'.

The mass media cannot:

- Convey complex information, e.g. the relative risks of different kinds of fat in the diet
- Teach skills, e.g. how to negotiate safer sex
- Shift people's attitudes or beliefs; if messages are presented which challenge basic beliefs, it is more likely that the message will be ignored, dismissed or interpreted to mean something else
- Change behaviour in the absence of other enabling factors.

Communication tools

A majority of patients actively seek information about how to cope with health problems, of whom three-quarters cite their doctor as the most important source of health information. About a third use the internet and a quarter look for information in leaflets and books (Coulter et al 2006). Leaflets and pamphlets have been used to educate the public since the beginning of the 20th century. When the Central Council for Health Education was established in 1927 it listed the provision of better and cheaper leaflets as its main aim. The greatest use of written material is to support one-to-one interactions with clients and patients. As only 50% of information can be recalled by patients 5 minutes after a consultation, this seems an effective use of leaflets. There is some evidence that written information can not only improve patients' understanding and recall, but also provide reassurance.

Multimedia tools and other new technologies offer many new opportunities for the dissemination of information. The worldwide web offers the possibility of interactive dialogue and for the public to select the information they require at a time convenient for them. These new forms of media are very popular. A survey in 2001 found that almost 100 million American adults regularly visit health-related websites (Wilson 2002). Telemedicine, including the helpline NHS Direct, offers a two-way dialogue allowing people who are unable to access primary care to ask questions and get feedback about their symptoms. These new technologies offer a simulation of human interaction – conversations, the café, support groups – all of which can be harnessed to link health information with the important element of sociability.

The proliferation of avenues of communication does not necessarily mean that people are better informed about health issues today. Quality control is often absent (e.g. in much of the worldwide web), and even when it exists, the criteria used are often not explicit. Commonly agreed criteria include being up to date, using reliable sources of information and information that is reliable, relevant, accurate and accessible (e.g. as assessed by readability tests) (Shepperd et al 1999; Coulter et al 2006).

Conclusion

The mass media is a significant partner and resource for health, but one that needs to be understood and used according to its own priorities. To expect a mass-media campaign to produce large shifts in behaviour and contribute directly to reduced morbidity and mortality is unrealistic. But the media can work for health by supporting individual and social change.

On an individual level, the mass media can supplement, but not substitute for, one-to-one education and advice. Even with sophisticated marketing and audience research, the mass media remains a fairly blunt instrument with little opportunity for feedback or clarification. However, the media can raise awareness, provide information and motivate people to change if their environment is supportive. The media can also be used to advocate for public health by shifting public opinion and encouraging the formation of healthy public policies. The media can also be used for social marketing, to promote attitudes, beliefs and behaviours that are conducive to health. Other forms of media, such as leaflets and posters, can provide a useful supplementary communication tool to inform, educate and advise people about health issues.

Questions for further discussion

- How could you use the media to raise public awareness of a health issue and get the issue discussed in a way which is health-promoting?

- Plan a media advertising campaign on a topic of relevance to you, e.g. breast-feeding, binge-drinking, accident prevention, healthy eating. Whom would you target? What media would you use? What message?

- How could you evaluate the use of health education materials such as leaflets and posters in doctors' or dentists' surgeries?

Summary

This chapter has looked at the ways in which the media, especially the mass media, is used to promote health. It has discussed different strategies, including information-giving, advertising as part of a planned campaign, media advocacy and the marketing of health messages. There is now greater awareness of how to use the mass media more effectively and this chapter looked at how media coverage can be generated and used to influence public opinion. It has reviewed evaluation studies that demonstrate how effective communication combines information with the key element of interaction.

Further reading

Corcoran N (ed) 2007 Communicating health: strategies for health promotion. Sage, London. *Chapter 4 examines the role of mass media in health promotion and engages with practical issues of how to design mass media campaigns. Social marketing and media advocacy are also discussed.*

Harrabin R, Coote A, Allen J 2003 Health in the news. Kings Fund Publications, London. *A study investigating how health is reported in the news and mass media.*

The relative invisibility of public health issues is documented, analysed and discussed.

Naidoo J, Wills J 2005 Public health and health promotion: developing practice, 2nd edn. Baillière Tindall, London. *Chapter 8, on information, education and communication, discusses how to target health messages so that they are effective, and how to use a social marketing approach.*

References

Atkin C K 2001 Theory and principles of media health campaigns. In: Rice R E, Atkin C K (eds) Public communication campaigns, 3rd edn. Sage, London, pp. 49–68.

Barth J, Bengal J 2000 Prevention through fear? The state of fear appeal research. Federal Centre for Health Education, Cologne.

Beattie A et al 1993 The changing boundaries of health. In: Beattie A, Gott M, Jones L (eds) Health and wellbeing: a reader. Macmillan/Open University, Basingstoke.

Cantril H 1958 The invasion from Mars. In: Maccoby E E, Newcombe T M, Hartley E L (eds) Readings in social psychology. Henry Holt, New York.

Chamberlain M A 1996 Health communication: making the most of new media technologies – an international overview. Journal of Health Communication 1: 43–50.

Chapman S 2004 Advocacy for public health: a primer. Journal of Epidemiology and Community Health 58: 361–365.

Chapman S, Dominello A 2001 A strategy for increasing news media coverage of tobacco and health in Australia. Health Promotion International 16: 137–143.

Chapman S, Lupton D (eds) 1994 The fight for public health: principles and practice of media advocacy. BMJ Publishing, London.

Coulter A, Ellins J, Swain D et al 2006 Assessing the quality of information to support people in making decisions about their health and healthcare. Picker Institute, Oxford.

Dobkin L, Kent C, Klausner J et al 2007 Is text messaging key to improving adolescent sexual health? Journal of Adolescent Health 40: S14.

Elder R W, Shults R A, Sleet D A 2004 Effectiveness of mass media campaigns for reducing drinking and driving and alcohol-involved crashes. A systematic review. American Journal of Preventive Medicine 27: 57–65.

Franklin V L, Waller A, Pagliari C et al 2006 A randomized controlled trial of Sweet Talk, a text-messaging system to support young people with diabetes. Diabetic Medicine 23: 1332–1338.

Gatherer A, Parfit J, Porter E et al 1979 Is health education effective? Health Education Council, London.

Grey A, Owen L, Bolling K 2000 A breath of fresh air: tackling smoking through the media. National Institute of Health and Clinical Excellence, London.

Grilli R, Ramsay C, Minozzi S 2002 Mass media interventions: effects on health services utilisation. Cochrane Database Systematic Reviews 1. CD000389

Harrabin R, Coote A, Allen J 2003 Health in the news. Kings Fund Publications, London.

Hastings G, Stead M, Webb J 2004 Fear appeals in social marketing: strategic and ethical reasons for concern. Psychology and Marketing 21: 961–986.

Joffe H, Haarhoff G 2002 Representations of far-flung illnesses: the case of Ebola in Britain. Social Science and Medicine 54: 955–969.

Katz E, Lazarsfeld P 1955 Personal influence: the part played by people in the flow of mass communication. Free Press, Glencoe, Illinois.

Lasswell H 1948 The structure and function of communication in society. Institute for Religious and Social Studies. New York. Sourced in Fiske J 1990 Introduction to communication studies, 2nd edn. Routledge. London

Lefebvre R C, Flora J A 1988 Social marketing and public health intervention. Health Education Quarterly 15: 299–315.

Lupton D 1994 Medicine as culture. Sage, London.

McKee M, Gilmore A B, Schwalbe N 2005 International co-operation and health: part 2: making a difference. Journal of Epidemiology and Community Health 59: 737–739.

McQuail D 2005 Mass communication theory, 5th edn. Sage Publications, London.

McVey D, Stapleton J 2000 Can anti-smoking television advertising affect smoking behaviour? Controlled trial of the Health Education Authority for England's anti-smoking TV campaign. Tobacco Control 9: 273–282.

Mendelsohn H 1968 Which shall it be: mass education or mass persuasion for health? American Journal of Public Health 58: 131–137.

Montazeri A, McGhee S, McEwan J 1998 Fear inducing and positive image strategies in health education campaigns. International Journal of Health Promotion and Education 36: 68–75.

Naidoo J, Wills J 2005 Public health and health promotion: developing practice, 2nd edn. Baillière Tindall, London.

Owen L, Youdan B 2006 22 years on: the impact and relevance of the UK No Smoking Day. Tobacco Control 15: 19–25.

Regidor E, de la Fuente L, Gutierrez-Fisac J L et al 2007 The role of the public health official in communicating public health information. American Journal of Public Health 97(Suppl. 1): S93–S97.

Reid D 1996 Health education via mass communications – how effective? Health Education Journal 55: 332–344.

Rogers E M, Scott K L 1997 The diffusion of innovations model and outreach from the national network of libraries of medicine to Native American communities. Available online at: http://nnlm.gov/archive/pnr/eval/rogers.html

Shepperd S, Charnock D, Gann B 1999 Helping patients access high quality health information. British Medical Journal 319: 764–766.

Smith B J, Ferguson C, McKenzie J et al 2002 Impacts from repeated mass media campaigns to promote sun protection in Australia. Health Promotion International 17: 51–60.

Stuart H 2006 Media portrayal of mental illness and its treatments: what effect does it have on people with mental illness? CNS Drugs 20: 99–106.

Tay R S 2005 Mass media campaigns reduce the incidence of drinking and driving. Evidence-Based Healthcare and Public Health 9: 26–29.

Tones K 1993 Changing theory and practice: trends in methods, strategies and settings in health education. Health Education Journal 52: 126–139.

Tones K, Tilford S 2001 Health promotion: effectiveness efficiency and equity, 3rd edn. Oxford University Press, Oxford.

Wallack L, Dorfman L 1996 Media advocacy: a strategy for advancing policy and promoting health. Health Education and Behaviour 23: 293–317.

Wammes B, Oenema A, Brug J 2007 The evaluation of a mass media campaign aimed at weight gain prevention among young Dutch adults. Obesity 15: 2780–2789.

Weinreich N K 1999 Hands-on social marketing: a step by step guide. Sage, London.

Wilson P 2002 How to find the good and avoid the bad or ugly: a short guide to tools for rating quality of health information on the internet. British Medical Journal 324: 598–600.

World Health Organization (WHO) 2004 Promoting physical activity: international and UK experiences. World Health Organization, Geneva.

Part 3

Settings for health promotion

This part is concerned with the settings which can promote health. It is in settings that we live our lives – at school, at work, in neighbourhoods, in our contact with health services or in prisons. How can these settings be made more effective?

Introduction

Health promotion has been carried out in particular settings for many years. Workplaces and schools, for example, have provided established channels to reach defined populations. The concept of a settings approach to health promotion, however, is quite distinct and first emerged in the 1980s. The settings approach seeks to make systemic changes to the whole environment. This contrasts with using the setting as a convenient route to access individuals and provide traditional health education messages. The Ottawa Charter (World Health Organization 1986, p. 3) stated that 'health is created and lived by people within the settings of their everyday life: where they learn, work, play and love'. One of the five key action areas identified in the Ottawa Charter was creating supportive environments. As we have seen in this book the focus of health promotion activity is moving away from identifying the diseases and conditions contributing to ill health and the groups at risk, to identifying the complex interplay of factors which create health. It is in settings – at school, at work, in our neighbourhood, in hospital or in prison – that we live our lives and it is these contexts or settings which need to be made more conducive to health.

The settings approach builds a concern for health into the fabric of the system and makes sure that the routine activities of the system are committed to and take account of health. Adopting a healthy-settings approach is fundamentally different to carrying out a one-off short-term health promotion project within a particular setting, which is referred to as 'health education in a setting' as opposed to a 'settings for health' approach (Tones & Green 2006). The settings approach is a long-term one.

In most cases it is being implemented through defined projects which are designed to:

- Introduce specific interventions to create healthy working and living environments
- Develop health policies
- Integrate health into quality, audit and evaluation procedures to build evidence of how health can make the system perform better.

The first and best-known example of settings-based health promotion is the Healthy Cities project. Originally this was a small project initiated by the World Health Organization in 1986 to put the Ottawa Charter and Health for All principles (World Health Organization 1985, 1986) into practice. It has subsequently expanded to become a worldwide movement incorporating over 1200 cities in more than 30 countries in the European region (www.euro.who.int/healthy-cities). Parallel initiatives have been developed and are coordinated by European Networks in schools, hospitals, workplaces, prisons and universities. The UK health strategies have all referred to the importance of settings. *The Health of the Nation*, published in 1992, stated that settings 'offer between them the potential to involve most people in the country' (Department of Health 1992). Schools, neighbourhoods, workplaces and prisons are also identified in *Choosing Health: Making Healthy Choices Easier* (Department of Health 2004) as key settings through which inequalities in health should be tackled.

The settings approach is complex and is characterized by several unique factors (Dooris 2005):

- An ecological model of health promotion that conceptualizes health as determined by a range of socioeconomic, organizational, environmental and personal factors
- A focus on health and well-being rather than illness
- A focus on populations rather than individuals
- A holistic view of health rather than a mechanistic reductionist view
- A systems perspective that sees settings as complex systems interacting dynamically with their environment

- A whole-organization focus that seeks to change from within the organization.

The benefits of such an approach are hard to quantify but appear to be significant. Benefits include encouraging partnership working and collaboration, embedding health in organizational structures and systems and taking account of broader determinants of health. Perhaps not surprisingly, given the complexity of this approach, evaluation and evidence for the effectiveness of the settings approach are rather scanty:

'The settings approach has been legitimated more through an act of faith than through rigorous research and evaluation studies … much more attention needs to be given to building the evidence and learning from it' (St Leger 1997, p. 100).

Dooris (2005) proposes the use of theory-based evaluation to build a stronger evidence base for the settings approach.

Part 3 looks at health promotion in five key settings:

1. Workplace
2. Schools
3. Neighbourhoods
4. Hospitals
5. Prisons.

Each setting is addressed in a separate chapter but it is important to remember that the settings are not discrete but coexist as part of a wider independent system. Schools, workplaces and hospitals are all in neighbourhoods and there is a constant flow of people within and between the settings. Prisons, although more separated from their neighbourhood, are also sited in a specific locality and impact upon that locality in terms of employment and transport. There are many other settings where health promotion interventions may be delivered e.g. night clubs or barbers' shops. Tones & Tilford (2001) have argued that the healthy-settings approach is unlikely to have any long-term impact on population health until 'different settings have congruent aims and operate synergistically'.

Each of the following chapters examines why the setting is appropriate for health promotion, identifying the factors of the settings which affect health and outlining some health-promoting initiatives which have been developed in that setting.

References

Department of Health 1992 The health of the nation. HMSO, London.

Department of Health 2004 Choosing health: making healthy choices easier. Stationery Office, London.

Dooris M 2005 Healthy settings: challenges to generating evidence of effectiveness. Health Promotion International 21: 55–65.

St Leger L 1997 Health promoting settings: from Ottawa to Jakarta. Health Promotion International 12: 99–101.

Tones K, Green J 2006 Health promotion: planning and strategies. Sage, London.

Tones K, Tilford S 2001 Health promotion: effectiveness, efficiency and equity, 2nd edn. Chapman & Hall, London.

World Health Organization 1985 Targets for health for all. WHO Regional Office for Europe, Copenhagen.

World Health Organization 1986 Ottawa charter for health promotion. WHO, Geneva.

Chapter Thirteen

Health promotion in schools

- The school setting
- Relationship between schools, education and health
- The context for health promotion in schools
- The health-promoting school
- Effectiveness of health promotion in schools

OVERVIEW

The view that schools can promote the health and welfare of children and young people has a long history. The development of a school health service, the requirement for school boards to provide meals and, more recently, the inclusion of physical education in the national curriculum and the setting of nutritional standards for school meals are examples of how the school was seen as a key setting in which a captive audience could be encouraged to adopt lifestyles conducive to good health.

The World Health Organization has defined a health-promoting school (HPS) as: 'one in which all members of the school community work together to provide pupils with integrated, positive experiences and structures which promote and protect health. This includes both the formal and informal curriculum in health, the creation of a safe and healthy school environment, the provision of appropriate health services and the involvement of the family and the wider community in efforts to promote health' (World Health Organization 1995). The school is seen as a total environment in which many aspects affect the health of its pupils and staff, including its organization, ethos and culture and its layout, in addition to any teaching about health issues and the provision of medical and nursing services. Schools also act as referral agencies, signposting children and parents to other health, welfare and voluntary services when appropriate.

This chapter looks at the physical, mental and social well-being of children and young people and how schools can be powerful agents in the promotion of good health through the curriculum and every day practices.

Why the school is a key setting for health promotion

Education is a resource for health. This is recognized by the World Health Organization, and the United Nations included 'achieving universal primary education' as one of its eight millennium development goals. Equally, health is a prerequisite for education: 'Children who face violence, hunger, substance abuse, and despair cannot possibly focus on academic excellence. There is no curriculum brilliant enough to compensate for a hungry stomach or distracted mind' (National Action Plan for Comprehensive School Health Education 1992).

School is seen as an important context for health promotion, principally because it reaches a large proportion of the population for many years. The emphasis on schools is also a recognition that the learning of health-related knowledge, attitudes and behaviour begins at an early age.

 Box 13.1

Reflect on your own experience of health promotion when you were at school. Do you regard your experience as adequate and appropriate?

Box 13.2

Consider each of the following statements about the aims for health promotion for young people and indicate how important you would rate each (very important/important/not very important/not important at all).

Health promotion should:

1. Provide information about how the body works.
2. Foster positive personal and social relationships.
3. Teach young people to keep fit and feel good.

4. Equip young people with the skills to make informed and responsible decisions.
5. Inform young people about local services and how to get help.
6. Teach young people about the dangers of certain behaviours, such as taking drugs.
7. Help young people to express their feelings and emotions.
8. Teach young people how to say 'no'.
9. Show young people the wonders of the human body so they do not damage it.
10. Put young people off unhealthy behaviour by emphasizing the risks to their health.
11. Prepare young people for parenthood.
12. Provide information about human sexuality, puberty and contraception.
13. Teach young people how to reduce their risk from drug-taking or sexual activity (safer sex and safer drug-taking).
14. Prepare young people to be active citizens.
15. Show young people how to cope with stress.
16. Equip young people with the skills to negotiate and be assertive in relationships.
17. Help to build young people's self-esteem.

Box 13.3

What factors would you identify as important in promoting a health-enhancing lifestyle for young people?

Childhood and adolescence is a time of great change, when young people often acquire lifetime habits and attitudes. One function of a healthy school environment is to enable children to develop healthy behaviours. Part of growing up is risk-taking, but problems arise when young people are unaware of the scale of risk involved. The effects of smoking, excessive alcohol consumption, drug use and low levels of exercise may not become apparent until later life. There is some evidence that risk-taking behaviour in one area can lead to risk-taking behaviour in other areas. A recent study of 15-year-olds found that the odds of someone having used cannabis in the last month were 12 times higher for those who had drunk alcohol in the last week compared with those who hadn't, and 8 times higher for those who had smoked in the last week (National Centre for Social Research and the National Foundation for Educational Research 2005). Similarly, two-fifths of sexually active 13- and 14-year-olds said they were under the influence of alcohol or cannabis the first time they had sexual intercourse (Wight et al 2000). Whilst adolescence is characterized by powerful peer group attachments, the school setting provides an opportunity to communicate with young people and provides learning opportunities and a safe environment to practise new skills.

 Box 13.4

In what ways might children's educational potential and attainment be influenced by their health?

There is a relationship between health and education and the ability to learn. Young people's experiences in school influence the development of their self-esteem, self-perception and their health behaviours. Pupils with low school performance and educational aspirations and high levels of absence from school are more likely to engage in earlier risk-taking behaviour such as drug use (Canning et al 2004). School attendance is particularly important and provision of food at school, e.g. through breakfast clubs, can improve attendance rates. Equally, health can have an impact on educational performance. There is evidence that providing good nutrition in school can improve attention, concentration and overall cognitive development (Powney et al 2000).

Health promotion in schools

The development of health education and promotion in schools has reflected many approaches to health promotion. Health education has tended to reflect the medical view of health and in many countries is almost exclusively concerned with hygiene, nutrition and fitness. In the 1960s education saw a swing to being child-centred and educational methods sought to develop autonomy and responsibility through discovery learning. Health education emerged as a complex theme of well-being and fulfilment of maximum potential. Health promotion in schools is now closely linked to personal and social development, and delivered in the curriculum as personal and social health education (PSHE). The aim is for young people to be in charge of their own lives and the role of the school is to develop self-esteem and self-awareness. Emphasis is placed on the *process* of education, and finding teaching and learning strategies which encourage reflection and personal awareness. The direction and organization of the health promotion programme also aim to reflect the needs of the children and young people. The provision of PSHE in schools remains patchy and often focuses on knowledge rather than skills and attitudes. There are many reasons for this, including the lack of training for teachers in this subject and mixed messages from government as to the importance of PSHE within the curriculum (PSHE is not mandatory but is strongly encouraged).

Alongside these attempts to promote autonomy and decision-making skills are more traditional information-giving approaches. Behind such an approach is the simple assumption that people are rational decision-makers whose behaviour will change once they have information about how to live more healthily. Much health promotion in schools therefore entails the provision of information about the health-damaging effects of certain behaviours, such as smoking and taking drugs.

The provision of sex education in schools reflects these views of health promotion. Sex education is now commonly referred to as 'sex and relationships education' in recognition of the need to move away from a focus on biology to a focus on emotional health, values and life skills.

 Box 13.5

Sex and relationship education

Following revisions to the English National Curriculum in 1999, a new personal social and health education (PSHE) framework for schools, and the Social Exclusion Unit's report on teenage pregnancy, schools were provided with specific guidance on the provision of sex and relationships education (SRE) in schools (Department for Children, Schools and Families 2000). The guidance requires that:

- SRE be firmly rooted within the National Curriculum and PSHE framework
- The aim of SRE is to support young people through their physical, emotional and moral development and to help them develop the skills and understanding needed to live confident, healthy and independent lives
- SRE is a core aspect of the National Healthy Schools Programme
- SRE will include teaching about the importance of relationships inside and outside marriage
- SRE will not encourage early sexual experimentation but will build knowledge and skills
- All schools must have a SRE policy developed in consultation with the whole school community. This policy is subject to inspection by Ofsted
- Teachers should deal openly, honestly and sensitively with sexual orientation and should not directly promote any particular sexual orientation.

The health-promoting school

The HPS is an international approach to addressing the health of pupils and teachers in a comprehensive and strategic manner (Fig. 13.1). If education for the health of young people is to focus on more than individual behaviour and be health *promotion*, it needs to acknowledge the influence of the school itself as a health-promoting environment and as part of a wider community.

The whole school context includes its ethos, organization, management structures, relationships and physical environment as well as the taught curriculum. In the HPS all these aspects will reinforce and support each other, leading to a synergistic effect. In reality, different aspects of the school often give conflicting messages. Many aspects of school can be health-promoting or health-inhibiting. Educationalists have long talked of a 'hidden curriculum' and the way in which messages can be transmitted through children and young people's daily experience of their surroundings and relationships at school. For example, the state of many school toilets might suggest that hygiene is not valued or that the pupils do not require (or deserve) cleanliness or care. Knowing that someone (e.g. personal tutor, school nurse) is always available to talk to about any personal concerns or incidents at school such as bullying or teasing is important for mental health and well-being.

The European Network of Health Promoting Schools (ENHPS) was launched in 1992 as an initiative of the World Health Organization. The principles of HPS have been identified as:

- Promotes the health and well-being of students
- Upholds social justice and equity concepts
- Involves student participation and empowerment
- Provides a safe and supportive environment
- Links health and education issues and systems
- Addresses the health and well-being issues of staff
- Collaborates with the local community
- Integrates into the school's ongoing activities
- Sets realistic goals
- Engages parents and families in health promotion (St Leger 2005).

In common with other settings, effective health promotion in schools happens when it is coordinated and takes place within structured frameworks. In the UK the National Healthy Schools Standard was launched

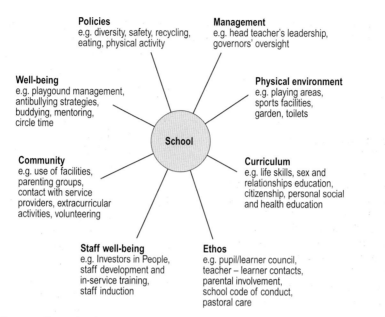

Policies
e.g. diversity, safety, recycling, eating, physical activity

Management
e.g. head teacher's leadership, governors' oversight

Well-being
e.g. playgound management, antibullying strategies, buddying, mentoring, circle time

Physical environment
e.g. playing areas, sports facilities, garden, toilets

School

Community
e.g. use of facilities, parenting groups, contact with service providers, extracurricular activities, volunteering

Curriculum
e.g. life skills, sex and relationships education, citizenship, personal social and health education

Staff well-being
e.g. Investors in People, staff development and in-service training, staff induction

Ethos
e.g. pupil/learner council, teacher – learner contacts, parental involvement, school code of conduct, pastoral care

Figure 13.1 • The health-promoting school.

in 2002. As with other award schemes for hospitals and workplaces, the scheme encourages institutions to work towards specific targets. A basic level is to ensure that systems are in place so that specific aspects of health can be incorporated into a school.

Box 13.6

The National Healthy Schools Programme (NHSP) is a government initiative to improve the health and achievements of children and young people. The NHSP focuses on four key themes:

1. Personal social and health education
2. Healthy eating
3. Physical activity
4. Emotional health and well-being.

The NHSP adopts a whole-school approach and aims to:

- Support children and young people to develop healthy behaviours
- Help raise the achievement of children and young people
- Help reduce health inequalities
- Help promote social inclusion.

The government has set a target that by 2009 all schools will be participating in the NHSP and that 75% will have achieved National Healthy School status (www.healthyschools.gov.uk).

Policies and practices

The policies that a school develops represent its values. Schools may have policies on equal opportunities, discipline and rewards, health and safety, bullying, healthy food and various curriculum issues, including sex education. Policies may be merely 'paper exercises' unless they have been influenced by wide consultation within the school and community, have been clearly written and disseminated and are consistently applied. The practices of a school can be evidenced in its daily life and the ways in which decisions are taken. Democratic participation by pupils is a key element in an HPS.

Box 13.7

The Ottawa Charter describes health promotion as a process of 'enabling people to take more control over and improve their health' (World Health Organization 1986). How can pupils in schools be enabled to make decisions about their education and their health?

Social environment

The quality of social interactions among pupils, between staff and pupils and between the staff contributes to the ethos or climate in a school. Increasingly, schools are recognizing that healthy schools which value positive relationships, prioritize learning and build self-esteem also drive up educational standards.

Curriculum

The formal curriculum includes knowledge and understanding of health-related topics (e.g. biology and nutrition) at a level appropriate for pupils' age, social and cognitive development. The informal curriculum refers to areas not formally taught or examined, including pastoral care and extracurricular activities in areas such as sports and arts. In the UK there is no statutory provision for health promotion and its integration into the curriculum is patchy.

Physical environment

The physical environment and layout of a school may be stimulating or depressing. Schools should provide a clean and safe environment with no litter or graffiti, clean toilets and a welcoming but secure entrance. There should be areas for play, for social interaction and for quiet study or reading. In many countries the provision of basic amenities such as sanitation, water availability and air cleanliness may be priorities.

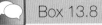

Box 13.8

Think back to your primary school and try to picture the playground area. Was it a health-promoting environment?

Links with the community

How well the school communicates and connects with its local community, where its pupils and their families live, is an important criterion for the HPS. Partnerships with parents may vary from information about school events and fund-raising requests, consultation about uniform or meals provision to the active involvement of all parents in decision-making about the curriculum, pastoral care and resource issues. Parents may also become involved in school life through reading schemes, practical parenting classes and breakfast clubs. A survey of parents' views on health education and promotion found that many parents did not know what schools were doing and had not been consulted about health promotion despite the fact that they saw school as a major influence on young people's health awareness (National Foundation for Educational Research 1997).

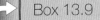

Box 13.9

'Society School'

A school in Belgium identified the need to integrate its diverse ethnic groups socially. One way to do this was to involve parents in school activities. The school took the approach of celebrating its multiculturalism by asking parents to prepare a snack food from their traditional foods for all the children in the school. Many parents participated, also providing decorations and music. All parents were invited to the school for a free meal. Parents reported that this project broke down their initial hesitation about coming into the school and enabled them to build relationships with other parents (European Network of Health Promoting Schools 1997).

Schools are also part of a wider community and should be open to that community. Many agencies and services can provide support to schools. For example, the police and emergency services often provide educational sessions concerning accident prevention.

Box 13.10

HPS and 'school connectedness' in Queensland, Australia

The Western Gateway project in Ipswich, Queensland aimed to encourage students' connectedness with school in order to promote mental health and act as a protective factor reducing the incidence of violence and substance abuse. Ten schools were supported over a 3-year period. Activities undertaken included health weeks, breakfast and lunchtime programmes, smoke-free toilet blocks, healthier tuckshops, comprehensive curriculum programmes, cultural days, parent information sessions and increased participation in physical activity within the school. Evaluation suggested activities improved pupils' connectedness with school and increased community participation and ownership in school activities (Queensland Government 2005a, b).

Box 13.11

Choose one of the following aims and make a list of indicators in the broad areas of policy, curriculum, social and physical environment and community links that would demonstrate that the school was health-promoting:

- Establishment of a safe and secure environment
- School ethos based on the promotion of mutual respect and understanding

- Promotion of physical activity
- An approach to food and nutrition which promotes the importance of healthy eating
- An informed and coherent approach to substance use
- An approach to sex and relationships that supports and informs pupils.

Effective interventions

Health promotion interventions in schools differ substantially in their nature, ranging from programmes providing physiological information to life skills to abstinence-oriented programmes, in addition to the comprehensive whole-school approaches outlined above. Many curriculum programmes aim to have outcomes relevant to risk reduction, such as increased knowledge or changes in behaviour. Programmes may thus be specific to a particular health issue (e.g. smoking education) or more generic life skills programmes aiming to develop self-esteem and social and communication skills. They may target pupils only, or extend their reach to include teachers, parents and the wider community.

Schools are dynamic communities and there are many varied influences on young people both within and outside the school setting, so demonstrating the particular effect of health promotion is extremely difficult. The majority of interventions aim to develop health-enhancing behaviours. These health outcomes will not be apparent until later in life. For example, the Australian 'no hat – no play' policy will not demonstrate an effect on skin cancer rates until well into adulthood. Evidence shows that increasing children's knowledge is feasible, but changing their attitudes and behaviour, even in the short term, is far more difficult (Lister-Sharp et al 1999). A recent study by the World Health Organization into the evidence of effectiveness of health promotion in schools and the HPS approach found that mental health promotion programmes were amongst the most effective. Factors associated with increased effectiveness included: long duration, high intensity and involvement of the whole school, a focus on the school environment, multifactoral interventions and peer-led health promotion (Stewart-Brown 2006). There is evidence that integrated, holistic and strategic programmes are more effective than classroom education programmes (St Leger 2005).

Box 13.12

Promoting mental health in schools

Schools should promote positive mental health and emphasize well-being as well as targeting those with particular needs. In this way, schools can help to disseminate the idea of mental health as everyone's business and tackle problems of stigma and denial. Research has shown that the following characteristics are associated with effective mental health programmes in schools:

- Provide a universal backdrop to promote mental health for all plus effective targeting of those with special needs
- Multidimensional and coherent
- Create supportive environments that promote warmth, empathy, positive expectations and clear boundaries
- Tackle mental health problems when they first become apparent and adopt a long-term approach
- Identify and target vulnerable at-risk groups and help them acquire life skills
- Involve service users and families
- Provide training for those who run programmes (Weare & Markham 2005).

Conclusion

Schools are widely seen as having a key role in health promotion. Young people are a key target group for the provision of information and encouragement of responsible and health-promoting attitudes and behaviour. The habits acquired in childhood and adolescence may prove influential for the rest of one's lifespan. Adolescence is also a time of development and risk-taking, and a fine balance needs to be struck

between encouraging the development of autonomy alongside responsible and health-promoting attitudes and behaviour. However health, personal and social education has always been marginalized within the formal curriculum. Currently PSHE is not a mandatory subject, although its inclusion is encouraged. Research suggests that narrow information-based programmes are less effective than broader programmes that address the school as a whole. This is the direction taken by the HPS initiative, which seeks to promote a whole-school approach, encompassing not just the formal curriculum but also the informal curriculum, the school's physical and social environment and its links with its community. The evolving evidence base suggests that the HPS approach is effective and contributes to children's and young people's health, education and welfare.

Questions for further discussion

- How can the core health promotion principles of collaboration, participation, empowerment and equity be incorporated into the school structure and management?
- What are the barriers to developing HPS?
- You are a newly appointed teacher in a failing secondary school in an inner-city area with an ethnically and culturally diverse intake of students. You are asked to produce a strategy to make your school an HPS. How would you go about this task? What areas would you prioritize, and why?

Summary

This chapter has examined the reasons why schools are a key setting for health promotion. Health and education have a reciprocal relationship, so that enhancing either one will impact favourably on the other. The holistic HPS approach has been identified as providing the most promising strategy. There is an accumulating evidence base to support the whole-school integrated approach.

Further reading and resources

The European Network of Health Promoting Schools is a useful resource and may be accessed via its website on http://www.who.int/school_youth_health/en.

The UK healthy school programme's website provides up-to-date news and resources and may be accessed via its website on www.healthyschools.gov.uk.

www.wiredforhealth.gov.uk provides information for teachers and schools with local case studies.

References

Canning U, Millward L, Raj T et al 2004 Drug use prevention among young people: a review of reviews. Health Development Agency, London.

Department for Children, Schools and Families 2000 Sex and relationships education guidance. HMSO, London.

European Network of Health Promoting Schools 1997 The health promotion school – an investment in education, health and democracy: conference case study book, Thessaloniki-Halkidiki 1–5 May. WHO, Copenhagen

Lister-Sharp D, Chapman S, Stewart-Brown S et al 1999 Health promoting schools and health promotion in schools: two systematic reviews. Health Technology Assessment 3: 22.

National Action Plan for Comprehensive School Health Education 1993 Working together for the future: 1992 comprehensive school health education workshop. Journal of School Health 63: 46–66.

National Centre for Social Research and the National Foundation for Educational Research 2005 Available online at: www.ic.nhs.uk/pubs/youngpeopledruguse-smoking-drinking2005/report/fi

National Foundation for Educational Research 1997 Parents' views of health education: summary of key findings from the ENHPS survey of parents. NFER, London.

Powney J, Malcolm H, Lowden K 2000 Health and attainment. SCRE, Glasgow.

Queensland Government 2005a Western Gateway health promoting schools grand scheme: final report. Available online at: www.chdf.org.au/i-cms_file?page=81/vh38.pdf

Queensland Government Western Gateway health promoting schools, community renewal 2005b Health promoting schools: a storybook of success stories. Available online at: health.qld.gov.au/ph/Documents/saphs/27008.pdf

Stewart-Brown S 2006 What is the evidence on school health promotion in improving health or preventing disease and, specifically, what is the effectiveness of the health promoting school approach? World Health Organization, Copenhagen.

St Leger L 2005 Protocols and guidelines for health promoting schools. Promotion and Education X11: 145–146.

Weare K, Markham W 2005 What do we know about promoting mental health through schools? Promotion and Education XII: 118–122.

Wight D, Henderson M, Raab G et al 2000 Extent of regretted sexual intercourse among young teenagers in Scotland: a cross sectional survey. British Medical Journal 6: 1243–1244.

World Health Organization 1986 Ottawa charter for health promotion. WHO, Geneva.

World Health Organization 1995 WHO expert committee on comprehensive school health education and promotion. WHO, Geneva.

Chapter Fourteen

Health promotion in the workplace

14

Key points

- The workplace setting
- Relationship between work and health
- Responsibility for workplace health
- Health promotion in the workplace

OVERVIEW

The workplace is significant both in affecting people's health and as a context in which to promote health. Employment rates in the UK have been rising. Statistics for the last quarter of 2007 show that 74.7% of people of working age, or 29.4 million people, were employed (www.statistics.gov.uk). Promoting health in the workplace will therefore reach a large percentage of the adult population, and will have an impact on a setting where many adults spend a considerable amount of their time.

This chapter looks at the workplace as a social system and ways in which it can contribute to ill health and health. It goes on to look at ways in which health promotion has been implemented in the workplace. Most health promotion interventions have tended to focus on individual lifestyle risk factors and employers' legal responsibilities to provide a safe working environment. Interventions that address the workplace

organization and culture as a whole are less common, but evaluation shows they are more effective. The different partners and stakeholders involved in workplace health promotion are identified and their contribution to interventions discussed.

Why is the workplace a key setting for health promotion?

There are four main reasons for prioritizing the workplace. First, the workplace gives access to a target group, healthy adults, especially men, who are often difficult to reach in other ways. Recent projections suggest that by 2020 32.1 million people will be economically active (Madouros 2006), which represents an increase of 6.7% from 2005. Employees in the workplace are a captive audience for health promotion. It is easy to follow up interventions and encourage participation in health programmes because there are established modes of communication. The cohesion of the working community also provides peer pressure and support. The second reason for promoting health in the workplace is to ensure that people are protected from the harm to their health that certain jobs may cause.

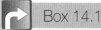

Box 14.1

Work-related ill health – U.K. statistics for the year 2006–2007

241 workers were killed at work (an 11% increase on 2005–2006)

141,350 employees suffered serious injuries at work

2.2 million people were suffering from an illness they believed was caused or made worse by their work. Of these, 646,000 were new cases in the last 12 months

36 million days were lost overall (1.5 days per worker), with 30 million due to work-related ill health and 6 million due to workplace injury (Health and Safety Executive (HSE) 2007).

Thirdly, there are economic benefits associated with healthy workplaces (Wanless 2004). American research studies provide evidence that workplace health promotion programmes are associated with lower medical and insurance costs, decreased absenteeism and enhanced performance, productivity and morale (www.uclan.ac.uk/facs/health/hsdu/settings/workplace/htm). The cost of sick leave and incapacity benefit averaged £476 per worker in 2002 (Dooris & Hunter 2007). Research has shown that employees who have three or more risk factors (e.g. smoking, overweight, excessive alcohol intake, physical inactivity) are likely to have 50% more sickness absence from work than employees with no risk factors (Shain & Kramer 2004). Investing in health and preventing ill health increase productivity and staff retention. The average cost–benefit ratio for a variety of health promotion programmes operated by large American companies is significant – just over a fourfold return on each dollar invested (Shain & Kramer 2004). Adopting

a healthy workplaces approach therefore makes sound business sense.

Box 14.2

Economic benefits of workplace health promotion programmes

Many evaluation studies of workplace health promotion programmes have reported positive results, including the following:

- Prudential Insurance Company reports that the company's major medical costs dropped from $574 to $312 for each participant in its wellness programme.
- A 2-year study by the DuPont Corporation reports that blue-collar employees involved in its comprehensive health promotion programme showed a 14% decline in sick leave compared to a 5.8% decline for controls.
- The Canadian Life Assurance Company demonstrated a 4% increase in productivity for workplaces with employee fitness programmes compared to controls. Nearly half (47%) of participants in the programme reported benefits, including enjoying work more, better rapport with coworkers, and feeling more alert

(www.uclan.ac.uk/facs/health/hsdu/settings/workplace/htm).

Fourthly, the workplace provides a resource for health that is relevant to a large percentage of the adult population. Creating a healthy environment at work will benefit employees' health and have positive spin-offs for their families and communities. The traditional focus on the workplace has centred on hazards and illnesses, but a health-promoting approach to the workplace has great potential.

The relationship between work and health

The relationship between work and health is complex. In general, attention has focused on the effects of work on health, although it is also acknowledged that poor health will have negative effects on the capacity for paid employment. There is evidence that paid work is good for your health and unemployment can be linked to ill health (Waddell & Burton 2006). Work is beneficial for health because it provides an income, a sense of self-worth and social networks of colleagues and friends. However, work may also harm health, and most research has concentrated on this aspect of the relationship.

Box 14.3

Think of a recent work experience.
- In what ways do you think work contributed to your health?
- In what ways do you think work had a negative impact on your health?
- Overall, would you say that work was a positive or a negative influence on your health?

The workplace can affect health in many different ways. Figure 14.1 provides a means of classifying these different kinds of relationship.

Box 14.4

Why do you think people do not always report injuries at work?

Hazards tend to be what people think of first when health in the workplace is mentioned. Most legislation is directed towards the containment of hazards, and safety legislation has been enshrined in numerous Factory Acts since the mid 19th century. Work that involves handling hazardous or toxic materials may have a direct negative effect on health (e.g. cancers caused by asbestos or occupational asthma). Work which provides easy access to hazardous substances is also linked to associated ill health. For example, doctors and pharmacists have high rates of suicide associated with drug overdose. In 2000 the government set out, for the first time, overarching targets for significant improvements in workplace health and safety. The statistics for workplace deaths and injuries for 2006–2007 are mixed (HSE

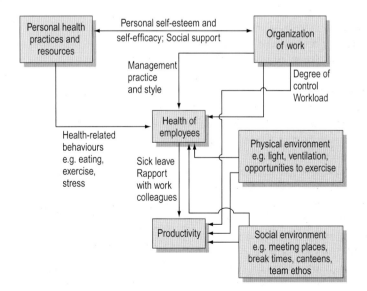

Figure 14.1 • The relationship between health and productivity in the workplace. From Shain & Kramer (2004).

2007; Health and Safety Commission 2007). Overall there has been progress in major injury reduction, but an increase in workplace deaths. Almost one-third of deaths occur in the construction sector, with agriculture, waste and recycling industries also implicated.

The workplace is characterized by fragmented information which is collected by different bodies (including the HSE and occupational health services). This poses obvious difficulties when trying to plan and implement a health promotion intervention. Health is often affected through risky behaviour or changed routines. Risky behaviour is the preferred explanation for most official accounts of accidents and injuries sustained in the workplace. There are extensive regulations to cover manual handling (Manual Handling Operations Regulations, amended in 2002) which require employers to provide training and equipment. Nevertheless, employees are expected to 'take reasonable care for the health and safety of themselves and any others who may be affected by their acts and omissions'. This approach extends to the workplace the victim-blaming ideology of some brands of health promotion. Behaviour which carries health risks may be an integral part of the job or part of the work culture. For example, bartenders have high rates of alcohol-related ill health because drinking heavily is associated with work (Wilhelm et al. 2004).

The general work environment and its effects on health are the most neglected aspects of the work–health relationship. This is due in part to ideological or political reasons, and in part to the fact that such a generalized relationship is hard to research or prove. Because the relationship between work and health is to a large extent indirect, it is often difficult to trace ill health to what happens in the workplace. This in turn leads to the true impact on health from work being underestimated. Focusing on the work environment instead of individual workers' behaviour shifts responsibility on to the employer and has resource implications.

Although the relationship is difficult to quantify, strong evidence implicating the importance to health of the general work environment is becoming available (Marmot & Wilkinson 2006). There is a body of research demonstrating that certain factors associated with some types of work, such as repetitive tasks, lack of autonomy and pressures to meet deadlines, have harmful effects on health. In particular, low control by workers over what they do and how they do it is associated with increased risk of ill health (Wilkinson 2006). Long-term exposure to stress results in poor health and may also lead to less healthy lifestyle choices, such as smoking. There is a growing acknowledgement of the impact of workplace stress on health:

- Work-related stress accounts for over a third of all new incidents of ill health.
- Each case of stress-related ill health leads to an average of 80.9 lost working days.
- 12.8 million working days were lost due to stress, depression and anxiety in 2004–2005 (www.hse.gov.uk/stress/why/.htm).

In response to this situation, the HSE (2005) has produced management standards to support employers who wish to tackle this issue.

Box 14.5

Stress in the workplace

A focus on individual stress can be counterproductive, leading to a failure to tackle the underlying causes of problems in the workplace. Evidence has shown that poor working arrangements, such as lack of job control or discretion, consistently high work demands and low social support, can lead to increased risks of CHD [coronary heart disease], musculoskeletal disorders, mental illness and sickness absence. The real task is to improve the quality of jobs by reducing monotony, increasing job control, and applying appropriate HR [human resources] practices and policies – organisations need to ensure they adopt approaches that support the overall health and well being of their employees (Department of Health 2004, Chapter 7 para 16).

There are two main ways in which workplace stress is being addressed. The traditional approach has been to see the individual as unable to cope with the demands and pressures and therefore in need of support. Many large workplaces offer stress management courses, counselling services and employee assistance programmes to help people adjust to new skills.

Organizational approaches to stress are still rare despite a growing literature linking stress with organizational factors, such as lack of control or lack of consultation over changes. These approaches start from the view that illness and stressed behaviour are responses to factors in the workplace, and of which individuals may not even be aware.

Box 14.6

Seven stressor areas that contribute to stress in the workplace have been identified:

1. **Demands** – workloads, work patterns
2. **Control** – how much of a say employees have over things that affect them
3. **Support** – encouragement, appreciation, sponsorship, resources
4. **Relationships at work** – managing conflict or unacceptable behaviour
5. **Role** – understanding of role and no conflicting roles
6. **Change** – how it is managed and communicated
7. **Culture** – management commitment and open and fair procedures (HSE 2001).

Task and work reorganization is the most successful form of intervention. It describes various system solutions to improve communication, the creation of autonomous work groups and whole-organization interventions to restructure relations between management and unions. These interventions do not obviate the need for individual support, but follow an earlier stage of raising staff awareness of stress and its causes.

Box 14.7

What could your organization do to reduce stress at work?

Responsibility for workplace health

The relationship between work and health may appear substantial but it is viewed in different ways by different groups of people. One of the defining characteristics of the workplace setting is that it brings together a variety of groups who have different agendas with regard to work and health. The key parties are workers or employees and their trade unions or staff associations, employers and managers, occupational health staff, health and safety officers, public health specialists and environmental health officers.

Workers

It has always been a priority for workers' organizations to ensure that employees are working in safe and healthy conditions. Membership of trade unions has, however, declined since the mid-1970s, when membership was just under two-fifths, to just over a quarter in 2006 (Department of Trade and Industry 2007). Changing patterns of employment also mean that part-time (mainly female) workers make up a significant percentage of the working population. So, although consultation with unions is an important means of reaching workers, it does not reach everyone. As the key target group, workers need to be fully involved as partners in decision-making processes. This is recognized by the European Network for Workplace Health Promotion (ENWHP), who state that effective workplace health promotion involves employees in decision-making processes and develops a working culture based on partnership (www.enwhp.org).

Employers and managers

Employers and managers have as their first priority the viability of the organization. Health is relevant in so far as it can be shown to be linked to organizational goals. Examples of 'hard' benefits are improvements in productivity due to lower rates of sickness, absenteeism and staff turnover, and improved recruitment and retention of trained staff. 'Soft' benefits, such as enhanced corporate image, are also influential.

Employers are responsible for the health, safety and welfare of all their employees under the Health and Safety at Work Act (1974). There is evidence of a shift in attitudes and awareness of health and safety issues in the workplace. A recent survey (Elgood et al 2004) found that between two-thirds and three-quarters of employees felt that employers take their responsibilities seriously. There was a high level of awareness and understanding about the HSE and its role, although this was less true within smaller organizations. The Investors in People standard is an example of the government's strategy to use awards to provide incentives for employers, and has been widely adopted. The Improving Working Lives standard is another example that sets a model of good human resources practice against which National Health Service employers can be measured. Leadership and commitment at senior management level have been shown to be vital for effective health promotion initiatives and the creation of healthy workplaces (Faculty of Public Health and Faculty of Occupational Medicine 2006).

Box 14.8

Employer responsibilities might be:
• Making healthy choices easy for staff
• Creating flexible working arrangements that are compatible with employees' home lives
• Ensuring a smoke-free environment.
Consider your current or a recent place of work. Can you identify ways in which each of these recommendations was carried out?

Occupational health staff

In many European countries occupational health is a statutory part of health care. In the UK there is no requirement for employers to provide an occupational health service, other than first aid. A recent survey (Institute of Occupational Medicine 2002) found that only 15% of all British firms provided basic occupational health support, and only 3% offered comprehensive support. Occupational health nurses (OHNs), who are specialist nurses with postqualification training, form an important element of the occupational health staff. OHNs are responsible for the health and well-being of employees in the workplace.

The main functions of an occupational health service are:
• Surveillance of the work environment, e.g. the effects of new technologies
• Initiatives and advice on the control of hazards
• Surveillance of the health of employees, e.g. assessment of fitness to work, analysis of sickness-absence
• Organization of first aid and emergency response
• Adaptation of work and the environment to the worker.

The workplace has experienced considerable change and uncertainty in the last 20 years. There has been a rapid growth in the service sector, a fragmentation of large organizations and a huge increase in information technology. The provision for health in companies thus needs to be seen alongside policies on employment, the work environment and overall company policy.

Box 14.9

Think of a workplace you are familiar with.
• In what ways were people expected to adapt to the job?
• In what ways was the job adapted to meet the health needs of people?
• Which approach is preferable, and why?

Health and Safety Officers and Environmental Health Officers

Health and safety officers and environmental health officers are responsible for ensuring that workplaces conform with safety legislation. They have powers to force workplaces to comply with health and safety regulations, and to impose penalties in the case of non-compliance. Responsibility for workplaces is divided between the HSE and environmental health officers employed by local authorities. There is now a developed body of European Union (EU) occupational health and safety legislation.

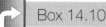 Box 14.10

Lighten the Load

The European Agency for Safety and Health at Work has organized the Lighten the Load campaign to promote an integrated approach to tackling musculoskeletal disorders (MSDs). MSDs are the most common form of work-related illness in Europe. In the EU 25% of workers suffer from backache and 23% from muscular pains. Nine organizations won good-practice awards in 2008. Winning projects included:

- Reducing manual handling in a greenhouse by introducing a load-moving system
- Developing an ergonomically designed sewing workstation
- Eliminating MSD problems experienced by handling heavy wooden pallets

(osha.europa.eu/press_room/news_article_CLEV_26_02_2008).

A recent consultation paper (Department of Trade and Industry 2007) documented the valuable role played by workplace safety representatives. Safety representatives prevent 8000–13 000 injuries and 3000–8000 work-related illnesses annually. The annual savings to industry and society as a whole are estimated as £578 million per year (at 2004 prices). Yet safety representatives are not universal. Only 46% of workplaces (92% of public sector and 39% of private sector) and 68% of employees (98% of public sector and 59% of private sector) are covered by employee representation.

Health promotion in the workplace

Several policy initiatives target the workplace as a setting for health promotion, e.g. the government's public health White Paper *Choosing Health: Making Healthy Choices Easier Choices* (Department of Health 2004) and *Health, Work and Wellbeing – Caring for our Future* (Department of Work and Pensions 2005). There are two approaches to health promotion in the workplace. The most common approach is to target individual lifestyles and behaviour within a workplace setting. This approach sees the workplace primarily as a site through which programmes can be delivered. The more challenging, but potentially more effective, approach is to target the workplace and its organization and culture. Health promotion in the workplace falls into the following categories:

- First aid and medical treatment
- Screening, e.g. bone density scanning
- Protection from accidents
- Control of hazards and infections
- Education and advice about healthy lifestyles and practices
- Policies and regulations to provide a healthier environment, e.g. catering choices
- Provision of services, e.g. exercise facilities, screening, counselling, smoking cessation.

Box 14.11

Examples of healthy workplace initiatives

- Provision of an online personalized health advice and information service
- Provision of an 'MOT' clinic at a railway station during rush hour, to encourage

women and especially men to attend for health check-ups

- Initiating physical activities in the workplace during lunch breaks, e.g. speed walks
- Encouraging healthy lifestyles through, for example, the provision of cycle racks, shower rooms, stair prompts to encourage staff to take the stairs rather than the lift, and healthy options in staff canteens and vending machines
- Changing the physical environment of the workplace to encourage exercise, e.g. situating key locations at an appreciable distance from one another (adapted from Dooris & Hunter 2007).

There is widespread acceptance of the require-ment to provide safe working conditions. Health promotion programmes in the workplace are still not widespread and are more likely in large work-places. Programmes include smoking cessation, alco-hol counselling, weight management, exercise and fitness interventions, general health screening and stress management courses.

 Box 14.12

A ban on smoking in all workplaces was introduced in England in 2007. Is legislation the most appropriate means to a healthy setting?

There is evidence that health promotion targeting the whole organization is more effective than tar-geting individual lifestyles (Noblet & LaMontagne 2006). Changing organizational culture and prac-tice, through more flexible working hours and break times, for example, has a more significant impact than programmes that assume individuals can make the necessary changes themselves, e.g. offering relaxation classes after working hours.

 Box 14.13

Workplace health promotion
The Director of Public Health and the Bristol North Primary Care Team worked collaboratively to introduce measures designed to help their staff cycle to work, and thereby embed physical activity in their daily routines. Measures included:
- New secure cycle parking facilities for 60 bikes (achieved through the removal of one car parking space)
- Provision of three 'pool' bikes and a web-based booking system
- Increase in cycle mileage rate to provide a financial incentive to cycle rather than drive
- Free cycling maps and advice on routes
- Annual bike-to-work events with free breakfasts

Within 1 year the number of employees cycling to work doubled, from 5% to 10% (Faculty of Public Health and Faculty of Occupational Medicine 2006).

The whole-organization approach has been recog-nized and endorsed at the highest level and by inter-national bodies. For example, the ENWHP adopted the Luxembourg Declaration on Workplace Health Promotion in 1997. The Declaration states that suc-cessful initiatives should follow these guidelines:
- Participation – all staff should be involved
- Integration – embedding health in all organizational areas, policies and decisions
- Project management – programmes to follow a problem-solving cycle of needs analysis, planning, implementation and evaluation
- Comprehensiveness – embraces individually focused and environmentally focused intitiatives.

In order to maximize the impact of workplace health promotion, the approach needs to shift from an exclusively individually focused lifestyle approach to a more comprehensive approach that includes whole-organization activities as well.

The evidence of effective health promotion inter-ventions in the workplace is building, although it remains rather scanty. The Department of Health (2004) has called for more rigorous evaluation of initiatives. A review of work-based health promotion programmes concluded that they have a positive impact, with a variety of risk factors including smoking being reduced amongst programme participants (Kreis & Bodeker 2004, cited in Department of Work and Pensions 2005).

Conclusion

The workplace is recognized as a key setting in which to promote health, due to both its reach (three-quarters of the working-age population are employed) and its importance in contributing directly and indirectly to people's health. Traditionally the focus has been on individually targeted programmes centred on hazards and the prevention of ill health. The challenge today is to broaden the focus to include the whole organizational setting and to move from ill health to positive health and well-being. There is a developing evidence base that demonstrates that such a comprehensive and multicomponent approach is effective. The proven benefits include not just better employee health, but also increased productivity and economic benefits to industry and society as a whole. Many different groups have a role to play in promoting health in the workplace, including workers, managers, employers, occupational health staff, health and safety officers and environmental health officers.

Questions for further discussion

- What are the potential benefits and limitations of health promotion in workplace settings?

- How should health promotion address the changes in work patterns in the 21st century (e.g. increased part-time working and short-term contracts, teleworking and home-working and increased information technology)?

- Think of a workplace with which you are familiar. Your task is to promote health within this workplace. What areas would you prioritize, and why? Who would you involve, and how?

Summary

This chapter has looked at the potential benefits to be gained from implementing health promotion within the workplace setting. The tension between interventions that focus on individual lifestyles and those that address the whole organization has been discussed. Evaluation studies have demonstrated that the whole-organization approach is more effective. The role of different partners in workplace health promotion has been identified and discussed.

Further reading

European Network for Health Promotion website is a useful resource for up-to-date information www.enwph.org.

The National Institute for Health and Clinical Excellence (NICE) has produced various documents synthesizing research evidence of effective health promotion practice in the workplace. Topics covered include smoking in the workplace, physical activity and mental health: www.nice.org.uk.

O'Donnell M P (ed) 2001 Health promotion in the workplace. Thomson Delmar Learning, Albany, New York. *This edited text provides a comprehensive overview of health promotion in the workplace, ranging from the practicalities of programme management and evaluation to discussion of the financial incentives.*

References

Department of Health 2004 Choosing health: making healthy choices easier. Stationery Office, London.

Department of Trade and Industry (DTI) 2007 Trade union membership 2006 report. HMSO, London.

Department of Trade and Industry Consultation Document 2007 Workplace representatives: a review of their facilities and facility time. HMSO, London.

Department of Work and Pensions 2005 Health, work and wellbeing – caring for our future. DWP, London.

Dooris M, Hunter D J 2007 Organisations and settings for promoting public health. In: Lloyd C E, Handsley S, Douglas J et al (eds) Policy and practice in promoting public health. Sage and the Open University, London. Chapter 4.

Elgood J, Gilby N O, Pearson H 2004 Attitudes towards health and safety: a quantitative survey of stakeholder opinion. Mori and HSE, London.

European Network for Workplace Health Promotion 1997 The Luxembourg Declaration on workplace health promotion in the European Union. European Network for Workplace Health Promotion, Luxembourg.

Faculty of Public Health 2005 Creating a healthy workplace: a guide for occupational safety and health professionals and employers. Available online at: www. fph.org.uk/policy_downloads/publications/reports/ healthy_workplaces_report_2006.pdf

Faculty of Public Health and Faculty of Occupational Medicine 2006 Creating a healthy workplace. FPH and FOM, London.

Health and Safety Commission 2007 Press release: HSC/E publishes health and safety statistics for 2006/07. Available online at: www.hse.gov.uk/press/2007

Health and Safety Executive (HSE) 2001 Tackling work related stress: a manager's guide to improving and maintaining employee health and well being. HSE Books, Sudbury.

Health and Safety Executive (HSE) 2005 Tackling stress: the management standards approach. HSE, London.

Health and Safety Executive (HSE) 2007 Achieving the 'Revitalising Health and Safety' targets: Statistical progress report, November 2007. Available online at: www.hse.gov.uk/statistics/pdf/prog

Institute of Occupational Medicine 2002 Survey of use of occupational health support. HSE Books, Sudbury, Suffolk.

Madouros V 2006 Projections of the UK labour force, 2006 to 2020. Labour Market Trends 114: 13–27.

Marmot M, Wilkinson R 2006 Social determinants of health, 2nd edn. Oxford University Press, Oxford.

Noblet A, LaMontagne A D 2006 The role of workplace health promotion in addressing job stress. Health Promotion International 21: 346–353.

Shain M, Kramer D M 2004 Health promotion in the workplace: framing the concept; reviewing the evidence. Occupational and Environmental Medicine 61: 643–648.

Waddell S, Burton A K 2006 Is work good for your health and well being? Occupational Health Review 24: 30–31.

Wanless D 2004 Securing good health for the whole population. Stationery Office, London.

Wilhelm K, Koves V et al., (2004) Work and Mental Health. Social Psychiatry and Epidemiology 39(11): 866–873.

Wilkinson R G 2006 The impact of inequality. Routledge, London.

Chapter Fifteen

Health promotion in neighbourhoods

Key points

- Definitions of neighbourhood
- Neighbourhoods as settings for health promotion
- Different aspects of neighbourhoods – physical, social, economic
- Evaluation of neighbourhood health promotion

OVERVIEW

As we have seen in other chapters in this part, healthy settings are physical and social settings, which serve as supportive environments for health and health promotion activities. This chapter examines the concept of neighbourhood and how different factors – physical, social and economic – contribute to the concept. The linked concept of social capital to describe neighbourly relationships and networks is explored. The popularity of neighbourhood in different policy and practice arenas in recent years, and the usefulness of the neighbourhood as a setting for health promotion, are discussed. Neighbourhoods include different levels or structures such as the neighbourhood environment, services and people, which may all be used as a springboard for health promotion. Examples of various initiatives which focus on the neighbourhood setting are given as examples of good practice. Evaluating such a multidimensional strategy poses many challenges,

and issues regarding the evaluation and evidence base for neighbourhood health promotion are discussed.

Healthy Cities are arguably the best known and largest of the settings approaches. The programme is a long-term international development initiative that aims to place health high on the agendas of decision-makers and to promote comprehensive local strategies for health improvement and sustainable development. The Healthy Villages programme addresses similar directives as the Healthy Cities programme in rural areas. Health is again defined by the area's residents; however, the generally accepted definition of a healthy village includes a community with low rates of infectious diseases, access to basic health care services, and a stable, peaceful social environment (see http://www.who.int/healthy_settings/types/en/index.html). In addition, the holistic and multifaceted linking of activities that characterizes the settings approach is used in schools, workplaces, hospitals (discussed in other chapters in this part) and also universities, markets, islands and homes. The neighbourhood provides a link between these and the other settings explored in this part. Neighbourhoods have been identified as important settings for health promotion in a number of English policy documents.

> *The environment we live in, our social networks, our sense of security, socio-economic circumstances, families and resources in our local neighbourhood can affect individual health* (Department of Health 2004, p. 77).

Box 15.1

The terms neighbourhood and community are frequently used. Are they the same thing?

Defining neighbourhoods

Box 15.2

- How would you define your neighbourhood?
- In what ways does your neighbourhood support health?
- In what ways does it compromise health?

Neighbourhoods are defined as small localities with a distinct identity forged by a community of people who know each other and the provision of essential services such as post offices, shops and health centres. Lay networks and support systems are an important element. Neighbourhoods will often be bounded by geographical features such as major roads, railways or green areas and may be urban or rural. The key factor is that residents define their local neighbourhood themselves and feel they have an investment in its future, the services provided and its appearance. In the modern world where transactions are increasingly fragmented and anonymous, and where the overarching symbols of community, such as religion and nationhood, are less cohesive and meaningful, the

role of the neighbourhood in promoting identity and self-esteem is more important. Neighbourhoods provide the immediate environment where people live, work and play, and for many more vulnerable groups, such as older people and those on low income, most of their lives are lived in one neighbourhood.

A recent research study (Robertson et al 2008) found that neighbourhood identity is established at an early stage in each neighbourhood's history and is resilient to change. Neighbourhood identity is largely based on residents' social class and status, which in turn is often based on men's employment patterns, as well as physical characteristics such as housing. Neighbourhoods are often internally differentiated and the sense of community is based on everyday social interactions and networks of friends, families and neighbours. Neighbourhoods therefore combine objective and subjective components.

There are many ways to get to know neighbourhoods, ranging from the objective gathering of statistics to the subjective collection of people's thoughts, feelings and memories. Local statistics on topics such as housing and crime are collected (see www.statistics.gov.uk) and can be used to compare different neighbourhoods. Community profiles or observation walks, where notes are taken of local facilities, the physical environment, transport routes and social networking opportunities, provide a more holistic picture of neighbourhoods.

Why neighbourhoods are a key setting for health promotion

Box 15.3

The public health White Paper *Choosing Health: Making Healthy Choices Easier* (Department of Health 2004) dedicates a chapter to communities (focusing on neighbourhoods) and makes a commitment to working through local communities to reduce inequalities in health. Why might neighbourhoods be identified as a key route through which to tackle health inequalities?

Neighbourhoods are a key setting for health promotion because they provide the infrastructure for health. Neighbourhoods are where the physical and social environments interact with service provision to provide an overall environment which has enormous potential to support people's health. Neighbourhoods include:

- *The physical environment*, e.g. the degree of air and noise pollution, quality of housing, amount of traffic and the availability of green space
- *The social environment* – the amount of social interaction between residents, the number of community or voluntary groups or organizations operating in the area and the extent of mutual self-help activities. The concept of social capital, which refers to relationships of trust and regard between people, and organizations they have contact with, is relevant to both the social environment and services provided
- *Services* provided in neighbourhoods include places such as shops, post offices, health services, places of worship, sports facilities, community halls, transport systems or outreach workers from statutory agencies, e.g. housing and welfare officers' weekly sessions held in the community hall.

Identifying what exactly it is about neighbourhoods that has an impact on well-being is difficult. Research suggests that people value neighbourhoods for their effect on quality of life, reflected through aspects such as friendliness, safety and quiet (Bowling et al 2006; Office of National Statistics 2007). In addition to providing the context for health, neighbourhoods are a popular setting because they are seen as a means to engage people in addressing their own health needs. A neighbourhood focus therefore fosters empowerment and independence, which are themselves health-promoting.

Box 15.4

Community development in Koonawarra
Healthy Cities Illawarra Australia is part of the World Health Organization Healthy Cities

programme launched in 1987. In 1999 the Koonawarra area was highlighted as having particular health and social issues and needs. Further research and collaboration with stakeholders (including residents, local MPs and service providers) led to a range of strategies. Achievements to date include:

- Breakfast programme launched and now self-funded by local business sponsors
- A Koori playgroup established and a local Koori family worker employed to run it
- A weekly gentle exercise programme
- Increased community participation in the Koonawarra Community Centre
- Community members developing skills and experience in, for example, running programmes, dealing with media and government (www.healthycitiesill.org.au).

The physical environment

Many aspects of the physical environment, such as buildings and land use, affect health. Transport patterns and car usage are linked to health. Cars contribute to climate change and have a negative impact on individuals' health. For example, in one rapidly developing area of China, those who bought a car gained 1.8 kg in weight (Rice & Grant 2007). Tackling issues such as dependence on private cars can seem a daunting proposition. UK car users, although a smaller percentage of the population than in other European countries, use their cars more frequently. However, the importance of weaning ourselves away from overdependence on cars has been recognized in a number of policies (Department for Transport 2000, Department of Health 2004) and strategies to combat this dependence and encourage active means of transport have been proposed (Department for Transport 2004, Department of Health 2005). Goals include ensuring the provision of high-quality routes for walkers and cyclists and making public spaces and the countryside seem more attractive.

Box 15.5

Walking the Way to Health

Walking the Way to Health was launched by the British Heart Foundation and Natural England to encourage people to take part in locally designed walks. Health care professionals are encouraged to 'prescribe' pedometers to act as an incentive. The benefits of this programme include:

- Promotes active lifestyles and physical exercise
- Improves self-image and social relationships
- Promotes neighbourliness and social interaction – helping to turn places into communities
- Tackles social isolation
- Discourages antisocial behaviour through more people being out and about
- Is a reason to conserve wildlife and enhance the character of local places (www.naturalengland.org.uk; www.whi.org.uk).

The impact of housing on health has been known since the 19th century and the role of housing as a key determinant of health is discussed in our companion volume (Naidoo & Wills 2005). Poor-quality housing is often sited in deprived neighbourhoods with few local amenities. Graffiti, litter, boarded-up premises and dog mess are all signs of a neglected environment which, in turn, affects people's perception of the safety of their neighbourhood, and hence their willingness to be active participants within it. These issues often rank high on community' agendas.

A national strategy on neighbourhood renewal included a 10-year programme to tackle unemployment, crime and poor physical environments, and to manage housing in neighbourhoods (the New Deal for Communities (NDC)). NDC areas are relatively disadvantaged and all NDC initiatives include integrated health programmes. The NDC strategy has a £50 million budget and covers 39 localities with populations of approximately 8000–10 000 people.

The social environment

The quality of life in a community is a powerful determinant of health. By studying several healthy communities, Wilkinson (1996) has identified several factors which contribute to that quality of life.

Box 15.6

Quality of life in communities

The small town of Roseto, Pennsylvania, USA (1600 people) is cited as an example of a community with markedly lower death rates from heart attacks than neighbouring areas. The population of Roseto is made up of Italian-Americans descended from migrants from the Italian town of Roseto in Southern Italy. It differed from other towns because it was 'remarkably close knit … with a sense of common purpose … [with] a camaraderie which precluded ostentation [and] … a concern for neighbours ensuring no one was ever abandoned … the family as the hub and bulwark of life provided a security and insurance against any catastrophe'. Roseto's considerable health advantage only seems explicable in relation to these social characteristics. As the younger people moved away, community and family ties broke down and people became more concerned with material values and conspicuous consumption (Bruhn & Wolf 1979, cited in Wilkinson 1996, p. 116).

Social capital refers to social cohesion and the cumulative experience of relationships, with both those known to us and those who are strangers, that are characterized by mutual trust, acceptance, approval and respect. People are social beings and the quality of social interaction is vital to both personal and communal well-being. Social capital provides the foundation for collective action in the public sphere for the public good. Although definitions of social capital vary, the main indicators are:

- Social relationships and social support
- Formal and informal networks

- Community and civic engagement, including voluntary associations
- Trust and neighbourliness.

Community networks may be built around activities associated with school, leisure or living in a particular locality. Parents, especially mothers, have been identified as particularly active in forging neighbourhood links (Robertson et al 2008). In addition to their primary purpose, buildings such as schools or leisure facilities are often used to house additional community events and networks. The closure of services such as schools and post offices therefore has a negative impact on neighbourliness, and this might help to explain the strength of feeling voiced whenever communities are threatened with the closure of such amenities.

There is evidence that building social capital is only possible above a certain threshold of income. If people are preoccupied with survival in its crudest meaning (i.e. ensuring they are fed, warm, sheltered and safe) they will be unable to focus beyond, on broader communal issues. The fact that social capital is not always benign also has to be acknowledged. Drug dealing and criminality on many housing estates rely on strong, closely integrated networks.

Box 15.7

The following criteria have been identified as central to the building of cohesive communities. To what extent are they evident where you live?
- A sense of belonging for all communities
- The diversity of people's backgrounds and circumstances is appreciated and valued
- Those from different backgrounds have similar life opportunities
- Strong and positive relationships are developed between people from different backgrounds (www.communities.gov.uk).

If social capital and trust are at the positive end of a neighbourhood quality-of-life spectrum, crime and fear of crime are at the opposite negative end.

Box 15.8

Research has linked poorer self-rated health with what have been called neighbourhood psychosocial stressors – fear of crime, feeling unsafe, nuisance from neighbours, drug misuse and youngsters hanging around (Agyemang et al 2007). What neighbourhood activities could be undertaken to improve health?
Effective measures might include:
- Preschool education, which has been shown to have a long-term effect on reducing criminal behaviour in adulthood
- Community policing, which involves local communities and may itself promote social cohesion
- Modifying the physical environment and increased surveillance, e.g. street lighting, concierge schemes
- Providing leisure activities for young people (e.g. drama, sports and music clubs) to occupy them and take them off the streets.

Both crime and the fear of crime are health hazards and are associated with negative effects, including depression and mental ill health. It has been suggested that negative effects are both direct, e.g. stress and depression, and indirect, e.g. mental health linked to social isolation and feelings of vulnerability. Acts of thoughtlessness and disregard, such as excessive noise or petty disputes, although less severe than violence or the threat of violence, can have a large impact on quality of life. The UK government has launched the Respect programme to tackle antisocial behaviour. It includes a range of actions, including working with 'problem families', keeping public spaces clean and safe and ensuring that victims and witnesses of antisocial behaviour are protected and supported.

Services

An adequate service infrastructure is essential to the health and life of a neighbourhood. If essential services, such as shops and post offices, are not available locally, people are forced to travel outside the area, leading to a loss of social contacts as well as incurring additional costs (time and travel). This has been recognized by many communities fighting to retain local schools or shops and by the Social Exclusion Unit (1998) in its NDC. However, many planning decisions appear not to recognize this fact. In particular, the increase in out-of-town supermarkets has had a severe impact on both small local shopping outlets and traffic rates.

 Box 15.9

Identify some examples of capacity building in a local community with which you are familiar.
 Examples that you might have included are:
- Managing services, e.g. tenants acting as housing managers
- Creating jobs, e.g. business start-up schemes
- Protecting the environment, e.g. recycling schemes
- Health and safety, e.g. community safety audits
- Responding to poverty, e.g. credit unions.

In all these examples the neighbourhood has become the focus for the creation of networks and for linking health and regeneration.

There is great potential in building health into community activities, such as adult education, leisure activities and cultural activities. The following example shows how community arts can collaborate with health workers to promote neighbourhood health.

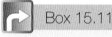 Box 15.10

Bolton street library
Residents of a Bolton estate took part in a 2-week project to create a 'street library'. The library was created by interviewing people about the book they would like to write or make. Interviews were recorded and transcribed and then printed as mini-books with a card cover. Participants commented on their sense of achievement and the opportunity to get to know their neighbours (www.beacons.idea.gov.uk).

It could be argued that any neighbourhood development work has the potential to promote health by increasing social contacts and trust, or social capital. Additional spin-offs in terms of direct support for healthy lifestyles are common, as the following example shows.

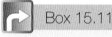 Box 15.11

Community gardens
Community gardens exist in many nations and in both urban and rural areas. They may fulfil a number of functions, including leisure gardens, child and school gardens, healing and therapy gardens, demonstration gardens and those concerned with ecological restoration. They are actively supported by specific communities, reflecting some form of mutual aid and communal reciprocity, probably having had a fair degree of altruism in getting them started and, very often, supported by charitable or municipal grant aid. They may also be grassroots initiatives aimed to revitalize low- to moderate-income neighbourhoods in urban settings. Community gardens have been shown to improve health by increasing participants' access to fruit and vegetables, providing the opportunity for regular exercise and communal interaction, and enabling economic self-reliance through using the gardens for training and recreation purposes and selling surplus produce (McGlone et al 1999; Ferris et al 2001).

Evaluating neighbourhood work

 Box 15.12

You have been asked to evaluate a neighbourhood development programme that has included reconfiguring local transport networks in order to encourage active forms of transport and neighbourliness. The programme includes different elements: setting up cycle routes and road-calming measures (e.g. speed bumps and narrowing of roads), a walk-to-school project and walking buddies to encourage older people to exercise. How would you go about evaluating such a programme? What challenges would you have to address?

Evaluation of neighbourhood and community work is extremely difficult for several reasons. Firstly, neighbourhood work involves long-term processes to promote social cohesion and regeneration. Funding long-term evaluation projects, and maintaining continuity of focus and resources, is difficult. Many projects are set up under time-limited funding initiatives, which then compromises their sustainability (e.g. Healthy Living Centres were funded through lottery money). Projects may find they are diverted from their core business into fund-raising in order to keep going. Funding streams may also specify certain activities or outcomes, leading to the neglect of long-term activities to build community capacity and networks.

In any consideration of the effect of neighbourhood on health it is very difficult to separate the effects of compositional factors (those relating to the kinds of individual being studied, including their socioeconomic status and lifestyles) from the effects of contextual factors (those relating to the environment) (Kawachi & Berkman 2003). There is a clear bias in research towards considering the impact of compositional factors. The complexity of relationships between individuals and environments, plus the long timescale in which effects become apparent, militates against research into contextual factors. There are some attempts to carry out research into contextual factors, including multilevel analysis, but it remains very difficult to attribute cause and effect in neighbourhood work.

Finally, the complexity of neighbourhood work is also a factor leading to difficulties in evaluation:

Responding to diverse evaluative expectations, while sustaining research integrity and rigour, requires a pragmatic multi-methods approach, responsiveness to local context, regular communication between funders, community stakeholders and evaluators, and flexible, reflective practice (Adams et al 2007).

However, even given these caveats, the evidence base for neighbourhood work having a positive impact on health is rather thin. Notions such as deprivation amplification (whereby low social class leads to poor access to amenities) have been challenged by the literature, which finds that the reverse can be the case (Macintyre & Ellaway 2003). Reviews differ as to the extent of area effects on health from modest to significant (Pickett & Pearl 2001; Riva et al 2007).

Conclusion

The neighbourhood provides a valuable setting for accessing many vulnerable groups, including older people and people on low income. Neighbourhoods are real-life settings with the potential for priorities to be defined by residents rather than professionals. Addressing health on a neighbourhood basis is attractive because it means addressing core determinants of health, such as the social fabric and quality of people's lives. It is important that in the new focus on neighbourhood settings the opportunity to address people's self-defined needs is taken. It would be easy to use neighbourhoods merely as a means of professional outreach work, but this would be to neglect one of the great strengths of this setting.

Box 15.13

Many members of the primary care team (especially health visitors and GPs) regard themselves as working with neighbourhood communities. How might their role change if they were to focus on community capacity building and building social capital?

Whilst there are many advantages to working within a neighbourhood setting, it is not a universal panacea. Many factors which affect people's lives are determined at national level, e.g. level of benefit entitlement or availability of employment. However, the neighbourhood setting does offer opportunities for creative and imaginative ways of working which support the core principles of health promotion – participation, equity, empowerment and collaboration.

Questions for further discussion

- What health promotion resources can neighbourhoods offer?

- What are the advantages and limitations of using a neighbourhood setting for health promotion?

Summary

This chapter has identified neighbourhoods as a key setting for health promotion and discussed reasons for its popularity. Government initiatives focusing on neighbourhoods, such as NDC, have been considered. Examples of innovative practice centred on neighbourhood work have been given and the problems of evaluating such work discussed.

Further reading

Gowman N 1999 Healthy neighbourhoods. Kings Fund, London. *Although a little dated, this is a useful summary of the arguments for neighbourhoods as a healthy setting. The document can be downloaded from http://www.kingsfund.org.uk/publications/kings_fund_publications/healthy.html.*

Macintyre S, Ellaway A 2003 Neighbourhoods and health: an overview. In Kawachi I, Berkman L F (eds) Neighbourhoods and health. Oxford University Press, Oxford, pp. 20–43. *A useful summary of the evidence for neighbourhoods impacting on health, covering both theoretical and methodological issues.*

Stewart M 2007 Neighbourhood renewal and regeneration. In Orme J, Powell J, Taylor P et al Public health in the 21st century: new perspectives on policy, participation and practice. McGraw Hill/Open University Press, Berkshire, pp. 170–184. *An account of the development of neighbourhood intitiatives, exploring their role in tackling inequalities and building social capital and partnership working.*

Useful websites include the following:

www.jrf.org.uk/knowledge/findings/housing is the website for the Joseph Rowntree Foundation, which conducts research into neighbourhoods and communities.

www.neighbourhood.gov.uk is the government website for neighbourhood renewal.

www.renewal.net is a guide to neighbourhood renewal.

Issues of definition and measurement of social capital at http://www.nice.org.uk/page.aspx?o=502681

References

Adams J, Witten K, Conway K 2007 Community development as health promotion: evaluating a complex locality-based project in New Zealand. Community Development Journal 10.1093/cdj/bsm049

Agyemang C, van Hooijdonk C, Wendel-Vos W et al 2007 The association of neighbourhood psychosocial stressors and self-rated health in Amsterdam, The Netherlands. Journal of Epidemiology and Community Health 61: 1042–1049.

Bowling A, Barber J, Morris R et al 2006 Do perceptions of neighbourhood environment influence health. Journal of Epidemiology and Community Health 60: 476–483.

Department of Health (DoH) 2004 Choosing health: making healthy choices easier. DoH, London.

Department of Health (DoH) 2005 Choosing activity: a physical activity action plan. DoH, London.

Department for Transport 2000 Transport 2010: Meeting the local transport challenge. DfT, London.

Department for Transport 2004 Walking and cycling: an action plan. DfT, London.

Ferris J, Norman C, Sempik J 2001 People, land and sustainability: community gardens and the social dimensions of sustainable development. Social Policy and Administration 35: 559–568.

Kawachi I, Berkman L F (eds) 2003 Neighbourhoods and health. Oxford University Press, Oxford.

Macintyre S, Ellaway A 2003 Neighbourhoods and health: an overview. In Kawachi I, Berkman L F (eds) Neighbourhoods and health. Oxford University Press, Oxford, pp. 20–43.

McGlone P, Dobson B, Dowler E et al 1999 Food projects and how they work. Joseph Rowntree Foundation, York.

Naidoo J, Wills J 2005 Public health and health promotion: developing practice. BaillièreTindall, London.

Office of National Statistics 2007 West of Scotland twenty-07 study NOS, London (see details at: http://www.sphsu.mrc.ac.uk/studies/2007_study/).

Pickett K E, Pearl M 2001 Multilevel analyses of neighbourhood socioeconomic context and health outcomes: a critical review. Journal of Epidemiology and Community Health 55: 111–122.

Rice C, Grant M 2007 The potential of car-free developments: practicalities and health impacts. WHO collaborating Centre for Healthy Cities and Urban Policy, Bristol.

Riva M, Gauvin L, Barnett T A 2007 Toward the next generation of research into small area effects on health: a synthesis of multilevel investigations published since July 1998. Journal of Epidemiology and Community Health 61: 853–861.

Robertson D, Smyth J, McIntosh I 2008 Neighbourhood identity: people, time and place Joseph Rowntree Foundation, Available online at: http://www.jrf.org.uk/bookshop/eBooks/2154-neighbourhood-identity-regeneration.pdf.

Social Exclusion Unit 1998 Bringing Britain together: a national strategy for neighbourhood renewal. Stationery Office, London.

Wilkinson R G 1996 Unhealthy societies: the afflictions of inequality. Routledge, London.

Chapter Sixteen

Health promotion in primary care and hospitals

Key points

- The concept of a health-promoting hospital
- Promoting the health of patients
- Promoting the health of staff
- Hospitals and their community
- Hospitals as a health-promoting organization
- Health-Promoting Hospital movement.

OVERVIEW

To change a large and complex organization such as a hospital from being a place of treatment to one where health gain is valued and seen as part of its purpose is a challenging process. Health-promoting hospitals (HPHs) incorporate a variety of different projects, but with the same overall aims:

- To make the hospital a healthier working and living environment for its large workforce and for patients
- To expand self-management, recuperation and rehabilitation programmes
- To encourage participation by staff and patients
- To provide information and advice on health issues
- To act as a community resource and agent of social cohesion

- To act in a socially responsible manner especially in relation to environmental impact.

A hospital, like a school or a workplace, is a social system with its own procedures, culture and values. The process of developing an HPH will thus involve the adaptation of management structures, top-level political commitment and the facilitation of greater participation by staff and patients.

Defining a health promoting hospital

Settings can normally be identified as having physical boundaries (including geographical), a range of people with defined roles and an organizational structure. As we have seen earlier in this part, a settings approach is not about doing a health promotion project such as a display for No Smoking Day nor is it about delegating health promotion to specific departmental or staff 'champions' (Johnson & Baum 2001), although both activities may be used as part of wider development. The settings approach to health promotion focuses on bringing about holistic organizational and practice changes to create a more health-promoting environment. The challenge lies in convincing hospital authorities that health promotion does not constitute an additional burden but is very much part of the core business and approach.

The World Health Organization (WHO) definition (Nutbeam 1998) provides a useful starting point for understanding what is required:

> A health-promoting hospital does not only provide high quality comprehensive medical and nursing services, but also develops a corporate identity that embraces the aims of health promotion, develops a health-promoting organizational structure and culture, including active, participatory roles for patients and all members of staff, develops itself into a health-promoting physical environment, and actively cooperates with its community.

The hospital as a setting for health was validated by the launch of the Health Promoting Hospitals (HPH) initiative in 1990 by the WHO Regional Office for Europe. This network now includes 669 institutions in 39 countries. In this chapter, the potential of the hospital setting to promote health is examined and examples of good practice are given to illustrate what can be achieved.

Why hospitals are a key setting for health promotion

Many health practitioners assume that health promotion has always been a core task of medicine in general and hospitals in particular. Yet health promotion can be at odds with the hospital context which is based on a medical model of care with an orientation towards cure and treatment. The expectation of the patient role has been one of 'passivity, trust and a willingness to wait for medical help' (Latter 2001, p. 78):

- Staff competence, job remit, and time are mainly dedicated to clinical work and care.
- Patient contact with the hospital staff is generally based on brief 'consultations' related to their particular disease.
- Patients in hospital are at a late stage in their disease and highlighting prevention may make them feel responsible and blameworthy.
- Hospitals are not in themselves healthy environments.

Yet hospitals are also a natural focus for health promotion:

- 20% of the population will visit a local hospital as a patient within a single year, and a further percentage will visit the hospital as family and friends.
- Hospitals are often the biggest employer in their community. In Europe, at least 3% of the entire workforce is employed at one of the 30 000 hospitals.
- Contact is with patients at a time of heightened awareness about health and illness, when they may be motivated to make major lifestyle changes.
- Staff are respected and credible.

Box 16.1

What might be the benefits of being an HPH?

There has been a shift in recent years away from an emphasis on the compliant patient to one which is more patient-centred that acknowledges patients' concerns and their own expertise (see Chapter 9 for an outline of the Expert Patient programme). Considerable evidence exists to show that patient outcomes are much improved when patients are involved in their own care and have adequate explanations and time to discuss their concerns (Coulter 2002;

Coulter & Ellins 2007 and see www.pickereurope. org). Researchers from Denmark, for example, showed in various randomized controlled trials that complications and length of stay after surgery were reduced when smokers or heavy drinkers underwent cessation programmes before surgery (Moller et al 2002). A major proportion of hospital admissions are related to patients suffering from one or more chronic diseases. These patients require support to cope with their disease and to achieve some changes in lifestyle, adherence to possibly complicated drug and nutrition regimes and management of their condition. There is evidence that patients are more receptive to information and advice in situations of acute ill health. Although hospitals may appear to be 'downstream', the hospital thus provides a 'window of opportunity' for patients to understand the potential benefits of behaviour change.

Box 16.2

Emergency care
The role of an Emergency Department (ED) or Accident and Emergency (A&E) unit is to provide treatment and care for the acutely ill and injured promptly at any time. This downstream focus paradoxically enables the ED to be a suitable setting for health promotion because it is an established entry point to the health system and because it tends to have good links into the community. Bensburg & Kennedy (2002) offer numerous examples of health promotion strategies from risk assessment (young people and alcohol) to health information (triage nurses providing information to carers who are high users of emergency paediatric services, including a follow-up appointment after discharge), to health education (asthma management training and follow-up telephone calls and using the waiting room to promote reading and literacy to children).

An HPH will also have benefits for its staff and community. Staff sickness/absence rates are likely to be lower, and staff retention is likely to be better. Local communities will benefit from having a large, responsible and responsive employer in their area. HPHs will bring income into local communities (through workforce wages), demonstrate how large organizations can be environmentally aware (through, for example, recycling and local sourcing of food) and provide an accessible and local source of expertise regarding health matters.

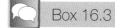

Box 16.3

Existing performance management measures for hospitals relate to productivity such as number of emergency admissions, unnecessary procedures and inpatient bed stays. What might be indicators of an HPH?

An HPH would be evident in the following core principles, outlined in the Vienna Recommendations (WHO 1997):

- Acknowledges differences in the needs, values and cultures of different population groups
- Promotes dignity and empowerment
- Forms as close links as possible with other levels of the health care system and the community.

Although hospitals will always be places of treatment and the pressure to reduce length of stay may limit health education opportunities, they are still numerous ways in which the setting can be more conducive to health.

The WHO HPH movement focuses on four areas (Pelikan et al 2001):

1. Promoting the health of patients

2. Promoting the health of staff

3. Changing the organization to a health-promoting setting

4. Promoting the health of the community in the catchment area of the hospital.

Promoting the health of patients

The main focus of most health promotion in hospitals is disease management and prevention for patients (Johnson 2000). But even in case of severe diseases, patients are always partly healthy (whether emotionally, socially, spiritually) when they enter the hospital and these aspects (e.g. of self-care, psychological well-being or social contact) can be maintained.

In many health care settings, including hospitals, health promotion strategies are often referred to as opportunistic when a chance has arisen to offer health education or other preventive action during a clinical visit. There are, however, opportunities for more coordinated intervention strategies such as risk assessment for alcohol-related problems or the offer of Chlamydia screening.

Professionals play a minor role in promoting the health of their patients however; the major contributors to patients' health are themselves, their relatives and friends. Empowering patients to get involved as partners and (co)producers of their health in decision-making and diagnostic and therapeutic processes, through the provision of information and education, is therefore an important health promotion strategy.

Box 16.4

Describe how the following activities might be implemented in hospital:
- Risk assessment
- Health information
- Health education and counselling
- Maximizing choice
- Promoting involvement and participation
- Reducing social isolation
- Tackling inequalities.

Actions such as co-designing pre-admission information with patients, offering computer-based decision aids for treatment options and patient involvement in infection control illustrate how health promotion principles of being equitable, empowering and participatory can become the basis of hospital practice. Maintaining patients' positive health with greater consideration of their quality of life and psychosocial functioning includes:

- Securing personal privacy (e.g. data protection, curtains around beds)
- Providing animal therapy
- Providing offers and options to encourage psychosocial activities of patients (e.g. cultural activities, religious services, patient libraries, discussions, patient internet café)
- Bringing humour into the hospital, e.g. by clown doctors
- Using the arts or art as therapy
- Providing adequate visiting hours for family members, friends or peers, lay carers
- Providing the possibility for caring relatives or friends to stay in the hospital (especially for very vulnerable groups of patients, e.g. children, terminally ill patients)
- Organizing visiting and lay support services for unattended patients
- Providing psychological and social assistance to cope with stress or anxieties related to the hospital stay or to the patient's specific disease (e.g. cancer, terminal illness) or to the patient's general life situation (e.g. loss of work due to disease) by specialized personnel (e.g. clinical psychologists, social workers, pastoral carers) (http://www.hph-hc.cc/Downloads/HPH-Publications/wp-strategies-final.pdf).

One of the poorer aspects of hospital care that is frequently cited by patients is the provision of food.

Box 16.5

Food in hospital
Intake of nutritious food is crucial for patients recovering after surgery or medical interventions.

Yet over the past few years there has been considerable concern about patient malnutrition, poor-quality food and poor hygiene standards amongst hospital food suppliers. The Council of Europe passed Resolution ResAP (2003) on food and nutritional care in hospitals. In the UK the Better Hospital Food programme was launched in 2001 (www.nhsestates/better_hospital_food).

National Health Service (NHS) trusts spend about £250 million a year on food alone, or £500 million on food, contract and catering staff costs. They serve about 300 million patient meals a year in about 1200 hospitals, as well as several million meals to staff and visitors. According to the Kings Fund (Jochelson et al 2005), food procurement in the NHS is still driven by price. Some hospitals spend only £2 a day on food per patient. Poor-quality food that is overcooked or lukewarm by the time it reaches patients often ends up in the bin. Uneaten meals cost about £18 million a year. If food preparation waste and labour are included, the price of uneaten food rises to over £144 million a year. In Europe organic and local food procurement is commonplace. The UK is slowly adopting the concept of corporate social responsibility which includes sustainability for the NHS (Department of Health 2004, pp. 60–68).

Accessing health care is also a concern for patients. 1.4 million people miss, turn down or do not seek hospital appointments because of problems with transport. Of those without a car, 31% have difficulties travelling to their local hospital, compared to 17% with a car (Social Exclusion Unit 2003). With the concentration of acute facilities into fewer and larger units, such problems are likely to increase. Others may not access care because of barriers of language or fears of discrimination. A low service uptake may be due to a service not meeting needs and not being adapted to take account of diverse cultures and religions. The articulated needs of minority groups focus on communication, information, account to be taken of religion, dietary preferences and consent (Bhopal 2007).

Promoting the health of staff

The hospital as a physical and social setting also has an impact on the health of staff. Hospitals are potentially dangerous workplaces, encompassing physical risks (e.g. exposure to biological, chemical, nuclear agents), mental risks (e.g. stress, night shifts) and social risks (e.g. night shifts have a negative impact on social life, bullying, violence against staff).

Box 16.6

Shift work

Shift work is a feature for all hospital staff. The Hospital at Night project was introduced to find ways of reducing trainee doctors' working hours to comply with the European Working Time Directive (WTD). The law states that, by 2009, junior doctors must not work more than 48 hours a week. Hospital at Night redefined how medical cover is provided in hospitals during the out-of-hours period. It moved away from cover defined by professional demarcation and grade, to cover that is defined by competency.

Other aspects of the environment that affect the health of staff are less addressed. For example, patients, staff, visitors and the local community are also affected by the physical environment of the hospital setting, including its functionality and aesthetic design. In 1859 Florence Nightingale commented:

People say the effect is on the mind. It is no such thing. The effect is on the body, too. Little as we know about the way in which we are affected by form, colour, by light, we do know this, that they have a physical effect. Variety of form and brilliancy of colour in the objects presented to patients is the actual means of recovery.

For many of today's patients, visitors and staff, however, the hospital environment remains soulless, drab and depressing. One report (Commission on Architecture and the Built Environment 2004) highlighted the following as key factors in the poor working environment:

- Fluorescent lighting
- Noise
- Lack of independent control over ventilation
- No facility for exercise.

Gardens have long been attached to hospitals for therapeutic uses. In one study Ulrich (1984) found that the surgical patients who had a window view of the outdoors were discharged earlier, took fewer painkillers and received fewer negative evaluations from nurses than matched patients in similar rooms that faced a brick wall. Similarly, staff frequently cite the lack of access to a green space in which to relax as a feature of their poor work environment. Johnson & Baum (2001) reported on the activities of Adelaide Hospital which sought to address this through lunchtime walking groups and staff aerobic classes. These activities were organized by the corporate services division of the hospital, which wished to be seen as a caring employer, rather than any coordinated vision of an HPH.

Box 16.7

Violence against health care staff is increasingly common and may include verbal abuse, threats and physical assaults. Those working in A&E and psychiatry are most likely to suffer abuse. What could a hospital do to protect the health of its staff?

The most common response is one of zero tolerance, a message which is promoted through publicity campaigns and education programmes for staff who are encouraged to report violent incidents with formal protocols for documentation of violent episodes. Although such programmes are seen to be protecting the health of staff, they are not tackling the systemic issues that give rise to these events.

Early studies of nursing, for example, focused on the profession's lack of power. The explanation for this was said to lie in nursing's predominantly female workforce, its function as the alleged hand-maiden to medicine, and because it had absorbed the values of its own activities which assumed a level of passivity and compliance.

Box 16.8

Kanter (1977) suggests that organizations can be empowering or disempowering and there are key tools which help to generate power which include:
- Access to information
- Support
- Resources
- Opportunity (e.g. for further learning).
How empowered do you consider hospital nurses?

The hospital and the community

The hospital also has an impact on the health of people living and working in the surrounding neighbourhood. The largest capital development programme in the history of the NHS means large car parks, energy-intensive air conditioning, heating and lighting as well as huge quantities of waste. Sustainability is central to the development of an HPH.

Hospitals can further promote health in their community by:

- Systematically contributing to health reporting (e.g. frequency and causes of accidents on roads help to create a data linkage with transport and planning)
- Organizing specific action programmes (e.g. information, counselling, training) in cooperation with schools, other health care providers and local community groups, e.g. dump campaigns (getting rid of unused medicines), promoting baby car seats, asthma management
- Being a responsible, health-promoting and ethical employer.

Organizational health promotion

The hospital is however not just a site for health promotion activities but a social entity that creates health. An HPH must therefore incorporate the vision, concepts, values and basic strategies of health promotion (equity, empowerment, participation and collaboration as well as sustainability) into the structures and culture of the hospital and thus health becomes its outcome (Figure 16.1).

Box 16.9

An ecological social systems approach of developing a healthy setting requires both change from the top in relation to organizational development and political commitment and change from the bottom from high-visibility innovative projects, engagement of all users of the setting and establishing the values of HPH into the institutional agenda and core business. HPH could be linked and combined with other strategies of hospital development (e.g. health education, patients' rights, self-help movements, health at work, hospital hygiene, the ecological and sustainable development movement, strategies for personal and organizational development, quality management) Dooris (2006).

Box 16.10

In pairs practise the following role play in which one of the pair is the Chief Nurse who has been asked to address the hospital board and must give five reasons why the hospital should become an HPH. The other partner is the hospital Chief Executive who must give five reasons why an HPH is not a good idea.

The HPH movement

The HPH network, launched by the WHO European Regional Office in 1990, now operates in 39 countries on all continents. This initiative seeks to promote good practice by developing concepts and strategies, developing and disseminating model projects and networking via conferences and newsletters (www.healthpromotinghospital.org). The HPH focuses on the health of staff, patients and its local community.

Hospitals accepted into the HPH network have to meet certain conditions (WHO 2004):

- Develop a written policy for health promotion; develop and evaluate an HPH action plan to support the introduction of health promotion into the culture of the hospital/health service during the 4-year period of designation
- Identify a hospital/health service coordinator for the coordination of HPH development and activity; and pay the annual contribution fee for the coordination of the International HPH Network
- Share information and experience on national and international level, i.e. HPH development, models of good practice (projects) and the implementation of standards/indicators.

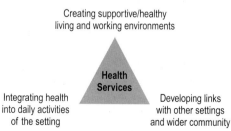

Creating supportive/healthy
living and working environments

Health
Services

Integrating health
into daily activities
of the setting

Developing links
with other settings
and wider community

Figure 16.1 • Health-promoting health services.

Box 16.11

Think of a hospital with which you are familiar. Does it promote health in the ways outlined above? What do you think might be barriers to extending its health-promoting role?

- Is there evidence to support a patient education programme?
- What are the key elements of such a programme – diet, exercise, stress management, medication?
- Are staff trained and motivated to deliver such a programme?
- Does everyone know about the programme and understand their role in supporting it?
- Is the ward and hospital environment supportive for both staff and patients, e.g. are there healthy food options on menus?
- Do patients and their families participate in rehabilitation programmes and are their concerns acknowledged and addressed?
- Are links made with local communities and services to support patients when they leave hospital?

The complex organizational structures of many hospitals and the fact that most health professionals in the hospital setting do not readily associate health promotion as part of their role make the HPH a challenging setting. Whitehead (2004) argues that the hospital setting is the least visible of all the Ottawa Charter settings and 'there is little empirical evidence of a measurable health impact' of policies focused on creating healthy environments as part of HPH (Dooris 2006, citing McKee 2000). In order to realize its full potential, the HPH strategy needs to be implemented not only within limited projects, but also embedded as an integral aspect of hospital service (quality) management systems (WHO 2004). Many hospitals now define themselves as an HPH, employ a coordinator, have specific projects (e.g. being smokefree or migrant-friendly) and endeavour to be learning organizations.

Conclusion

Although core activities of hospitals remain focused on medical diagnosis and treatment, the HPH concept has taken root and there are many examples of hospitals embracing health promotion principles. Health-promoting initiatives occur at all levels, from individual practitioners using checklists to include health promotion systematically in client contacts, to hospital-wide initiatives to increase service user participation and reduce environmental impact. In between lies a range of activities at ward or departmental level, including the use of arts therapies and the provision of healthy locally sourced food. All initiatives are guided by core health promotion principles: a holistic concept of health, empowerment, participation, intersectoral collaboration, equity and sustainability.

The HPH needs to be supported by an organizational structure: support from management, a budget, specific aims and targets and action plans for implementing health promotion into everyday business. All hospital staff need to make health promotion their business. This can be a challenge, particularly for staff in acute settings who are trained in other (diagnosis and treatment) priorities (Latter 2001). Treating health promotion as one specific quality aspect to be monitored can aid its incorporation into core processes. Integrating health impact assessments into all decision-making within the hospital will also help to advance the HPH.

Questions for further discussion

- Take one of the core health promotion principles (equity, collaboration, participation and empowerment) and consider how activities built on this principle could be integrated into a hospital with which you are familiar.

- What are the advantages and disadvantages of health promotion in hospital settings?

Summary

This chapter has looked at the reasons for prioritizing hospital settings for health promotion. Recent national and international policy developments which affect the delivery of health promotion in health service settings, and the range of professionals involved, have been identified. Ways in which health promotion principles may be applied in health service settings have been discussed and illustrated with examples.

Further reading

Gröne O, Garcia-Barbero M (eds). Evidence and quality management. WHO, Copenhagen2005. *Summarises evidence on HPH and knowledge on implementation of the concept implementation.*

Scriven A, Orme J (eds). Health promotion: professional perspectives. Macmillan/Open University Press, Hampshire2001. *Section 2 on the health service looks at the potential for health promotion in different health service settings including primary health care and hospitals.*

World Health Organization 1991 Budapest declaration on health promoting hospitals. *First policy paper on HPH; outlines target groups, basic principles and action areas.*

World Health Organization 1997 Vienna recommendations on health promoting hospitals. Adapted HPH policy to the structure of national/regional networks. Available online at: http://www.euro.who.int/document//IHB/hphviennarecom.pdf.

World Health Organization 2004 Standards for health promotion in hospitals. WHO office for Europe, Copenhagen. Available online at: http://www.euro.who.int/document/e82490.pdf

World Health Organization 2006 Putting HPH policy into action: working paper. WHO Collaborating Centre on Health Promotion in Hospitals and Health Care, Vienna. *Theory-driven background paper on 18 HPH core strategies, including examples and selected evidence.*

World Health Organization 2007 Integrating health promotion into hospitals and health services. Concept, framework and organization. WHO Office for Europe, Copenhagen.

Health Promotion Hospital websites: www.euro.who.int/healthpromohosp; www.hph-hc.cc

References

Bensberg M, Kennedy M 2002 A framework for health promoting emergency departments. Health Promotion International 17: 179–188.

Bhopal R 2007 Ethnicity, race and health in multicultural societies. Oxford University Press, Oxford.

Commission on Architecture and the Built Environment 2004 The role of hospital design in the recruitment, retention and performance of NHS nurses in England. Available online at: www.cabe.org.uk or www.healthyhospitals.org.uk

Coulter A 2002 The autonomous patient: ending paternalism in medical care. Nuffield Trust/TSO, London.

Coulter A, Ellins J 2007 Effectiveness of strategies for informing educating, and involving patients. British Medical Journal 335: 24–27.

Department of Health 2004 Choosing health: making healthy choices easier. Department of Health, London.

Dooris M 2006 Healthy settings: challenges to generating evidence of effectiveness. Health Promotion International 21: 55–65.

Jochelson K, Norwood S, Hussain S et al 2005 Sustainable food and the NHS. Kings Fund, London.

Johnson J 2000 The health care institution as a setting for health promotion. In: Poland B, Green L, Rootman I (eds) Settings for health promotion: linking theory and practice. Sage, London, pp. 175–216.

Johnson A, Baum F 2001 Health promoting hospitals: a typology of different organizational approaches to health promotion. Health Promotion International 16: 281–287.

Kanter R M 1977 Men and women of the corporation. Basic Books, New York.

Latter S 2001 The potential for health promotion in hospital nursing practice. In: Scriven A, Orme J (eds) Health promotion: professional perspectives. Macmillan/Open University Press, Hampshire.

McKee M 2000 Settings 3 – health promotion in the health care sector. In: International Union for Health Promotion and Education. The evidence of health promotion effectiveness. Shaping public health in a new europe. Part two: evidence book. ECSC-EC-EAEC, Brussels.

Moller A M, Villebro N, Pedersen T et al 2002 Effect of preoperative smoking intervention on postoperative complications: a randomised clinical trial. Lancet 359: 114.

Nightingale F 1859 Notes on nursing. What it is and what it is note 84. Lippincott, Williams and Wilkins, Philadelphia.

Nutbeam D 1998 Health promotion glossary. WHO, Geneva.

Pelikan J M, Krajic K, Dietscher C 2001 The health promoting hospital (HPH): concept and development. Patient Education and Counseling 45: 239–243.

Social Exclusion Unit 2003 Making the connections. SEU, London.

Ulrich R S 1984 View through a window may influence recovery from surgery. Science 224: 420–421.

Whitehead D 2004 The European health promoting hospitals (HPH) project: how far on?. Health Promotion International 19: 259–267.

World Health Organization 1991 The Budapest declaration on health promoting hospitals. WHO, Copenhagen.

World Health Organization 1997 Vienna recommendations on health promoting hospitals. WHO, Vienna.

World Health Organization 2004 Standards for health promotion in hospitals. WHO, Copenhagen.

Chapter Seventeen

17

Health promotion in prisons

Key points

- Prisons as a healthy setting
- Reasons for prioritizing health promotion in prisons
- Barriers to using prisons as health-promoting settings
- Interventions and evidence of their effectiveness

OVERVIEW

Prisons have been identified as a health promotion setting in a variety of policy documents, ranging from the World Health Organization to the continental European Union to the UK and other countries. Within the last 25 years the idea of a prison setting for health promotion has taken root and spread. Over 30 European countries are now members of the Health in Prisons Project (HIPP) network. Prisons have been identified as a key setting for health promotion for several reasons. Prisoners are one of the most socially excluded groups in society, so addressing their health is a means of addressing health inequalities. However there are also challenges to promoting health within prisons, and there are many features of prison life that would seem to militate against a healthy lifestyle. There is a range of possible interventions and a growing body of evidence for their effectiveness. As with all settings, the evidence suggests that an integrated whole-systems approach works best within the prison setting to promote the health of prisoners, staff and the wider community.

Why prisons have been identified as a setting for health promotion

There are several reasons why prisons have been identified as a suitable setting for health promotion:

- Prisoners are a socially excluded group with demonstrable health inequalities.
- The prison population is a 'captive audience'.
- Prisoners typically comprise the 'hard-to-reach' and 'needy' segments of the population.
- Focusing on the prison setting will also have an impact on the deprived families and communities of prisoners, and prison staff.

Box 17.1

Prisoners – a socially excluded group

The following statistics clearly demonstrate that 'many prisoners have experienced a lifetime of social exclusion' (Condon et al 2006, p. 20).

- Prisoners are 13 times more likely than the general population to have been in care as a child and to be unemployed.
- One-third of prisoners were not in permanent accommodation prior to their imprisonment.
- Almost three-quarters suffer from two or more mental disorders.
- Half of women prisoners have suffered domestic violence and a third sexual abuse.
- Half of male prisoners have no qualifications.
- Nearly half of all prisoners' reading age is at or below the level expected of an 11-year-old.
- Prisoners are more likely than the general population to engage in high-risk behaviours such as smoking, hazardous drinking and unprotected sex.

Imprisonment tends to exacerbate social exclusion and mental ill health, and increase the risk of some behaviours such as shared use of needles for drug injections. Overcrowding is an ongoing problem within prisons. A recent estimate suggests that 12 000 prisoners (out of a total prisoner population of around 75 000) are being held two to a cell designed for one (Howard League for Penal Reform 2005). Overcrowding leads to unsafe and degrading conditions, increases the risk of transmission of infectious diseases and impedes prisoners' access to purposeful training opportunities, exercise and fresh air. From a health inequalities perspective prisoners are a key target group.

Box 17.2

Is there a contradiction between using prisons as a penal system to remove people's liberty, and using prisons as a health promoting setting?

Box 17.3

List all the characteristics you can think of that differentiate the prison from other health-promoting settings and make it unique. Then take each characteristic in turn and discuss whether and in what ways this: (1) promotes and (2) inhibits health. Then take all the health-promoting aspects and identify what resources you would need to turn their potential into reality.

Barriers to prisons as health-promoting settings

Prisons are by their nature closed communities. For some this may mean the use of prisons as a health-promoting setting is a contradiction in terms, as key principles of health promotion such as free choice and empowerment are severely restricted (De Viggiani 2006a). The prison regime allows prisoners little opportunity to make decisions, exert their autonomy or become empowered. The monotony and boredom of prison life may predispose some prisoners towards risk-taking behaviour, such as smoking or drug use. Prison culture is known for its bullying, victimization and violence – all factors that contradict health promotion principles. It has been argued that preventive measures in prison, such as mandatory drug testing, may backfire, as prisoners may switch from cannabis to heroin (which cannot be so easily detected) or use other harmful methods to conceal their drug use (such as ingesting bleach) (Smith 2000). Instead of empowering prisoners, health promotion initiatives may become punitive.

Other commentators however see the nature of the prison setting as an advantage, as it guarantees access to prisoners and a long-term stable environment where any changes will have a direct impact on inmates (Ramaswamy & Freudenberg 2007). The prison population would normally be considered 'hard to reach', so their accessibility within the prison setting is unique. Prisoners have very high rates of physical and mental ill health and risky behaviours (Smith 2000). In all, 90% of prisoners have a diagnosable mental health problem or a substance misuse problem or both. A total of 80% of prisoners smoke and 24% have injected drugs, making them a key target group for health promotion.

Targeting prisoners also potentially enables health promotion programmes to reach out beyond the prison to prisoners' families and deprived communities. There are an estimated 1 million relatives affected by imprisonment each year (Williams 2006). The imprisonment of one family member often leads to emotional, psychological and financial stress for the rest of the family. Conversely, providing health promotion for prisoners can have a positive effect on their families and communities. For example, providing health education about human immunodeficiency virus (HIV) transmission for prisoners has been shown to diffuse outwards to their family (Scott et al 2004). It is likely that in the long term this reduces the demand on services, and therefore represents sound economic sense (Curd et al 2007).

Finally, targeting the prison as a setting enables interventions to reach prison staff as well. Prison staff are an important, if neglected, target group in their own right. The positive health and well-being of staff can also be expected to have a favourable impact on the prisoners in their charge.

Health-promoting prisons

A focus on the health of prisoners and the prison setting is a relatively new phenomenon. The first ever seminar on prison health, organized by the Council of Europe and the Ministry of Justice in Finland, was held in 1991. A European programme, HIPP, was first launched by the World Health Organization in 1995. HIPP identified three key priority areas: communicable diseases, mental health and drugs. HIPP also stated some of its underlying principles:

All prisoners have the right to health care, including preventive measures, without

discrimination and equivalent to what is available in the community (World Health Organization/UNAIDS 1998).

Box 17.4

Health in Prisons Project (HIPP) strategies

- To integrate public health and prison health systems in order to reduce health inequalities and promote overall public health
- To encourage prisons to operate their services within recognized international and national codes of human rights and medical ethics
- To use prison health services to contribute towards prisoners' rehabilitation and resettlement, especially with regard to drug addiction and mental health problems, and thereby reduce reoffending
- To reduce prisoners' exposure to communicable diseases
- To ensure that the standard of all prison health services, including health promotion services, is equivalent to those in the wider community (World Health Organization Regional Office for Europe 2004).

The World Health Organization Healthy Prisons Project (World Health Organization 1998) is an international strategy that has been endorsed in England and Wales (Department of Health 2002). The strategy has three priorities: health-promoting policies, environments supportive of health and access to preventive health care. In 2005 the World Health Organization launched its 10-year Prison Public Health Plan (World Health Organization 2005). Prison health was identified as a key public health target in New Labour's *Choosing Health* (Department of Health 2005), although it was conceptualized rather narrowly as access to health services. In 2005 prison health care services were reformulated as a new arm of the NHS, providing both opportunities and challenges (Department of Health 2005). In the UK primary health care teams and practitioners are now responsible for the health of prisoners. The change in accountability follows evidence that prison health services were extremely variable and in many cases did not provide the same standard of service as the NHS.

The challenge is to use the prison setting to tackle long-term inequalities in health, and to go 'upstream' to address the social and systemic determinants of health (De Viggiani 2006b). Although integrating the prison health system within the NHS might ensure comparability of service provision, it does not facilitate this movement upstream towards the determinants of health. The wider determinants of health, e.g. low educational attainment, poor literacy and little work experience, need to be tackled by a whole-prison approach. An example of such an approach is the strategy document *Health-Promoting Prisons: A Shared Approach* (Department of Health 2002) and the accompanying prison service order set out the need to:

- Develop the physical, mental and social health of prisoners and staff as part of a whole-prison approach
- Prevent the deterioration of prisoners' health during or because of custody
- Help prisoners adopt healthy behaviours that can be taken back into the community.

Box 17.5

The concept of decency has been identified as an important foundation for promoting health. What do you understand by this concept?

It has been argued that decency underpins all aspects of prison life (Wheatley 2001). Decency includes clean facilities, attending promptly to prisoners' concerns, protecting prisoners from harm, and fair and consistent treatment by staff (Figure 17.1).

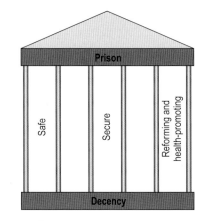

Figure 17.1 ● Prison decency.
Source: From Wheatley (2001) Crown copyright material is reproduced with the permission of the Controller Office of Public Sector Information (OPSI).

Examples of effective interventions

The novelty of the prison as a health-promoting setting means that the evidence base for effective interventions is rather scarce. However, in common with the settings approach as applied to other settings, theory suggests that a whole-systems approach, involving the prison social and physical environment as well as individual behaviours, is likely to prove most effective. Developing a whole-prison approach involves three components:

1. Policies that promote health, e.g. no-smoking policy, prevention of communicable diseases

2. Environment that is supportive of health, e.g. the opportunity to undertake meaningful work

3. Prevention and health education programmes, e.g. avoiding sexually transmitted infections, anger management, immunization against tuberculosis and hepatitis B.

Dissemination of what works is also important. The World Health Organization has launched an awards programme to recognize best practice within prisons, and to encourage networking and the dissemination of successful programmes (see Example 17.6). What evidence there is suggests prisons can be an effective setting for health promotion. For example, a review of evidence of the effectiveness of needle exchange programmes in prisons concluded that such programmes were effective and did not undermine institutional safety or security (Lines et al 2005). There is also evidence that substitution therapy is beneficial, and that together these measures can reduce the spread of HIV and help support the health of drug-addicted prisoners (Gatherer et al 2005). Smoking cessation services targeted at prisoners have achieved quit rates equal to, or better than, rates for other groups in the community (Braham 2003).

 Box 17.6

Prison Healthy Living Centre
The World Health Organization awarded Swinfen Hall Prison and Young Offenders Institution (YOI) one of only 14 best-practice awards for health in prisons in 2007. Rethink's innovative Healthy Living Centre (HLC) develops communication and builds mutual respect and understanding between staff and prisoners. The HLC is funded by the local primary care trust and offers nine places on each 12-week programme. The programme is integrated into the prison's reducing reoffending action plan. The programme leads to raised self-esteem and confidence, which enable the young offenders to reflect on how their behaviour affects their health and to identify positive changes they can make (http://www.rethink.org).

A coordinated approach is necessary to address the multiple determinants – individual, social and environmental – that affect prisoners' health. This in turn requires an infrastructure, including supportive policies, senior support and leadership, coordination of efforts and engaging with both staff and prisoners.

Conclusion

The prison setting poses many challenges for health promotion, yet it also presents an opportunity to tackle health inequalities and address a socially marginalized and excluded group in conditions of relative security and predictability. Over the last 25 years the prison setting has been identified as a health-promoting setting by the World Health Organization, the continental European Community and the UK in a number of policy and strategic documents. A number of projects tackling health behaviours have been launched, but evaluation suggests the most effective programmes are those that address the whole prison system, including the prison culture, physical and social environment. Funding prison health promotion programmes is likely to be a sound economic investment, as it will help prevent reoffending as well as improve health.

Summary

This chapter has examined the reasons why the prison has been identified as a health-promoting setting and outlined some of the most important policies and strategies. The barriers to promoting health in prisons have been identified and discussed. Some examples of successful projects have been given to illustrate the potential for the prison as a healthy setting.

Further questions

- 'Prison health is a key strategy to tackle health inequalities.' Discuss.

- 'Health promotion in prisons is a contradiction in terms.' Construct an argument either for or against this proposition.

- You are part of a voluntary group trying to negotiate access and resources to implement a positive mental health project in your local low-security prison. How would you try to persuade the prison governor to allow your project to go ahead? What arguments would you use to persuade the local community that your project would be beneficial?

Further reading

Baybutt M, Hayton P, Dooris M 2007 Prisons in England and Wales: an important public health opportunity?. In: Douglas J, Earle S, Handsley S et al (eds) A reader in promoting public health: challenge and controversy. Open University Press/Sage, London, pp. 237–245. *An up-to-date review of recent advances in prison health promotion, both internationally and within the UK.*

Department of Health 2002 Health promoting prisons: a shared approach. Department of Health, London. *This document includes numerous examples of interventions tackling mental health promotion, substance use, smoking prevention and healthy lifestyles.*

De Viggiani N 2006 A new approach to prison public health? Challenging and advancing the agenda for prison health. Critical Public Health 16: 307–316. *A persuasive proposal to advance prison health through moving 'upstream' to address the determinants of health.*

References

Braham M 2003 Acquitted best practice guidance for developing smoking cessation services in prison. Department of Health, London.

Condon L, Hek G, Harris F 2006 Public health, health promotion and the health of people in prison. Community Practitioner 79: 19–22.

Curd P R, Winter S J, Connell A 2007 Participative planning to enhance inmate wellness: preliminary report of a correctional wellness program. Journal of Correctional Health Care 13: 296–308.

Department of Health 2002 Health-promoting prisons: a shared approach. Department of Health, London.

Department of Health 2005 Choosing health: making healthier choices easier Cm 6374. Stationery Office, London.

De Viggiani N 2006a Surviving prison: exploring prison social life as a determinant of health. International Journal of Prisoner Health 2: 71–89.

De Viggiani N 2006b A new approach to prison public health? Challenging and advancing the agenda for prison health. Critical Public Health 16: 307–316.

Gatherer A, Moller L, Hayton P 2005 The World Health Organization European Health in Prisons Project after 10 years: persistent barriers and achievements. American Journal of Public Health 95: 1696–1700.

Howard League for Penal Reform 2005 Prisons are incapacitated by overcrowding. Press Release 11/03/2005.

Lines R, Jurgens R, Betteridge G et al 2005 Taking action to reduce injecting drug-related harms in prisons: the evidence of effectiveness of prison needle exchange in six countries. International Journal of Prisoner Health 1: 49–64.

Ramaswamy M, Freudenberg N 2007 Health promotion in jails and prisons: an alternative paradigm for correctional health services. In: Greifinger R B, Bick J, Goldenson J (eds) Public health behind bars. From prisons to communities, Springer, New York, pp. 229–248.

Scott D P, Harzke A J, Mizwa M B et al 2004 Evaluation of an HIV peer education program in Texas prisons. Journal of Correctional Health Care 10: 151–173.

Smith C 2000 Healthy prisons: a contradiction in terms? Howard Journal of Criminal Justice 39: 339–353.

Wheatley P 2001 Prison service conference speech. HM Prison Service Internal Communications Unit. Available online at: www.hmprisonservice.gov.uk

Williams M 2006 Improving the health and social outcomes of people recently released from prisons in the UK. The Sainsbury Centre for Mental Health, London.

World Health Organization 1998 Promoting health in prisons – a good practice guide. World Health Organization, Geneva.

World Health Organization Regional Office for Europe 2004 Strategic objectives for the WHO Health in Prisons Project: 2004–2010. World Health Organization, Copenhagen.

World Health Organization 2005 Prison public health plan. World Health Organization, Geneva.

World Health Organization/UNAIDS 1998 HIV/AIDS, sexually transmitted diseases and tuberculosis in prisons; Joint consensus statement. World Health Organization, Geneva.

Part 4

Implementing health promotion

This final part is concerned with the practical task of how to implement health promotion. Good practice depends on the coexistence of many factors: adherence to core health-promoting principles, personal skills and training, and the use of suitable models and frameworks to guide action. Health promotion programmes and activities should be guided by the following principles:

- Empowering, to enable individuals and communities to take control over the factors affecting their health
- Participatory, involving all concerned in all stages of the process of development and evaluation
- Equitable and guided by a concern for social justice
- Intersectoral, involving the collaboration of many sectors and agencies
- Sustainable such that any change can be continued once initial funding has ended
- Multistrategy, including policy development, legislation and regulation, organizational change, community development, advocacy, communication and education in combination (Rootman et al 2001).

Good practice also depends on a systematic and structured approach to interventions, which is the focus of this part. There are three major stages in carrying out interventions: needs assessment, planning and evaluation. In this final part we consider each of these stages in turn, devoting a chapter to each. Chapter 18 explores how needs – whether identified by communities or practitioners or researchers – underpin the actions we take. The process of assessing needs includes soliciting subjective perceptions from clients as well as accessing objective factual indicators such as mortality, morbidity or service use statistics. Needs assessment methods should be health-promoting in themselves, including a variety of participatory methods to support empowerment and capacity building, and a focus on equity of inputs and outputs. Resource and organizational constraints tend to prioritize disease reduction targets, but understanding the determinants of health will help orient health promotion activities to 'upstream' interventions.

A systematic approach to planning will help the health promoter to analyse clearly the problem or area of need, set appropriate aims and objectives, and identify an appropriate plan of action. Chapter 19 discusses the factors that need to be taken into account when planning a health promotion intervention at any level (individual intervention; project or strategy). Planning is an important tool for the practitioner, enabling a structured and rational approach to one's workload. Planning enables transparency and accountability, allowing all stakeholders to assess the proposed plan and monitor its progress. Planning also contributes towards reflective practice, enabling practitioners to develop their expertise and build their capacity to promote health.

Evaluation has long been recognized as fundamental to good practice but is often neglected. From the point of view of practitioners, reviewing progress and making changes to ensure a project or intervention proceeds as envisaged is all part of sound planning and professional practice. For other stakeholders, evaluation is a means to have their voice heard, and their values and priorities recognized. Evaluation

helps to build an evidence base identifying interventions that are not only effective and cost-effective but also acceptable and sustainable. Such evidence should inform decision-making, but is often missing in the field of health promotion. Evaluation is therefore a vital stage in developing professional health promotion practice. Chapter 20 discusses the importance of identifying appropriate outcomes and indicators of success and how practitioners may evaluate their health promotion activities.

Together these three chapters provide a reflective and critical account of the practice of health promotion, combining 'how to' information with a critique of underlying assumptions and values. The intention is to help practitioners develop effective and reflective practice that operationalizes core health promotion principles, produces the desired results and helps build a solid evidence-base for health promotion.

Reference

Rootman I, Goodstadt M, Hyndman B et al 2001 Evaluation in health promotion. Principles and perspectives. WHO Europe, Copenhagen.

Chapter Eighteen

18

Assessing health needs

Key points

- Concepts of need
- Needs assessment strategies
- Relating needs to strategic planning
- Problems in assessing needs

OVERVIEW

The first phase in health promotion planning is an assessment of what a client or population group needs to enable them to become healthier. Health care usually takes the individual as its starting point. Public health concerns the health and welfare of people in groups. Practitioners do not assess individuals in isolation from the communities in which they live. As we have seen in previous chapters the health experiences of individuals are affected by where they reside. The local knowledge of practitioners about the range of local services, facilities and networks is an important part of needs assessment. Within a neighbourhood there will be people in settings such as schools and workplaces and population groups with specific health needs. Practitioners need to know how to assess individuals, how to manage their care and how to encourage healthier lifestyles. They also require an understanding of people's ways of life and the health problems and opportunities they experience and they

need to know how to use this understanding to assess the needs of people in groups systematically. The term needs assessment describes the process of gathering information. It has been defined as a 'systematic method of reviewing the health needs and issues facing a given population leading to agreed priorities and resource allocation that will improve health and reduce inequalities' (Cavanagh & Chadwick 2005). The purpose of health needs assessment at national, regional or local level is twofold:

1. To identify which actions to improve health should have greatest priority

2. To choose which particular groups or communities should have priority and so help in targeting interventions and commissioning services.

Recognition of the right to participate in defining health needs and health care was acknowledged in the 1978 World Health Organization (WHO) Alma Ata Declaration, and one of the underlying principles of Health For All is community participation (WHO 1985).

National Health Service (NHS) reforms have emphasized the participation of local people in setting priorities, signalling a philosophical shift from a paternalistic medical model to a participatory consumer-led model. This chapter considers the ways in which local health needs are assessed and applied in planning for health promotion. It should be read in conjunction with Chapter 3, which outlines the principal sources of information about health status.

Defining health needs

The concept of need is widely used but often not well understood. People may believe they 'need' a new coat because someone observed that their old one is worn out, or because it looks old compared to other people's coats, or simply because they would like one. A need may thus be something people want or something that is lacking in comparison to others.

 Box 18.1

How would you distinguish between a need, a want and a demand?

There are two different understandings of what constitutes a health need. It can be seen as:

1. A subjective, relative concept which is judged by an expert or professional and is influenced by whether the need can be met

2. An objective and universal concept which is a fundamental right.

Box 18.2

Make a list of 10 important human needs:
• Are some more fundamental than others?
• Are these needs relative to a particular country or are they universal?

Economists tend to avoid the use of the term needs altogether, arguing that it is overlaid with emotion and what is really meant by a health need is actually a matter of people's wants and demands, and these are limitless (Cohen 2008). Identifying health needs is therefore a question of identifying priorities.

An alternative view is that there are universal needs. Maslow's hierarchy of needs (Maslow 1954) suggests that all human needs are in fact health needs (Figure 18.1).

For a person to be self-actualizing, physical, social and emotional needs must be met. Doyal & Gough (1992) have similarly argued that the ultimate goal of human beings is to participate fully in society and to do this the basic needs for physical health and for autonomy must be met. These needs are not relative to a particular country or period of time but are fundamental rights and include the prerequisites for health – peace, shelter, education, food, income, a stable ecosystem, sustainable resources, social justice and equity (WHO 1986). But these needs are not undisputed. How healthy do people have to be before we can say that their needs have been met? Bradshaw (1972), in a widely used taxonomy, distinguished four types of health and social need:

1. Normative needs, as defined by experts or professional groups

2. Felt needs, as defined by clients, patients, relatives or service users

3. Expressed needs, when felt needs become a demand

4. Comparative needs, identified when people, groups or areas fall short of an established standard.

Normative needs

Normative needs are objective needs as defined by professionals, who also identify the ways in which these needs can be met. A normative need reflects a professional judgement that a person or persons deviate from a required standard. This may be against some external criteria such as occupational or legal

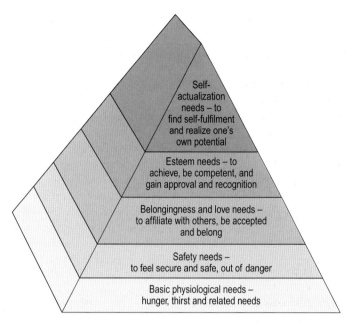

Figure 18.1 • Maslow's hierarchy of needs.

requirements. Thus the manager of a restaurant is in need of training because she has not completed a course in food hygiene. Or it may be that a person deviates from what is defined by medical staff as the range of 'clinically normal' physiological indicators.

Box 18.3

Normative need: child development
A health visitor decides that, according to a growth chart, an infant has failed to gain weight for some time and has fallen below the third centile. She deems the infant to be in need of supplementary feeding and suggests this is done by additional bottle-feeding. Yet expectations of child development vary according to the place and time. This infant would not be regarded as failing to thrive in the USA or in pre-war UK.

Normative needs are not absolute or objective 'facts' – they reflect the judgement of professionals which may be different from that of their clients. Health care workers will judge a need relative to what they are able to provide. The ability to judge normative needs also contributes to the notion of professionalism and the authority and status of professionals.

Felt needs

Felt needs are what people really *want*. They are needs identified by clients themselves which may relate to services, information or support which can be termed service needs. Moves towards bottom-up approaches in health and social care have meant a greater acceptance of service users' views. (Chapter 6 in our companion volume (Naidoo & Wills 2005) discusses some of the policy drivers to patient and public involvement.) Needs may be limited by the perceptions of an individual. Individuals may not believe themselves to be in need simply because they do not know what is available in terms of treatment or services.

Box 18.4

A GP practice is aware that a lot of patients are seeking consultations for their concerns about not getting pregnant. The practice decides to hold an evening talk on preconceptual care. The talk is advertised in the surgery. No one attends.

- On what grounds did the practice decide that there was a need?
- Why did the practice decide the need was for preconceptual care?
- What other needs might patients have in this area?
- What other response might the practice have to this patient need?

This is an example of a need identified by professionals. No consultation was involved. The intervention was planned in the expectation that it would result in a saving of GP time, not as part of a programme to prioritize infertility. The intervention was poorly presented with no marketing, and no attempt to make it accessible for clients.

Expressed need

Expressed need arises from felt needs but is expressed in words or action – it has become a *demand*. Thus clients or groups are expressing a need when they ask for help or information, or when they make use of a service. Expressed need is often used to measure the adequacy of service provision, even though it is not a comprehensive or complete measure. There are also objective needs which exist but are not expressed. Only a proportion of patients make contact with health services and they are merely the tip of an iceberg of potential need, as illustrated in Figure 18.2.

Sometimes people will use a service because it is all that is available, even if it does not adequately meet needs. The best example of expressed need (and unmet demand) is the waiting list. Some needs are not expressed, perhaps because of an inability or unwillingness to articulate the need. This could be due to language difficulties or a lack of knowledge.

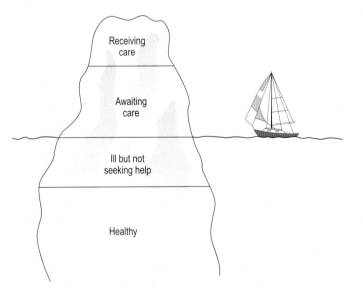

Figure 18.2 • Iceberg of health care needs.

Expressed needs should not be taken as an indicator of demand because they also exclude needs which are felt but not expressed. Tudor Hart's inverse-care law has been of vital importance in showing that just because a service or treatment is used less does not mean that it is needed less (Tudor Hart 1971). Those who could most benefit from a service are often those least likely to use it. People may express different needs, and there is a tendency to listen to those with loud and powerful voices, such as views which come from an established group or views which appear to express a popular need. Responding to expressed needs may also therefore have the effect of increasing inequalities in service provision.

Comparative needs

Individuals or groups are said to be in need if their situation, when compared with that of a similar group or individual, is found wanting or lacking with regard to services and resources. For example, if a person with schizophrenia in area A was living in sheltered accommodation and receiving day care, but in area B this was not available, we would say that schizophrenics in area B were in need. In the NHS, although people may be assessed to be in absolute need (normatively), in practice comparative needs assessment will often dictate whether their needs will be met. Areas may be compared on the basis of provision of services or length of waiting lists to see if the health needs of their populations are being met. In a sense, then, comparative need is about equity. It is about equal provision for equal need. This kind of analysis of need does, of course, assume that those in receipt of a service are receiving adequate provision and that their needs are being met.

Bradshaw's work (1994) is useful in showing that different groups in society hold different definitions of need. We can see that needs are not objective and observable entities to which we must just match our interventions. The concept of need is a relative one and is influenced both by values and attitudes and by other agendas.

Box 18.5

Consider these interventions available to women in childbirth. Has medicine created these needs or are they needed improvements in technology?
- Prostaglandin to induce labour
- Epidural to reduce pain
- Electronic fetal monitoring
- Belt monitoring of contractions
- Elective caesarean section.

At first sight, these developments may be seen as the consequence of medical advances. However, medical interventions in childbirth can also be seen as an attempt to establish doctors' control over that of midwives. The range of interventions may, on the one hand, alienate women and make childbirth an uncomfortable and distressing experience and, on the other hand, the very availability of these services may create a need for them.

A very different list of needs may be compiled by pregnant women, including for example:
- The same known midwife to be present throughout labour and birth
- Water births
- Partner to be present during birth
- Home births.

These felt or expressed needs may or may not be acknowledged and provided for by service providers. Consider the following questions:
- How are these different needs communicated?
- If these needs conflict, which would take priority and why?

What is clear from the above discussion is that definitions of need vary depending on whose interpretation and values are used. People's health needs are not the same as those of 20 years ago – the nature and prevalence of diseases may change, as do the expectations of the population and the capacity of health services to meet them. The NHS uses the term health gain in association with health needs to

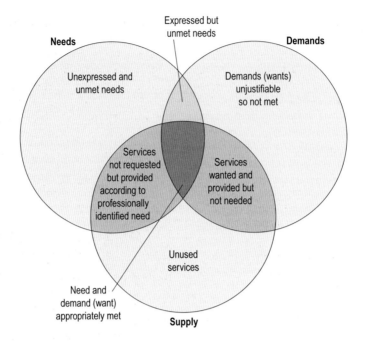

Figure 18.3 • Needs, wants, supply and demand.

signal that the meeting of needs is related to a person's ability to benefit. Health gain is defined as:

- Adding years to life by reducing premature mortality
- Adding life to years by enhancing the quality of life and improving well-being.

The concept of health gain is rooted in a medical model which sees health as the absence of disease. Consequently, health needs tend to be defined as problems which may be successfully met by services or treatment. Because need is seen as infinite and resources as limited, health authorities confine themselves to what is known to be effective care. Yet community surveys often show that the public define ill health far more broadly than simply problems requiring treatment by health services. Many priorities for health go beyond the narrow outcomes encompassed by adding 'years to life' and require health authorities to take account of the structural influences on health, such as housing, community safety and transport links. The meeting of needs is also related to what can be offered (what the state can supply). These differing interpretations are illustrated in Figure 18.3.

The purpose of assessing health needs

The process of assessing needs is nothing new. As we shall see in the next chapter, understanding needs is integral to a basic process approach to planning. Needs assessment including the collection of data is the first step, from which subsequent aims will be derived. Assessing the health and social needs of local populations is a means of obtaining accurate and appropriate information on which to base priorities and ensures that decisions are based on solid information and evidence. This overall purpose can be broken down into different stages as follows.

First stage: help in directing interventions appropriately

Within clinical practice assessing needs is routine and accepted. Assessment takes place to determine what care is required through the gathering of data about:

- The individual, e.g. age
- Health history, e.g. medical, surgical, activities of daily living
- Current health, e.g. self-reported symptoms
- Current health measurement, e.g. blood pressure, pain assessment, oxygen saturation.

An integrated care pathway gives a single record of assessment for all the many professionals and agencies who may be involved with a patient but it also provides a map of care for all patients with a similar set of symptoms or diagnosis. It is intended to reduce variations in interpretations of need and treatment offered.

For those practitioners who work with individual clients, there is increasing recognition of the importance of client participation in the assessment of needs. Nursing practice, for example, has frequently been criticized for being too inflexible and routine – doing things *to* people rather than *with* them. Prescription has now given way to negotiation alongside the move from sick nursing to health nursing. Understanding the thoughts, feelings and experiences of individuals has become an important part of the therapeutic and nursing process.

Box 18.6

For what reasons might clients find it difficult to express their needs in a clinical situation?

Increasingly, health care workers seek to identify clients' views and perceptions about their health as part of their assessment. What they often find is that their perception differs from that of the client. Clients' need for information is often underestimated and in health care settings this may mean that information is confined to ward or clinic routines. Despite the greater emphasis on being client-centred, practitioners tend to assess needs in relation to the service they provide. Practitioners may interpret client needs as information needs because it is possible to provide this, whereas the satisfaction of physical needs (as in Maslow's hierarchy) may seem beyond their scope.

Box 18.7

A male patient who is young and fit has a heart attack. The nurse on the ward offers the patient advice on cardiac rehabilitation and information on healthy eating, exercise and safe drinking.
- Is the nurse meeting the patient's needs?
- Is health education information an appropriate intervention?

The medical and individualistic approach is adopted because it is a well-understood part of the nurse's professional role. The nurse understands coronary heart disease prevention as focusing on risk factors even though they are not relevant to this situation. The patient may have other health needs such as a concern about getting back to work or when he might be sexually active again. Assessing individual health needs means starting with the patient's own concerns.

Second stage: identifying population needs and reducing inequalities

To meet community health needs it is essential to have a clear understanding of what the needs are, what capacity communities have for addressing these needs, and whether particular groups face specific challenges in meeting their needs. Health equity audit is a requirement of planning in which local strategic partnerships and other organizations systematically review the role of inequities in the causes of ill health and the access to services for defined population groups. Health equity audits show whether different categories of people (categorized by socioeconomic group, geographical area, age, sex, disability or minority ethnic group) are having their needs met in an equal manner and whether the most appropriate services are being provided (http://www.nice.org.uk/niceMedia/documents/equityauditfinal.pdf).

Box 18.8

Consider the following information about a ward (Easttown) in a local borough (Townsville). What are its health needs?

Rates of mortality (SMR*)	Easttown	Townsville
All causes	144.6	133.4
Circulatory disease	201.4	153.2
Cancer	84.5	110.4
Coronary heart disease	244.2	153.1

*An SMR (standardized mortality rate) of 100 indicates that the ward has average mortality. Higher than 100 indicates higher than average mortality.

A population such as Townsville that has significantly above-average rates of coronary heart disease could be said to be in need of more health service provision, including hospital beds, defibrillators, appropriate medication, e.g. statins and health promotion programmes. On the other hand, such statistics may be interpreted as revealing a community-wide need for an infrastructure to support healthier lifestyles, including aspects such as transport, food security, exercise and access to health services.

Third stage: identifying and responding to the specific needs of minority groups and socially excluded groups

There are recognizable social, demographic or identity-based groups who have traditionally avoided or been excluded from service needs assessments. Such harder-to-reach groups may think that services don't care about them, don't listen or are irrelevant. For example, studies of the health of gypsies and travellers have shown that:

> There are widespread communication difficulties between health workers and gypsy travellers, with defensive expectation of racism and prejudice. Barriers to health care access were experienced with several contributory causes, including reluctance of GPs to register travellers or visit sites (Parry et al 2004 p 8).

Box 18.9

How might health practitioners attempt to meet the needs of hard-to-reach clients?

A first step might be an audit to compare caseloads with the local population. If particular groups are underrepresented, involving members of such groups in discussion about service provision would be useful. This might involve practitioners going out to community venues and networks, e.g. community or religious centres. Other strategies might involve addressing obvious barriers such as language by the translation of information materials or the use of interpreters. If particular groups have specific health risks (e.g. coronary heart disease amongst Asians and stroke amongst African-Caribbeans), opportunistic screening and monitoring might be encouraged. Providing mobile services in people's communities has also been used successfully, e.g. to provide sexual health services for young people.

Fourth stage: targeting risk groups

Targeting may be done in terms of diseases, life cycles, lifestyles or social groups. The concept of risk groups has emerged as a means of directing health promotion activities to people who are most in need. A risk group may be defined as a population group vulnerable to certain diseases or conditions. A risk group's vulnerability may be due to genetic, lifestyle, economic, social or environmental characteristics. Normative needs derived from epidemiological research, which identifies groups with poorer than average health, are often used to establish target groups. For example, lower socioeconomic groups at most risk from ill health and premature death are a commonly identified risk group. Comparative need is used to identify at-risk groups who have low take-up rates of services.

However, a focus on high-risk groups can lead to 'victim-blaming'. Health problems are seen as specific to particular groups who may also be seen as responsible through their behaviour for their own ill health (Naidoo & Wills 2005). For example, young people are the subject of numerous targeted health promotion campaigns. Yet it is not being young that is a risk but certain activities. Many health promoters also reject the notion of targeting because they prefer to work in partnership with groups and communities on the issues *they* define as important.

Fifth stage: allocating resources

The NHS was predicated on the notion that there was an untreated pool of sickness that, once treated by a national health service, would diminish. Experience shows that there can be unlimited demand for health care. As health care is provided, so expectations rise; as technology improves, people with disabilities and chronic diseases live longer and demand more health care. General improvements in health and living conditions have led to people living longer and an increase in the percentage of older people in the population. It will not be possible to meet all these needs as resources are limited.

Most doctors and health care workers accept that some kind of priority-setting or rationing of health care is inevitable. There have always been waiting lists but rationing is a more far-reaching concept. It entails decisions about how much money should be put into different forms of care or treatment. Not only does this raise issues about justice and equity, it also poses the huge dilemma about who decides the priorities for investment. Public views may be very different from those of doctors. For example, infertility treatment may have a high value to individuals but not to society as a whole. Osteoporosis screening (bone density measurement) may be rated highly by the public but not by doctors who have access to more information and are therefore able to question its effectiveness.

While the 'postcode lottery' of accessing drugs such as Herceptin on the NHS is frequently highlighted, there are also considerable variations in spending by primary care trusts (PCTs). This is only partly explained by the age and needs of the population and the local cost of services. For example, Islington PCT in inner-city London spends four times as much as Bracknell PCT on the outskirts of London on mental health, even after adjustment for needs (Kings Fund 2006).

In Oregon in the USA a health commission of health care workers and the public devised a complex formula to prioritize health services and decided there were certain services that they would not provide (www.oregonhealthdecisions.org/index.htm#welcome). In the UK health care may no longer be free and available to all who need it. PCTs are beginning to consider particular services which will not be provided as part of the NHS. Cosmetic surgery, for example, is not provided free for cosmetic reasons alone, but may be allowed for the correction of congenital abnormalities and injuries and other special criteria determined by PCTs locally. Many primary care organizations elicit public views on health care priorities and changing provision to primary care, day-case surgery and the care of the mentally ill in the community.

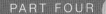

 Box 18.10

PCTs have limited resources. Consider the following typical costs of interventions (not actual amounts). What factors would you take into account in deciding priorities?

Home visit by community psychiatric nurse	£50
Tonsillectomy	£250
Hip replacement	£1000
Place in group home for someone with learning difficulties	£30 000 per year
Pregnancy termination	£200
Brief intervention of psychotherapy (10 weeks)	£1500
Day care for an older person with mental ill health	£200 per week

Some of the factors you might take into account are:
- Costs – the relative costs of different services, and the opportunity costs (i.e. if the money is spent on this, what is it not being spent on)
- Numbers – how many people will benefit from the service and will it provide the greatest good for the greatest number?
- Effectiveness – what are the likely outcomes of providing care or treatment? Will it promote health, prevent ill health, improve or cure ill health?
- Quality – what areas of health-related quality of life (physical, mental, social, well-being, perception of pain, self-care) will be most affected by the service?

Health needs assessment

Needs assessment can be carried out from the perspectives of professionals, the lay public and key informants (members of the community with a particular viewpoint, such as teachers or police officers). It can be carried out at different levels from that of the individual to specific groups (e.g. population groups, such as older people or people with specific health problems) to local geographic communities to national populations. It can inform general practice profiles, community profiles, intervention planning or service design.

Wright (1998) describes three approaches to health needs assessment:

1. Epidemiological (the focus is on the size and nature of the problem)

2. Corporate (the focus is on the views of stakeholders)

3. Community (uses a variety of methods to enable communities to identify, prioritize and decide what actions to take to meet health needs).

In all cases health needs assessment is a systematic and explicit process identifying issues affecting a population that can be addressed.

Health needs assessment should be guided by these common questions:
- What information is needed?
- How can I find out this information?
- What am I going to do with the information when I obtain it?
- What scope is there to act on the information?

What information is needed?

The first step in a needs assessment is to define the relevant population group or community, including its demographic and social characteristics; behaviours, values and lifestyles; cultural environment and historical circumstances. Community nurses are often involved in compiling community profiles to identify the health of a community and what resources are needed to enable the community to achieve health and stay healthy. A community profile has been described as:

A comprehensive description of the needs of a population that is defined, or defines itself, as a community, and the resources that exist within a community, carried out with the active

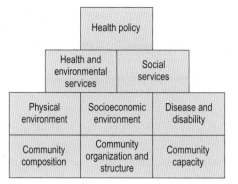

Figure 18.4 • Community information profile. From Annett & Rifkin (1990).

involvement of the community itself, for the purpose of developing an action plan or other means of improving the quality of life in the community (Hawtin & Percy Smith 2007, p. 5).

Community profiles do not follow a standard format. Figure 18.4 shows a schematic representation of the main elements:

- The composition of the community, e.g. its age profile, social networks, the way the community is organized and its capacity in relation to skills, organizations
- Socioecological environment, e.g. extent of economic activity and unemployment, private car ownership, housing, transport links, green areas, air pollution
- Availability, effectiveness and impact of health and social service provision
- Local strategies for health, e.g. health improvement programmes, regeneration projects.

 Box 18.11

For each of these elements, list the main sources of information that would need to be accessed to complete a community profile. What are the strengths and limitations of each information source in providing a picture of the community?

Information that is required for planning will include indicators of the state of health and well-being of the population, the factors that determine or influence health and the capacity of the population to meet identified needs. Some of this information is routinely collected and already exists, some will be known by stakeholders (e.g. health professionals, policy-makers, key members of the community) and the community members themselves will have views on what their needs are and how they wish them to be met. Chapter 3 outlined some of the indicators of health status and where this information is available, including:

- Self-reported health
- Life expectancy
- Mortality rates and cause
- Morbidity (sickness)
- Services available and their use.

Gathering information

Routine information that is already available (e.g. census, NHS and local authority data) will give a picture of the potential needs of a community and what is available to meet those needs. It may give an idea of areas of unmet need and identify groups experiencing inequities of health care provision. Information on effective interventions is also available (see Chapter 20). The community's perceptions of its own health needs and expectations of services or interventions are a vital part of planning, as are the views of professionals about the nature of health needs, best practices and existing service delivery.

The NHS reforms of the 1990s emphasized the need to involve local people in the shaping of local services. Our companion volume (Naidoo & Wills 2005) discusses this shift to patient and public involvement. There are many reasons for this:

- Ethical – people have the right to a voice
- Pragmatic – where people have identified the solution it is more likely to be appropriate and used
- Political – experts and professionals may have vested interests in a particular provision and limited understanding of people's needs.

The gathering of community knowledge can take place in different ways. Chapter 10 discusses this in more detail. There may be a formal exercise of consultation conducted in a top-down way. Frequently the consultation is confined to issues relating to patient satisfaction with services and particularly the hotel aspects of care.

Ong & Humphris regard this as inadequate:

> It is not sufficient to see users as consumers who are satisfied or dissatisfied with services. The place of users is in the joint definition of need, priority setting and evaluation. This approach means a paradigm shift whereby the community perspective will be used as the guiding principle for setting priorities in health care (Ong & Humphris 1994, p. 80).

Consultation in this way is not always successful. It often views people as the passive providers of information and not as active participants in the process. The results of consultations may seemingly be ignored. The timing, location and publicity for public meetings may lead to a poor turnout. Those consulted may not be representative of the community or may be token representatives of particular groups.

Many health and local authorities are using a range of methods to achieve a wider picture of community needs than one-off consultations. These approaches represent a move away from traditional epidemiological data-gathering towards techniques which reflect the importance of social and environmental factors and the involvement of the community in data collection. These include:

- Public meetings and forums
- Interviews with users and key informants
- Focus groups
- Using local media such as radio phone-ins
- Community health panels and citizens' juries
- Research techniques such as rapid appraisal, ethnographic studies and observation.

Rapid appraisal is a research technique applied to both urban and rural settings. It is geared to quickly identifying the health needs and priorities of a target population without great expense. It uses secondary data already available and then researchers interview people with knowledge of the area to identify problems and solutions. Key informants are:

- People who work in the community and have a professional understanding of the local issues (e.g. teachers, health visitors, police)
- People who are recognized community leaders and represent a section of the community (e.g. religious leaders, councillors, leaders of self-help groups)
- People who are important in informal networks and play a role in local communication (e.g. shopkeepers, bookmakers, lollipop persons).

Box 18.12

List some of the advantages and disadvantages of rapid appraisal as a method of community needs assessment.

Rapid appraisal is useful if virtually nothing is known about the needs and priorities of the target population. It can give a deep understanding of the problems and issues in a community and provide a sense of local ownership. But it does not provide the quantitative analysis of the size of the problem which many public health departments require. It may also be difficult to get beyond personal agendas to find out the community's views.

Participatory appraisal uses members of the community as data-gatherers. A range of methods may be used to capture the ways in which people describe local issues, e.g. mapping, community walks, timelines, photography, life histories. These techniques focus on mapping community assets and resources.

Whose needs count?

Moves to participation either in community affairs or health care cannot involve everyone. There will be individuals and groups who are not able to take advantage of opportunities for expression. These include potential and future users of a service; those who are not part of an established group; and those who are not deemed sufficiently rational to have a view, e.g. children, people with mental ill health and people with learning difficulties. Participation obviously favours those with the most influence and loudest voices.

 Box 18.13

- What reasons can you think of to explain why certain groups are harder to reach?
- Can you think of groups that might be harder to reach?

It is very difficult to get a cross-section of a community and there are some groups of people who are harder to reach. These include homeless people, unemployed people and people from Black and minority ethnic groups. Some groups comprise individuals who may have a similar experience of health services because of a defining characteristic of being unemployed or homeless, but who do not have a collective voice or means of expressing their views. Other groups may be informal with no recognized meeting place. Many groups may be wary of formal and statutory bodies.

Setting priorities

Within the NHS the criteria used for setting priority areas are:

1. The issue should be a major cause of premature death or avoidable ill health in the population as a whole or amongst specific groups of people.
2. There are marked inequalities in those who suffer ill health or premature death.

3. Effective interventions should be possible, offering scope for improvements in health.

In addition, there may be locally determined priorities of specific health issues, such as diabetes, or particular population groups, such as older people.

We have seen in this chapter that people's identified needs may also be taken as the first step in the planning process. However, this subjective interpretation may be tempered by economic priorities. People may express a need for interventions or treatment, the effectiveness of which is in doubt, e.g. antibiotics for simple colds or ear infections. For health promoters, therefore, a simple needs assessment may not be an adequate basis for setting priorities. There is a range of other influences which may determine what is included in a local health promotion plan:

- National targets of reducing disease
- A national theme, e.g. World Aids Day
- A major determinant of health in the area, i.e. age or poverty
- Pragmatism on the basis of available skills and interests
- Cost and staffing
- Longer-term strategy
- Existing activity
- Cost-effectiveness and what is amenable to change and evaluation
- Client choice
- Professionals' views.

Box 18.14

Questions to ask when planning a needs assessment: guide for practitioners

- What is your area of interest which defines the scope of the health need to be addressed? Are you interested in a whole population or a particular subsection such as older people or women?

- What is the size of the problem? How many people share the health need?
- What are the views of patients, carers and the local community? What is known from previous work? Who do you need to talk to locally?
- How do your figures compare with local and national averages? How important is the problem in your practice compared with others?
- What interventions are you already making? Do you have a response to the problem? What are other agencies doing?
- What has worked elsewhere? Is there any relevant literature available or projects which can be visited? Are there examples of best practice in the area you are interested in?
- What could and should you be doing in future? Consider all options, prioritize, develop an action plan.

Conclusion

There are many ways of measuring needs and no consensus as to the best method. The selection of a method or methods to measure needs will depend on the purpose and context. The process of encouraging consumerism and participation in public services by identifying and understanding individual and community needs has led to attempts to make such services more flexible. So we find, as part of the nursing process, clients being encouraged to identify aspects of their situation that they deem harmful to their health. We find health organizations using a variety of methods to ascertain the views, beliefs and health behaviours of their population in addition to the objective measures yielded by epidemiology. We find voluntary and community groups being required as part of their funding to monitor not only their clients' use of the service but also their health needs.

The public sector, including the NHS, is seeking to integrate public views into the planning process. However, most of the information used to assess needs is gathered from a professional perspective which assumes a direct relationship between certain indicators and needs and which is embedded in a medical model of health. For example, if health statistics show an above-average incidence of coronary heart disease, local health planners may well assume a need for greater provision of cardiac treatment and rehabilitation services and a health promotion programme to address risk factors for coronary heart disease. Health promoters have an important role to play in ensuring that needs assessment which feeds into planning takes account of public views and self-defined needs, and uses indicators to measure a social model of positive health.

For those with client caseloads, it is a vital task to know the health status of patients/clients and how this may differ from the broader community in order to plan appropriate interventions.

Assessing health need is important then both in terms of promoting health and in determining priorities. For health promoters the process of identifying needs is not however the only basis for setting priorities. Resource constraints will limit what is available and what is deemed amenable to change. Professional views, practice wisdom and existing activity will provide boundaries to what is considered possible.

Questions for further discussion

- How useful is the concept of need as a basis for planning health promotion interventions?
- How would you go about assessing the needs of:
  – Women who inject drugs?
  – Young asthmatics?
  – Carers of older people?

Summary

This chapter has discussed the ways in which need is defined. We have seen that perceptions of need vary according to whether these are client or professional views, and how the assessment is made – clients' expressed views; levels of service use; epidemiological and social data. The chapter concludes that need is relative, and influenced by values and attitudes as well as the historical context. It also considers the role of health promotion in identifying and meeting certain needs.

Further reading

Health Development Agency 2005 Clarifying approaches to health needs assessment, health impact assessment, integrated impact assessment, health equity audit and race equality impact assessment. HDA, London. *Practical guides to assessing health needs to inform decisions and assess impact through auditing provision, access and outcomes.*

Robinson J, Elkan R 1996 Health needs assessment: theory and practice. Churchill Livingstone, Edinburgh. *A clear and readable account of the issues in health needs assessment. It looks at epidemiological approaches and locality commissioning.*

Tones K, Green J 2004 Health promotion planning and strategies. Sage, London. *A useful text illustrating approaches to promoting health. Chapter 5 discusses needs assessment.*

References

Annett H, Rifkin S 1990 Improving urban health. WHO, Geneva

Bradshaw J 1972 The concept of social need. New Society 19: 640–643

Bradshaw J 1994 The conceptualisation and measurement of need: a social policy perspective. In: Popay J, Williams G (eds) Researching the people's health. Routledge, London

Cavanagh S, Chadwick K 2005 Health needs assessment: a practical guide. Health Development Agency, London. Available at http://www.nice.org.uk/media/150/35/Health_Needs_Assessment_A_Practical_Guide.pdf

Cohen D 2008 Health economics. In: Naidoo J, Wills J (eds) Health studies; an introduction. Palgrave/Macmillan, Basingstoke

Doyal L, Gough I 1992 A theory of human need. Macmillan, London

Hawtin M, Percy-Smith J 2007 Community profiling: a practical guide, 2nd edn. Open University, Buckingham

Kings Fund 2006 Local variations in NHS spending priorities. Kings Fund, London

Maslow A H 1954 Motivation and personality. Harper & Row, New York

Naidoo J, Wills J 2005 Public health and health promotion: developing practice. Baillière Tindall, London

Ong B N, Humphris G 1994 Prioritising needs with communities: rapid appraisal methodologies in health. In: Popay J, Williams G (eds) Researching the people's health. Routledge, London

Parry G, Cleemput P V, Peters J 2004 The health status of gypsies and travellers in England. Department of Health, London

Tudor Hart 1971 The inverse care law. Lancet 1: 405

Wright J (ed) 1998 Health needs assessment in practice. BMJ Publishing, London

World Health Organization 1978 Report on the Primary Health Care Conference: Alma Ata. World Health Organization, Geneva

World Health Organization 1985 Targets for health for all. WHO Regional Office for Europe, Copenhagen.

World Health Organization 1986 Ottawa charter. WHO, Geneva

Chapter Nineteen

Planning health promotion interventions

- Systematic planning and its advantages
- The principles of planning
- Strategic planning
- Project planning
- Ewles & Simnett planning model
- PRECEDE planning model
- Quality and audit

OVERVIEW

We have seen in Chapter 18 how needs assessment and targeting may be carried out, and the importance of carrying out this process and being clear about the context in which this is done. This chapter builds on the discussion of the first stage of planning – needs assessment – in Chapter 18. Firstly, definitions of planning are given and the reasons for planning discussed. Planning at different levels, from broad strategic planning through project planning to small-scale health education planning, is considered. The Ewles & Simnett (2003) and PRECEDE–proceed models (Green & Kreuter 2005) are reviewed in detail. Quality and audit issues and how this relates to planning are then considered.

Definitions

Planning is one of those terms which is used in many different ways. Other related terms are used in equally imprecise ways, so that often the same activity is labelled in different ways by different people. There are no hard and fast rules about the way terms are used, but the following definitions are presented as a means of clarifying the differences between related activities. These are the definitions we shall be using in this chapter.

- *Plan* – how to get from your starting point to your end point and what you want to achieve
- *Strategy* – broad framework for action which indicates goals, methods and underlying principles. It derives from evidence, identified needs and

experience. It may be used at all levels as in a programme strategy or an implementation strategy

- *Policy* – guidelines for practice which set broad goals and the framework for action
- *Programme* – overall outline of action. The collection of activities in a planned sequence leading to a defined goal or goals
- *Priority* – the first claim for consideration
- *Aim* or *goal* – broad statement of what is to be achieved
- *Objective* or *target* – specific and precise statements of the intended outcomes that will contribute to the achievement of the aim
- *Stakeholders* – all those individuals or groups who have an interest in the programme

---

Box 19.1

Policy development

Judy has been given a remit to develop a health promotion *programme* with the aim of reducing the suicide rate. Her health authority's *policy* includes a commitment to equal opportunities. She decides her *priority* will be unemployed people, who are known to be at increased risk of suicide. She consults with *stakeholders*. Judy's *objectives* are: (1) to set up a support group for unemployed people; and (2) to provide specialist counselling services. Her *strategy* is to network with existing community groups, and to recruit and train volunteer counsellors.

Reasons for planning

Health promoters usually have no problem in finding things to do which seem reasonable. Work areas are inherited from others, delegated from more senior members of the workplace or demanded by clients. It is possible to be kept very busy reacting to all these pressures, and planning health promotion interventions may seem a luxury or a waste of time.

However, there are sound reasons for planning health promotion or being proactive in your work practice:

- It ensures a systematic and logical approach to establishing priorities.
- It helps direct resources to where they will have most impact.
- It makes clear what is to be achieved, the methods and how success will be demonstrated.

Planning takes different forms and is used at different levels. It may be used to provide the best services or care for an individual client, as in the nursing process, or planning may be for group activities, such as antenatal classes. Planning may also refer to large-scale health promotion interventions targeted at whole populations.

The degree of formality of the planning process also varies. When planning a one-to-one intervention, the process is informal and may involve no one else. Planning for a group intervention may involve liaising with other professionals as well as the target group, to find out what their aims and objectives are and what sorts of methods and resources are available and acceptable. A written plan may be produced to act as a guide and a statement of agreed outcomes and methods. Planning a large-scale intervention will usually involve more long-term collaborative planning. Often a working group (or taskforce or local forum) will be established early on to identify interested groups and gain their support and expertise. A written plan will usually be produced, outlining not only objectives and methods but also a timescale of what is to be achieved when; funding details and a budget; who is responsible for which tasks; and how the intervention will be evaluated and the findings reported back.

There has been much greater emphasis on systematic planning in recent years due to a need for greater economic accountability, more focus on targets and their achievement, and the need to include evidence as part of project development. It is particularly important for practitioners to be clear about the rationale for interventions, the goals and the approach adopted.

Health promotion planning cycle

Planning involves several key stages or logical stepping stones which enable the health promoter to achieve a desired result. The benefit is being clear about what it is you want to achieve, i.e. the purpose of any intervention. Planning entails:

1. An assessment of need.

2. Setting aims – what it is you intend to achieve

3. Setting objectives – precise and measurable outcomes

4. Deciding which methods, interventions or strategies will achieve your objectives

5. Evaluating outcomes in order to make improvements in the future.

Some planning models are presented in a linear fashion. Others show a circular process to indicate that any evaluation feeds back into the process, as illustrated in Figure 19.1. This seemingly rational and simple approach describes how decisions should be made. It does not take into account that there may not be agreement on objectives or the best way to proceed and that in real life, planning is often piecemeal or incremental. There is no grand design, but circumstances dictate many small reactive decisions.

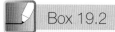

Box 19.2

What do you think would be the best starting point for planning an intervention or programme? Why? Think of any planned activities you have been involved with. What was the starting point? Why?

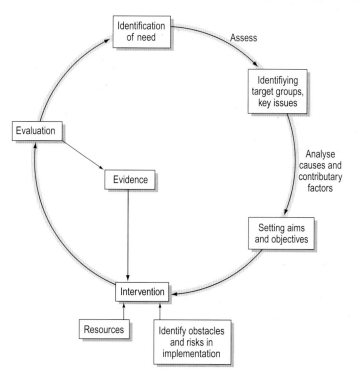

Figure 19.1 • Health promotion planning cycle.

Figure 19.1 suggests that the planning cycle begins with a needs assessment through which the programme's focus and any specific target groups may be identified. The underlying causes and contributory factors that led to the problem and the areas that will need to be addressed are then identified. Figure 19.2 shows how understanding the effects of a problem can help to identify indicators and desired outcomes from an intervention. Turning the problem, in this case antisocial activity by young people in a neighbourhood, into a positive statement gives a purpose for the intervention. Addressing the causes of the problem identifies outputs and activities. The aims and objectives can then be clearly stated. This provides a number of options for intervention and at this point many other issues come into play such as resource availability, capacity and potential obstacles. These issues will then be considered alongside any evidence of effective interventions. The actual intervention or programme and its methods can then be selected. The practicalities of implementation will need to be explored and the evaluation and monitoring plans put in place. This simple model can be applied to all levels of planning activities, from large-scale strategic planning, to middle-scale project planning and small-scale interventions with clients.

Strategic planning

Strategy tends to be used as an umbrella term to cover a broad programme. It may therefore have several different objectives and projects. Practitioners often do not start with a blank sheet and have to work in a wider policy context where issues are determined nationally. For example, all primary care trusts are required to have a strategy to tackle obesity. Strategies may be local as well as national and involve many stakeholders. A stakeholder analysis helps to identify relevant partners and their interests regarding the issue. For example, local area agreements (LAAs) require consultation between statutory and voluntary agencies and local populations to draw up agreed plans to promote health in a defined locality. LAA plans include:

- Detailed specification of services, projects and activities
- Identification of costs, inputs and quality standards
- Targets for what will be achieved.

Box 19.3

Developing a local obesity strategy
Read the extract below from a local obesity strategy. What actions can you identify?
To ensure the long-term commitment of all stakeholders and to try to develop a robust action plan, an extensive consultation process has been undertaken within Torbay during the development of this strategy. Opinions have been sought with regards to both the prevention and management of obesity from stakeholders and members of the general public living in Torbay. Furthermore, a resource mapping exercise has also been undertaken. Alongside the mapping of current practice and the recording of both public and stakeholder opinion regards priorities for action, the evidence for the effectiveness of a broad spectrum of interventions was researched at length. This, alongside local and national policy, was used to help prioritise potential actions. Furthermore, those actions known to have evidence of effectiveness reaching those individuals at greatest potential risk were given largest priority ... Work to improve the health of the population is by no means the sole responsibility of the health service and increasingly local responsibility for the health of communities is being shared between the agencies that make up Local Strategic Partnerships (LSPs) and with the communities themselves (Torbay Care Trust 2006).

There are several stages in developing a strategy:

1. *Getting people involved.* Identifying likely partners and developing a team

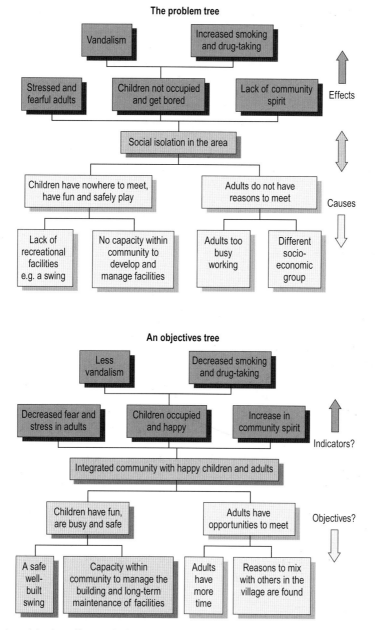

The problem tree

Effects

Causes

An objectives tree

Indicators?

Objectives?

Figure 19.2 • Developing objectives (Centre for International Development and Training 2006).

2. *Where are we now?* Analysing the current situation and building an information baseline

3. *Where do we want to go? What outcomes do we want? What do other people want?* Consultation with stakeholders. Analysing evidence from needs assessments. Prioritizing and setting objectives

4. *How do we get there?* Identifying activities

5. *What may stop us getting there?* Understanding the factors that may affect what we want to achieve

6. *How will we know if we have got there?* Evaluating the effects of activities and mapping these against stated objectives.

These stages correspond to those of a rational planning model: assess–plan–do–evaluate.

Project planning

Project planning is a smaller-scale activity and refers to planning a specific project which is time-limited and aims to bring about a defined change. Examples of small-scale health promotion projects include a project to raise the awareness of university students about meningitis, a project to train school nurses in presentation skills and a project to map safe routes to school for young children.

Box 19.4

You are involved in a working group drawing up a local strategy to reduce alcohol use. Who would you want to be involved in the working group? What broad goals would be appropriate?
Broad goals might be framed in terms of:
- Reducing availability of alcohol, e.g. alcohol-free policies in leisure places and workplaces, refusing licences for additional pubs or bars, clamping down on alcohol sales to young people

- Reducing the promotion of alcohol, e.g. banning advertisements for alcohol on local-authority premises
- Reducing alcohol-related antisocial behavior, e.g. use of local byelaws to prevent drinking in public
- Protecting young people from alcohol-related harm, e.g. sessions in youth clubs and community centres
- Promoting alcohol awareness at work, e.g. supporting workplaces to develop alcohol policies
- Promoting health practitioners' awareness via sessions for GPs and practice nurses on early identification and referral
- Increased health promotion coverage in local mass media linking alcohol to increased risk of accidents and violence.

The working group would need to involve a variety of partners in order to maximize its effectiveness. You might have identified representatives from the local authority, mass media, occupational health services covering workplaces, primary health care practitioners, mental health practitioners, teachers and youth workers, licensed victuallers, magistrates, the police service and voluntary agencies dealing with alcohol-related problems. The success of this strategy will depend on the different partners working together to achieve aims.

Ewles & Simnett (2003) define project stages as:

1. Start

2. Specification

3. Design and implementation

4. Implementation

5. Evaluation, review and final completion.

The start of the project is agreement that the project should take place, its overall aims and the allocation of a budget to support the project. Often the start is signalled by the formal adoption of a project proposal, indicating that an organization has given support for the development and implementation of a project. Specification means setting objectives and quality criteria for how the project is to be delivered. Setting objectives is considered in more detail below. Quality and audit are discussed later in this chapter. Design is the detailed planning of the training intervention. A Gantt chart (set out as an example in Figure 19.3) is a useful tool to use at this stage. A Gantt chart plots tasks and the people responsible for these tasks against a timescale in which these activities need to be undertaken. It portrays in a graphical form the interdependence of project tasks and how each single task contributes to the whole. Implementation is the project activity, e.g. training sessions. Evaluation, review and final completion report on project outcomes and assess whether objectives have been met. It is useful to have a time lag between completing the project and the final review in order to assess long-term as well as immediate outcomes.

Box 19.5

The strategy outlined in Activity 19.4 includes a project centred on training GPs and practice nurses to identify problematic use of alcohol at an early stage. This project, which is part of the overall alcohol reduction strategy, would require careful and detailed planning, including:

- Setting appropriate objectives. For example, would it be appropriate to set an objective of reducing problem drinking in the practice population? Why not?
- How might objectives best be achieved? For example, should training be unidisciplinary or multidisciplinary? Should the training be accredited? Who would be the best person to run the sessions? What venue, day and time would be most acceptable? How would the sessions be funded? How long will the project last?
- How would you evaluate the project? What criteria would you use to demonstrate success?

The kind of planning most health practitioners will be involved in will be on a much smaller scale. For example, you may want to plan a health education session with an individual client, or a series of sessions with a small group around a specific issue. Using the example above, you might want to plan a single session in detail. This would require you to:

- Set detailed objectives for participants to achieve by the end of the session, e.g. being aware of symptoms and behaviours (for example, poor attendance and time-keeping at work, especially in the mornings) which might be due to problematic alcohol use
- Investigate the range of resources available and select resources to use in the session
- Plan the session showing different activities and time allocated for each
- Plan a means of evaluating the session.

Planning models

Planning, whatever the scale of the activity, requires systematic working through a number of stages. There are a number of different planning models that have been developed, two of which are now discussed in greater detail.

Ewles & Simnett (2003) planning framework

The Ewles & Simnett (2003) planning framework (Figure 19.4) is a useful generic framework which can be adapted to a number of situations.

Stage 1: identify needs and priorities

This may need local research and investigation, or may be the selection of particular clients from a caseload. Researching needs may require additional investigation. For example, local community profiles and local agencies might provide information on pressing local needs. Consultation with community

	March	April	May	June	July	August	September	October
Marketing and publicity	H and A							
Recruit participants		A						
Plan sessions				H	H			
Accreditation			H and A					
Pre-course needs assessment questionnaire				H and R				
Prepare materials, collect resources					H and A			
Check venue, timing, refreshments						A		
Action: training sessions							H	
Post-course sessions								H and R
Evaluation report								H and R

Three workers are involved:

H is a health promotor
A is an administrative officer
R is a researcher.

Figure 19.3 • Gantt chart: planning training project. Three workers are involved: H, health promotion specialist; A, administrative officer; and R researcher.

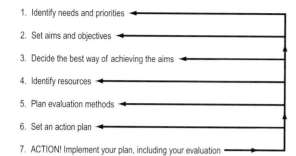

1. Identify needs and priorities
2. Set aims and objectives
3. Decide the best way of achieving the aims
4. Identify resources
5. Plan evaluation methods
6. Set an action plan
7. ACTION! Implement your plan, including your evaluation

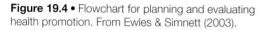

Figure 19.4 • Flowchart for planning and evaluating health promotion. From Ewles & Simnett (2003).

members may flag up their felt needs and priorities. Needs may already be defined for you, often on the basis of national or local epidemiological data reporting trends in illness and deaths. Chapter 18 discusses this stage in more detail.

Other planning models start at different points. For example, a stated health promotion goal can be analysed to determine an appropriate educational intervention. This intervention is modified by referring to the characteristics of the target group, and a detailed educational programme planned. For example, an accident reduction programme identifies education about hazards in the home as a priority. The target group is older people. Based on evidence of other interventions with older people, it is decided that interpersonal communication would be the most effective intervention. Specific objectives are formulated concerning education about lighting and mobility aids.

Stage 2: set aims and objectives

Aims are broad goals concerned with improving health in a particular area or reducing a health problem, e.g. reducing the amount of alcohol-related ill health. Objectives need to be specific and should be statements that define what participants will have achieved by the end of the intervention. Objectives therefore need to be measurable in some way. There is a balance to be struck between setting objectives which are realistic but also challenging. When

writing objectives it is recommended that they are SMART:

Specific
Measurable
Achievable
Realistic
Time-bound.

Health promotion objectives can refer to educational, behavioural, policy, process or environmental outcomes:

Educational objectives may be divided into three categories:

1. Knowledge objectives, concerning increased levels of knowledge

2. Affective objectives, concerning changes in attitudes and beliefs

3. Behavioural or skills objectives, concerning the acquisition of new competences and skills.

• Behavioural objectives include changes in lifestyles and increased take-up of services, e.g. reducing the amount of binge-drinking or the prevalence of drink-driving.
• Policy objectives include the development or implementation of policy, e.g. implementing alcohol-free policies in workplaces.
• Process objectives include the achievement of health promotion principles, e.g. participation and intersectoral collaboration.
• Environmental objectives include changing the environment to make it more health-promoting, e.g. restricting the advertising and sale of alcohol.

Box19.6

Setting objectives for a training programme

A project has the overall aim of improving the early identification of alcohol-related problems. One of the objectives is to raise the awareness of GPs and practice nurses to such problems in patients. One activity might involve a training session with the following educational objectives:

1. Increasing participants' knowledge of the range of harmful effects and symptoms associated with problematic alcohol use.
2. Increasing participants' knowledge of the extent of problematic alcohol use and its association with social and demographic factors, e.g. gender, age, employment status, occupation.
3. Investigating participants' attitudes towards alcohol and cultural depictions of alcohol use. Identifying the range between social drinker and alcoholic, with the many stages in between. Recognizing social, media and peer pressures to drink which contribute to many people's problematic usage of alcohol.
4. Enabling participants to use an assessment tool effectively to identify problematic alcohol use.
5. Enabling participants to use the Stages of Change model to identify problem drinkers and appropriate interventions.

Objectives also reflect perspectives about the determinants of health and values about what are the most important things to achieve. These perspectives and values may be your own or may be derived from your organization.

Stage 3: identify appropriate methods for achieving the objectives

Decisions about how to go about addressing the problem will depend on objectives but also available evidence of effective interventions, available funding and the expertise of practitioners. Certain methods go with certain objectives but would be quite inappropriate for other objectives. For example, participative small-group work is effective at changing attitudes but a more formal teaching session would be more effective if specific knowledge is to be imparted. Community development is effective at increasing community involvement and participation but would not be appropriate if local government policy change is the objective. The mass media is effective in raising people's awareness of health issues but ineffective in persuading people to change their behaviour. So the next stage in planning is deciding which methods would be the logical choice given your objectives. You may then find you have to compromise owing to constraints of time, resources or skills, but this compromise should concern the amount of input, or the use of complementary methods. It should not mean that you end up using inappropriate methods which are unlikely to achieve your objectives.

Box 19.7

Consider the different aims that may be included in a drug prevention strategy:
- To reduce the risks associated with drug use and enable clients who do choose to use drugs to do so safely
- To reduce levels of harmful drug use.

What values and views about the determinants of drug use are reflected in these different aims?

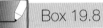

Box 19.8

A Sun Smart programme in Australia identifies a major health problem in children's exposure to ultraviolet light. A diagnosis of the risk factors for this identifies children not wearing hats and lack of shade in the playground. The contributory factors for children not wearing hats are their dislike of wearing them and the lack of any requirement to wear them. The contributory factors for the children's exposure to sun when in the playground are lack of funds to build shelters and lack of awareness by children of the need to keep out of the sun.

- What would be appropriate and SMART objectives for such a project?

Regulating to make the wearing of hats part of school uniform might make the healthy choice easier, so encouraging stakeholder involvement in a review of uniform requirements might be an objective. Making hats a fun and desirable part of clothing and raising funds to build a playground shelter might be other objectives.

Stage 4: identify resources

When objectives and methods have been decided, the next stage is to consider whether any specific resources are needed to implement the strategy. Resources include human resources, financial resources and materials and equipment.

 Box 19.9

What would you need to include in a budget plan for the training sessions for GPs and practice nurses on early identification of problematic alcohol use discussed in Box 19.4?

Funding is an important issue for larger-scale interventions which require additional inputs over and above existing services and staff. For larger-scale interventions you may need to prepare a budget which is a statement of expected costs. This includes direct costs, which relate to the project, and fixed costs, which happen anyway.

Direct costs include:

- Staff costs – salaries, superannuation, employer's National Insurance payments, annual increments
- Capital costs, e.g. computer
- Costs of specific activities, e.g. rental of community centre for training, buying resources to use in the training

- Telephone, postage, photocopying
- Travel and subsistence
- Training and conferences to support staff development.

Fixed costs include overheads to cover accommodation, heating, lighting and telephone rental.

A budget control system regularly monitors what is spent and what remains. This is usually done by monitoring the amount of money allocated, the amount of money spent and the variance between the two (underspend or overspend) under each budget heading every month.

Stage 5: plan evaluation methods

Evaluation must relate to the objectives you have set but can be undertaken more or less formally. For example, in relation to an educational session you might decide to ask participants their views at the end of the session, or spend some time noting your own perceptions of what went well and what could be improved next time. Or you might design a more formal means of evaluation, e.g. a questionnaire for participants to fill in anonymously, which is timetabled into the session. Project evaluation is discussed in more detail in the next chapter.

Stage 6: set an action plan

This is a detailed written plan which identifies tasks, the person responsible for each task, resources which will be used, a timescale and means of evaluation. You might also include interim indicators of progress to show if you are proceeding as planned. Many factors can threaten the sustainability of a project. Being clear about the external factors underlying the structure of the project and what assumptions are being made is a key requirement of most project plans, especially where large sums of money are being allocated. For example, projects may depend on achieving community involvement or successful funding bids.

Log frames (logistical frameworks) are widely used in international development projects to identify the

Project	Indicators of achievement	Means of verification	Important risks and assumptions
Goal • To reduce the harmful effects of binge drinking amongst young women			
Purpose (or objective) • To raise awareness of using safe taxi companies to get home			
Outputs • Purse cards with taxi numbers • Posters in bar and club toilets • Tannoy announcements in bar and club toilets			
Activities • Working with specified taxi companies to recruit women drivers • Working with bar and club owners			

Figure 19.5 • Example of a logistical framework for a project to reduce binge drinking.

activities of a programme and any inherent risks that might delay completion (see Figure 19.5). The benefit of a log frame is that it tests the assumptions of a project plan. Working from the bottom up, it tests the logic through 'if–then', i.e. if we do these activities, then this output will be achieved. If we deliver these outputs, then this purpose will be achieved. If the purpose is achieved then this will contribute to the goal. Flaws in logic might include having a purpose that is too far away from the outputs or a purpose that cannot be assessed.

Box 19.10

Complete the log frame, in Figure 19.5 above. What are the advantages of using this framework in project management?

Stage 7: action, or implementation of the plan

It is often useful to keep a log or diary to note unexpected problems and how you dealt with them, as well as unintended benefits. This information can then be fed into the evaluation process. You will also want to plan for the documentation and dissemination of the findings from the project, whether in the form of a report, a newsletter or presentation.

PRECEDE–proceed model

Figure 19.6 illustrates the PRECEDE–proceed planning model, one of the earliest and best-known models which has now been revised and simplified (Green & Kreuter 2005). PRECEDE stands for

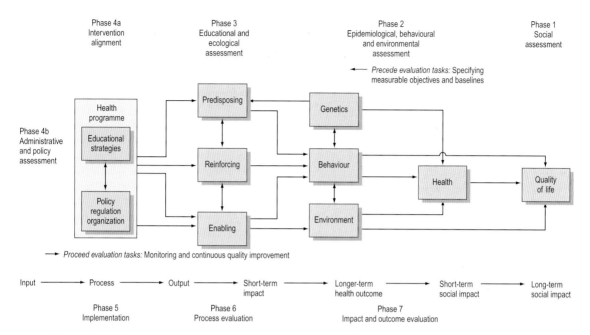

Figure 19.6 • PRECEDE–proceed planning model. From Green et al 2005.

predisposing reinforcing and enabling causes in educational diagnosis. This model recognizes the multiple determinants of health and starts with an assessment of the quality of life, which is the ultimate goal. Health contributes towards quality of life. The model then works backwards in a sequence of diagnostic phases to identify the environmental and organizational factors that influence health behaviour, including health service utilization. It considers the predisposing factors, those personal factors such as individual motivation, knowledge attitudes and beliefs; reinforcing factors, the attitudes and behaviours of role models, peers, employers; and enabling factors, resources and skills that either support or hinder change in behaviour or environment. As well as diagnosing what needs to be addressed, the capacity for implementation of a proposed programme is also considered.

The model may be broken down into phases, as illustrated in Box 19.11. Priority targets for

intervention are established through each phase of the assessment process (phases 1–4) on the basis of:

- their causal importance in the chain of health determinants
- their prevalence
- their changeability

The results of this assessment process guide the development of the intervention (phase 5). The evaluation (phases 6–7) then tracks the impact of the intervention on factors identified as important targets in the assessment process.

Box 19.11

Phases of the PRECEDE–proceed model

Phase 1: *Social diagnosis* – the identification of a population's felt concerns and problems relating to their quality of life e.g. unemployment, crime

Phase 2: *Epidemiological, behavioural and environmental assessment* – determines health issues associated with the quality of life, e.g. genetic risk factors, disability. Health practices linked to health problems are identified, e.g .compliance, preventive actions, service utilization, self-care and management, lifestyles and environmental factors

Phase 3: *Educational and ecological assessment* – the identification of three categories of factors which affect behaviour:

- Predisposing factors – beliefs, values and attitudes that affect motivation to change
- Enabling factors – skills and resources, social factors, e.g. income. Absence of enabling factors constitutes a barrier which will need to be overcome in order to enable behaviour change to occur
- Reinforcing factors – the feedback received from significant others, which may help or hinder the process of behaviour change

Phase 4: *Analysis* – of the phase 3 categories of factors and the selection of the most important factors

Phase 4: *Intervention alignment* follows automatically and is the decision of which factors are to be the focus of the intervention according to their severity and changeability. The type and extent of resources available will help inform this decision

Phase 5: Intervention development and implementation again follow logically from the previous phases. The management and administration of the intervention are also considered at this stage. Administrative diagnosis includes assessment of resources and organizational relationships, and the production of a timetable

Phase 6: *Evaluation of the intervention* assesses impacts and outcomes, although Green & Kreuter (2005) stress that this should be an integrated activity addressed throughout the planning process, as shown in Figure 19.6.

The intention is that using the PRECEDE–proceed model will guide the health educator to the most effective type of intervention. Using knowledge drawn

from epidemiology, social psychology, education and management studies, the health educator can arrive at an optimum intervention. The model is said to be based on a complementary mix of expertise drawn from these different disciplines. In practice, the model is often modified and is rarely used as illustrated (see Green's own website for an account of the application of the model: http://www.lgreen.net/precede.htm). For example, it is unusual to begin the process of planning with an agenda as open as 'quality of life'. Priority topics, target groups or settings are more often identified at the outset. For example, the *Saving Lives: Our Healthier Nation* targets (Department of Health 1998) focus on specific diseases. So in practice the use of the PRECEDE proceed model often begins at the behavioural diagnosis rather than the needs assessment phase.

The PRECEDE–proceed model may be criticized on several grounds. As a health education planning model it mirrors the medical world. The planning process is dominated by experts. The general public may be involved in identifying problems, but the ways and means of tackling these problems are to be determined by experts. The focus is on achieving behavioural change at the level of individuals or groups. The social, political and environmental context of health is systematically screened out by the model in phases 2 and 3. To some extent this may be explained by the PRECEDE proceed model being a health education rather than a health promotion planning model. A model developed specifically for health education cannot be expected to apply to other forms of health promotion but, for most people, education, even if it does not include changing the environment, does include clarifying values, beliefs and attitudes, facilitating self-empowerment and supporting autonomy. Using the PRECEDE-proceed model subordinates these activities to the primary aim of behaviour change. It could be argued that PRECEDE–proceed is a model dominated by social psychology and behavioural perspectives rather than educational perspectives, and that the label is therefore misleading. PRECEDE–proceed is, however, a highly structured planning model which ensures that certain issues are considered. If the objective is behaviour change, then PRECEDE–proceed is a useful model to follow.

Quality and audit

Assessing the quality of practice through quality assurance, quality management or audit is an important aspect of professional practice. It helps to improve standards, identify cost-effective activities, demonstrate worth to outside agencies and ensure that activities meet stakeholders' requirements. The introduction of commissioning of services and the placing of contracts have highlighted the need for specification of quality. There has also been an increased emphasis on audit of public sector activities and clinical audit is well established. Frameworks are established such as the protocols established by the National Institute for Health and Clinical Excellence (NICE) as well as National Service Frameworks and the Healthcare Commission in order to ensure high-quality health services. Continuous quality improvement, total quality management and the use of external standards all aim to improve services and also provide answers to the variability in programme development. The core principles of quality interventions in health promotion have been defined as (Speller et al 1997):

- Equity – that users have equal access and/or equal benefit from services
- Effectiveness – that services achieve their intended objectives
- Efficiency – that services achieve maximum benefit for minimum cost
- Accessibility – that a service is easily available to users in terms of time, distance and ethos
- Appropriateness – that a service is that which the users require
- Acceptability – that services satisfy the reasonable expectations of users
- Responsiveness – that services adapt to the expressed needs of users.

Quality expresses a notion of 'fit for the purpose' but also conveys a notion of excellence. Applying the notion of quality to work practice is difficult. One means of trying to do this is through quality assurance or audit which is a 'systematic process through which achievable and desirable levels of quality are described, the extent to which these levels are achieved is assessed, and action taken following assessment to enable them to be realised' (Wright & Whittington 1992).

Quality assurance is an ongoing process of continual assessment and improvement of practice, and therefore differs from evaluation, which focuses on outcomes at a specific point in time. A quality system may include elements of quality assurance and quality management. Quality assurance involves setting standards which specify quality and ensure consistency. Quality management applies the emphasis on quality to everyone through increasing their control over their performance. Quality assurance in health promotion is defined as:

the process of assessment of a programme or intervention in order to ensure performance against agreed standards, which are subject to continuous improvement and set within the framework and principles of the Ottawa Charter (Speller 1998, p. 79).

Quality is about doing things in the correct manner. Box 19.12 outlines the criteria in the European Quality Instrument for Health Promotion for supporting development of interventions, benchmarking and evaluation (Bollars et al 2005). It states that indicators of quality relate to appropriate design, good management and practice that accord with core principles.

Box 19.12

European quality instrument for health promotion

I. Framework of health promotion principles

This approach embraces the principles of health promotion, including a positive and comprehensive approach to health, attention to the broad determinants of health, participation, empowerment, equity and equality.

II. Project development and implementation

a. Analysis – the project is based on a systematic analysis of the health problem and its determinants and of the context in which it will be implemented

b. Aims and objectives – the aims and objectives of the project are clearly defined

c. Target group – the group of people the project intends to influence is clearly defined

d. Intervention – the strategies and methods for an effective intervention are clearly outlined

e. Implementation strategy – there is a clear description of the way the intervention will be carried out

f. Evaluation – the effects (effect evaluation) and quality (process evaluation) of the intervention will be assessed

III. Project management

a. Leadership – a person has been designated who is ultimately responsible for and capable of managing the project

b. Planning and documentation – the working plan and organization of the project are firmly established

c. Capacity and resources – are the expertise and resources available that are necessary to implement the project successfully?

d. Participation and commitment – the ways in which various parties will be involved and committed to the project are clearly outlined

e. Communication – the way in which all the participants (target group and stakeholders) will be informed about the project is clearly established

IV. Sustainability

The continuation of the project is ensured

(www.nigz.nl/gettingevidence and in full at http://ws5.e-vision.nl/systeem3/images/ Annexe%2010%20EQUIHP.pdf).

Audit is a systematic process of scrutinizing a service or programme in order to improve performance. Audit may focus on a particular aspect, e.g. organization and management or training. Part of the purpose of an audit is to build a picture, providing evidence of gaps and areas for improvement by comparing what is done with agreed best practice. A key part of an audit is to see if a service meets the needs of its users, so it may involve gathering and acting on local people's views. Audit may involve an internal review or scrutiny by an independent external auditor (e.g. the Audit Commission, Ofsted inspectors of schools).

Box 19.13

Identify one aspect of your health promotion work that would benefit from an audit. Using the above criteria and any others you think are important, draw up a list of standards that might be relevant.

Conclusion

There are sound reasons for adopting a planning model to structure health promotion interventions. Recognizing that health is a complex socially determined concept means that activities to promote health require careful planning, and often collaboration and working together with different agencies. Activities at different levels all benefit from planning, although the factors which need to be considered will vary according to the level of planned intervention.

The rationale for planning is summarized by the Centre for International Development and Training (2006) as follows:

- Relevant to agreed strategic objectives
- Key stakeholders are involved at the important stages of the project
- Relevant to the real problems and issues of target groups/beneficiaries

- Objectives are feasible and can be realistically achieved
- Successes can be measured and verified
- Benefits generated by projects are likely to be sustainable
- Decision-making is well informed at each stage.

Planning provides a standard framework in which projects/programmes/interventions are developed, implemented and evaluated. The planning cycle ensures that the results of a project are fed back into new projects and programmes. There are a variety of planning models for health promotion and they can help make explicit the various values, rationales and assumptions that are inherent in the decision-making process.

In reality, planning health promotion is a more complex process than the planning models suggest. This is because rational decision-making is only one factor in determining what happens. Many other factors are also important, including historical precedent, enthusiasms of key people and the political context. So it is unlikely that any health promotion intervention proceeds exactly along the lines indicated by a planning model, but this does not mean models are not useful. Models help structure activities and can act as a checklist to ensure that important stages are not missed out. They are there to be modified in the light of experience, not to act as straitjackets.

Chapter 20 goes on to discuss the evaluation stage. Evaluating interventions, and being able to determine to what extent health promotion is successful in achieving its objectives, is the key to establishing health promotion as a central plank of health work.

Questions for further discussion

- What factors would you take into account when planning a health promotion intervention?
- How could you assess the quality of your health promotion work?

Summary

This chapter has clarified the terminology used in the planning process and has discussed the reasons for planning health promotion interventions. Planning happens at different levels, and an account of this has been given. Two planning models which have been developed specifically for health promotion have been discussed in greater detail. The assessment and evaluation of planning have been discussed through reference to quality assurance and audit cycles.

Further reading

Bollars C, Kok H, Van den Broucke S et al 2005 European Quality Instrument for Health Promotion with User Manual Woerden: NIGZ *www.nigz.nl/gettingevidence. The important development of a quality tool for health promotion can be explored through the Netherlands Institute.*

Davies M, Kepford J 2006 Planning a health promotion intervention. In: Davies M, Macdowall W (eds) Health promotion theory. Understanding public health series. OUP, McGrawHill, Maidenhead. *A useful short summary of some key factors to take into account.*

Ewles L, Simnett I 2003 Promoting health: a practical guide 5th edn. Baillière Tindall, Edinburgh. *Chapter 7 gives further details and a practical guide to Ewles & Simnett's model. Chapter 8 discusses project planning in more detail.*

Tones K, Green J 2004 Health promotion. Planning and strategies Sage, London. *Chapter 4 provides a readable and detailed discussion of systematic approaches to planning and discusses various planning models.*

References

Bollars C, Kok H, Van den Broucke S et al 2005 European Quality Instrument for Health Promotion with User Manual Woerden: NIGZ

Centre for International Development and Training 2006 An introduction to multiagency planning using the logistical framework approach. CIDT, Wolverhampton

Department of Health 1998 Saving lives: our healthier nation. Stationery Office, London.

Ewles L, Simnett I 2003 Promoting health: a practical guide, 5th edn. Baillière Tindall, London.

Green L W, Kreuter M W 2005 Health program planning: an educational and ecological approach, 4th edn. McGraw-Hill Higher Education, New York.

Speller V 1998 Quality assurance programmes: their development and contribution to improving effectiveness in health promotion. In: Scott D, Weston R (eds) Evaluating health promotion. Stanley Thornes, Cheltenham.

Speller V, Evans D, Head M 1997 Perpectives. Developing quality assurance standards for health promotion in the UK. Health Promotion International 12: 215–224.

Torbay Care Trust 2006 Tipping the scales: an obesity strategy for Torbay. Torbay Care Trust, Torbay.

Wright C, Whittington D 1992 Quality assurance: an introduction for health care professionals. Churchill-Livingstone, London.

Chapter Twenty

20

Evaluation in health promotion

OVERVIEW

Evaluation is an integral aspect of all planned activities, enabling an assessment of the value or worth of an intervention. Evaluation also performs several other roles. For practitioners, evaluation helps develop their skills and competences. For funders evaluation demonstrates where resources can be most usefully channelled. For lay people, evaluation provides an opportunity to have their voice heard. There are additional reasons why evaluating health promotion is a key aspect of practice. As a relatively new discipline there is great pressure on health promotion to prove its worth through evaluation of its activities. In addition, the drive in the National Health Service (NHS) to ensure that all practice is

evidence-based affects health promotion as well as more clinical activities. In a situation where resources will always be limited, demonstrating the cost-effectiveness of interventions is important. There are thus many factors leading to a demand for evaluation of health promotion practice.

Evaluating health promotion is not a straightforward task. Health promotion interventions often involve different kinds of activities, a long timescale, and several partners who may each have their own objectives. Health promotion is still seen as belonging within the health services, where the dominant evaluation model is quantitative research centred on experimental trials, with randomized controlled trials (RCTs) as the preferred evaluation tool. Health promotion has had to argue its case for a more holistic evaluation strategy encompassing qualitative methodologies and taking into account contextual features.

The focus of this chapter is on evaluating health promotion interventions. Evaluation of research studies is also part of the health promoter's role and remit, and readers are referred to Chapters 2 and 3 in our companion volume (Naidoo & Wills 2005) for a detailed discussion of this topic. This chapter considers what is meant by evaluation, the range of research methodologies used in evaluation studies, its rationale, how it is done and the role of evaluation in building the evidence base for health promotion.

Defining evaluation

Evaluation is a complex concept with many definitions that vary according to purpose, disciplinary boundaries and values. A comprehensive definition of evaluation is: 'the systematic examination and assessment of features of a programme or other intervention in order to produce knowledge that different stakeholders can use for a variety of purposes' (Rootman et al 2001, p. 26). The above definition is useful because it also flags up the importance of the purpose of evaluation, and the fact that there can be many different reasons to evaluate. Evaluation can provide information on the extent to which an intervention met its aims and goals, the manner in which the intervention was carried out, and the cost-effectiveness of the intervention. It is important to be clear at the outset about the purpose of evaluation as this will determine what information is gathered and how information is obtained. The value-driven purpose of evaluation distinguishes it from research (Springett 2001). Evaluation uses resources which might otherwise be used for programme planning and implementation, so a clear purpose is also necessary in order to legitimate and protect this use of resources.

Box 20.1

You have a limited budget (from lottery money) and tight timescale to deliver a community

health promotion intervention designed to improve nutrition. Stakeholders include the funders, local schools, social housing and sheltered accommodation providers, community associations, primary health care staff, social care staff and the community. Your proposed plan of action includes an evaluation and you have suggested earmarking 5–10% of your budget and time for this purpose. A coalition of some of the stakeholders has approached you requesting that you omit the evaluation and concentrate all your resources on the intervention. How would you respond? What arguments might you use to defend the proposed evaluation?

From a practitioner's perspective, evaluation is needed to assess results, determine whether objectives have been met and find out if the methods used were appropriate and efficient. These findings can then be fed back into the planning process in order to progress practice. Evaluations of interventions are used to build an evidence base of what works, enabling other practitioners to focus their inputs where they will have most effect. From a lay perspective, evaluation helps to clarify expectations and assess the extent to which these have been met. Evaluation may also help determine what strategies had most impact, and why. Without evaluation, it is very difficult to make a reasoned case for more resources or expansion of an intervention. Even when a programme is rolling out an established and effective intervention, specific local features may have an unanticipated impact that will only become apparent in an evaluation. There are sound reasons for evaluating all interventions, although more innovative projects will require more substantial and costly evaluation.

Box 20.2

Principles to guide the evaluation of health promotion interventions
The World Health Organization (WHO) has identified four principles that should be used

to guide the evaluation of health promotion interventions:

1. **Participation** – all stakeholders should be involved in evaluation
2. **Multidisciplinary** – evaluation should combine quantitative and qualitative methodologies drawn from different disciplines
3. **Capacity** – evaluation should help to build the capacity of all stakeholders to address health promotion concerns
4. **Appropriate** – evaluation should be appropriate, taking into account the complexity of health promotion interventions and their long timescale (Rootman et al 2001).

Box 20.3

A well-man clinic is introduced in a primary health care practice. The aim is to monitor the health of middle-aged men and to provide information and advice enabling them to adopt healthier lifestyles, so that in the longer term health risks such as high blood pressure or smoking are reduced. Over a period of time, the practice nurse invites all men aged 40–65 into the practice for a half-hour session where she checks vital statistics (weight, blood pressure), asks about lifestyle (e.g. diet, smoking, alcohol and drug use, sexual activity, exercise) and gives individually tailored information and advice about adopting a healthier lifestyle. This intervention takes up a significant proportion of her time and workload.

How would you evaluate this programme, using the four criteria outlined above?

Evaluation covers many different activities undertaken with varying degrees of rigour or reflectiveness. At its simplest level, evaluation describes what any competent practitioner does as a matter of course, that is, the process of appraising and assessing work activities. This includes the process of informal feedback or more systematic review of health promotion interventions. In the example above, noting how the sessions have been received by the men, or soliciting their comments, or those of peers and colleagues, is part of the evaluation process. Evaluation is often used to refer to a more formal or systematic activity, where assessment is linked to original intentions and is fed back into the planning process. For the well-man clinic example, this might involve monitoring vital statistics and doing a before-and-after study of lifestyle behaviours. Health promotion evaluation should integrate core health promotion principles such as equity and participation into the evaluation process. In the well-man clinic example this might be achieved through asking the men what they wanted from participating in the programme and whether they achieved their goals. Comparing the socioeconomic status of participants and non-participants would help determine if the programme was reinforcing or challenging social and health inequalities.

Evaluation research methodologies

Box 20.4

A hospital nurse has set up a project to help cardiac patients to stop smoking. The intervention involved the identification of a key worker who was allocated time to interview patients to assess their smoking behaviour and draw up individual plans. After discharge, patients were followed up by a weekly telephone call for 6 weeks.

How could this project be evaluated so that any success in terms of smoking cessation in the target group could be shown to be due to the project?

What would be the strengths and limitations of the methods you identify?

1. An RCT would involve each smoking patient on arrival in the ward to be randomly allocated to either the experimental group (who receive the interview) or the control group (who do not receive the interview but get a care plan and general leaflet).

2. Case-study evaluation would interview patients about their involvement in the project and examine their knowledge, attitudes and reported behaviour.

Evaluation is often more formally conducted as research using a variety of different methods. The classic scientific method of proof, the experiment, relies on controlling all factors apart from the one being studied and can best be achieved under laboratory conditions. However, this is clearly impossible and unethical to achieve where people's health is concerned. The RCT is the next most rigorous scientific method of proof. The RCT involves randomly allocating people to an intervention or control group. Random allocation means that the two groups should be matched in terms of factors such as age, gender and social class which are all known to affect health. Any changes detected in the intervention group are then compared to those found amongst the control group. Those changes which occur in the intervention but not the control group can then be attributed to the health promotion programme.

In the well-man clinic example in Activity 20.3 an RCT study would involve randomly allocating all men in the target group to either the intervention group (invited for screening) or the control group (not invited). The two groups would then be compared after the intervention had taken place. If the intervention group showed statistically significant improvements in health status or health-related behaviour over and above those recorded for the control group the intervention would be deemed to be effective.

The degree of scientific rigour necessary to conduct an RCT is hard to achieve in real-life situations. Most health promotion programmes have spin-off effects and indeed are designed to do so. It is impossible to isolate different groups of people or to ensure that programmes do not 'leak' beyond their set boundaries. However, the RCT design does mean that changes detected in the input group may be ascribed to the health promotion programme with a greater degree of confidence.

Evaluation research may also use qualitative methods to focus on understanding the processes involved in change. This kind of evaluation provides details on what is happening in interventions and which features have been effective. This is achieved through the use of qualitative methodologies and methods, and the case study is one example of this approach. The health promotion intervention is the 'case' that is intensively studied using a variety of methods. This enables the evaluator to get a detailed picture of how the intervention has affected the people involved. Case studies are typically small-scale and findings are expressed in descriptive rather than numerical terms. Each case study is unique and findings cannot be generalized to other situations. Its strength as a method is that there is a high degree of confidence that identified effects are real and result from the programme.

In the well-man clinic example in Activity 20.3, a qualitative case-study approach might involve indepth interviews with a sample of men who took up the screening opportunity and the practice nurse. The interviews would aim to explore what motivated the men to accept the invitation to attend the clinic, how they found the experience and how (if at all) it has affected them.

Both the RCT and the case study are valid methods which can be used to isolate the effects of health promotion interventions. There are also many other methods that lie between these two extremes, e.g. surveys which aim to identify significant trends. In practice methods often overlap or are combined. The RCT fits into a scientific, quantitative medical model of proof, has higher status and is generally regarded as more respectable and credible than the case study.

Why evaluate?

Evaluation uses resources that could otherwise be used to provide services. Given that services are always in demand, there needs to be a strong rationale for devoting resources to evaluation rather than service provision. New or pilot interventions warrant a rigorous evaluation because, without evidence of their effectiveness or efficiency, it is difficult to argue that they should become established work practices. Other criteria that can be used to determine if evaluation is worth the effort relate to how well it can be done. If it will be impossible to obtain cooperation from the different groups involved in the activity, it is probably not worthwhile trying to evaluate. If evaluation has not been considered at the outset but is tacked on as an afterthought, the chances are that it will be so partial and biased as to be not worth the effort.

Evaluation is only worthwhile if it will make a difference. This means that the results of the evaluation need to be interpreted and fed back to the relevant audiences in an accessible form. All too often, evaluations are buried in inappropriate formats. Work reports may go no further than the manager, or academic studies full of jargon may be published in little-known journals.

Box 20.5

Reasons for evaluation
- To assess how resources were deployed (*effort*)
- To assess whether what has been achieved was an economically sound use of resources (*efficiency*)
- To measure impact and outcomes and whether the intervention was worthwhile (*effectiveness*)
- To judge the adequacy and relevance of the delivery of the intervention (*execution*)
- To assess the overall benefits of the intervention (*efficacy*)
- To inform future plans
- To justify decisions to others (O'Connor-Fleming & Parker 2001).

Results of evaluation studies will be relevant to many different groups and it may be necessary to reproduce findings in different ways in order to reach all these groups.

Box 20.6

A specialist community public health nurse has evaluated her health promotion activities. These include opportunistic one-to-one counselling and education, setting up a carers' support group, producing information leaflets on coping with dementia, and health surveys of people aged 75 and over.

How could she make her findings known to her clients, her manager, her nursing colleagues and other health and welfare workers?

What to evaluate?

Health promotion objectives may be about individual changes, service use or changes in the environment. Example 20.7 shows the range of possible objectives associated with smoking reduction interventions, each of which would need evaluation.

Box 20.7

Health promotion objectives for smoking reduction
- Increased knowledge, e.g. harmful effects of passive smoking
- Changes in attitudes, e.g. less willingness to breathe in others' smoke
- Changes in behaviour, e.g. stopping smoking
- Acquiring new skills, e.g. learning relaxation methods to reduce stress
- Introduction of healthy policies, e.g. funding to enable GPs to prescribe nicotine replacement aids for people on low income
- Modifying the environment, e.g. banning tobacco advertising and promotion, workplace no-smoking policies
- Reduction in risk factors, e.g. reduction in number of smokers and amount of tobacco smoked per person
- Increased use of services, e.g. take-up rates for smoking cessation clinics, number of calls made to quit-smoking telephone helplines

- Reduced morbidity, e.g. reduced rates of respiratory illness and coronary heart disease (CHD)
- Reduced mortality, e.g. reduced mortality from lung cancer.

Although all these factors relate to health, they are quite separate, and there is no necessary connection between, say, increased knowledge and behaviour change. It is therefore inappropriate to evaluate a given objective (e.g. increased physical activity) by measuring other aspects of an intervention (e.g. number of leaflets taken at a health fair or number of people reporting that they would like to exercise more). It is important to choose appropriate indicators for the stated objectives. This issue is discussed further in Chapter 19, where the log-frame model and the use of logic to select appropriate indicators are considered.

Process, impact and outcome evaluation

Evaluation is always incomplete. It is not possible to assess every element of an intervention. Instead, decisions are taken about which evaluation criteria to prioritize and also sometimes which objectives are to be assessed. A distinction is often made between process, impact and outcome evaluation. Process evaluation (also called formative or illuminative evaluation) is concerned with assessing the process of programme implementation. Outcomes can be immediate (impacts), intermediate or long-term (outcomes). Impact and outcome evaluation are both concerned with assessing the effects of interventions.

Box 20.8

Classify the objectives in Example 20.7 according to whether they refer to immediate, intermediate or long-term outcomes.

The following criteria have been proposed to guide evaluation in public health (Phillips et al 1994, cited in Douglas et al 2007):

- Effectiveness – the extent to which aims and objectives are met
- Acceptability – to the people concerned and society at large
- Appropriateness – relevance to need
- Equity – equal provision for equal needs
- Efficiency – cost–benefit ratio.

Box 20.9

Which of these criteria above apply to process evaluation? Which apply to impact and outcome evaluation?

Process evaluation

Process evaluation may be from the perspective of participants and/or practitioners and/or other stakeholders such as funders. Stakeholders' perceptions and reactions to health promotion interventions and facilitating or inhibiting factors may be sought. More objective data, such as whether targets were met and timescales and budgets adhered to, can also be included. The aims of process evaluation are practical – can the intervention be repeated, can it be refined, and can it be reproduced in similar or different settings with similar or different target groups (Parry-Langdon et al 2003)?

There are four main questions in process evaluation:

1. Is the programme reaching the target group (programme reach)?

2. Are participants satisfied with the programme (programme acceptability)?

3. Are all the activities of the programme being implemented (programme integrity)?

4. Are all the materials and components of the programme of good quality (programme quality) (Hawe et al 1994; Nutbeam 1998)?

Process evaluation employs a wide range of qualitative or 'soft' methods. Examples of such methods are interviews, diaries, observations and content analysis of documents. These methods tell us a great deal about that particular programme and the factors responsible for its success or failure, but they are unable to predict what would happen if the programme were to be replicated in other areas. Because process evaluation does not use 'hard' scientific methods, its findings tend to be more easily dismissed as unrepresentative. However, process evaluation is crucial to health promotion. We need to understand how health promotion interventions are interpreted and responded to by different groups of people and whether the intervention itself is health-promoting, and for this we need process evaluation.

Impact and outcome evaluation

Evaluation of health promotion programmes is usually concerned to identify their effects. The effects of an intervention may be evaluated according to its:

- *Impact* – the immediate effects or outputs such as increased knowledge or shifts in attitude
- *Outcome* – the longer-term effects such as changes in lifestyle.

The timing of an evaluation will affect what data can be collected and how confident we can be that the effects are due to the intervention. This is illustrated in the following example.

 Box 20.10

When to evaluate: impact and outcomes of a CHD prevention programme

A CHD prevention programme may have the following five effects:

1. Improves people's knowledge of the risk factors for CHD
2. Increases people's motivation and intention to take up CHD risk factor screening opportunities
3. Persuades more people to attend screening clinics
4. Increases media coverage of CHD
5. Reduces premature mortality rate from CHD.

An immediate postprogramme evaluation may identify the first and second effects, or the impact of the intervention. The third and fourth effects may only be apparent at a later evaluation, e.g. after 6 months, and are called outcomes. Twelve months after the programme, the increased attendance at screening clinics may no longer be discernible and attendance figures may have reverted to preprogramme levels. A reduction in the mortality rate may not be discernible for 5 years or more, by which time it will be difficult to attribute it to the health promotion programme. The assessment of the overall success or failure of a programme is therefore influenced by the timing of the evaluation.

Impact evaluation tends to be the most popular choice, as it is the easier to do. Impact evaluation can be built into a programme as the end stage. For example, a health promotion programme for secondary schools may include as the last session a review of the programme. Students may be invited to identify how they have changed since the programme began and how they think the programme will affect their future behaviour. Outcome evaluation is more difficult, because it involves an assessment of longer-term effects. Using the same example given above, outcome evaluation may be used to determine whether the programme did affect students' behaviour 1 year later. One way of ascertaining this would be to compare participants' health-related behaviour (e.g. smoking, alcohol and exercise) before and after the programme, but there are bound to be changes in students' behaviour over 1 year irrespective of any health promotion programme. So it would be better to compare the students to another group of similar students who did not receive the programme, to see if the same changes occur in both groups. The second or control group of students is necessary to avoid the danger of attributing all behaviour change to the health promotion programme and therefore of overestimating its influence.

Outcome evaluation is therefore more complex and costly than impact evaluation. Going back a year later to the same students and getting new information from them will take up time and resources, as will obtaining a matched group of students to use as the control group. However, despite these problems, outcome evaluation is often the preferred evaluation method because it measures sustained changes over time. Results using data on impact or outcome are often expressed numerically, and this again increases credibility. Quantitative or 'hard' data are seen as more concrete or factual than the 'soft' data used in process evaluation.

How to evaluate: the process of evaluation

In order to evaluate, decisions need to be taken about what information is needed and how it will be gathered. This needs to be done at the outset of an intervention, in order to ensure that relevant data are gathered at the appropriate time. Rootman et al (2001) propose an eight-stage framework for the evaluation of health promotion interventions:

1. Describe the programme, clarify aims and objectives.

2. Identify issues and questions of concern to all stakeholders.

3. Design the information-gathering process.

4. Collect the data.

5. Analyse the data.

6. Make recommendations.

7. Disseminate findings.

8. Take action.

Many commentators have argued that the evaluation process should adhere to health-promoting principles (Thorogood & Coombes 2004; Morgan 2006). Evaluation should involve the participation of all stakeholders and be an empowering experience. The evaluation of community health promotion interventions is particularly challenging as these are complex, context-specific programmes focusing on socioeconomic and environmental determinants of well-being.

Evaluation therefore involves several key aspects that need to be considered. These key aspects may be summarized as: what to measure? who evaluates? how to evaluate, including how to gather and analyse data? and what to do with the results? or putting the findings into practice. Each of these key aspects will now be considered.

What to measure?

Deciding what to measure to assess the effects of health promotion is not easy. In theoretical terms, the many meanings and definitions of the concept of health result in a lack of consensus about how best to evaluate it. For those who subscribe to the medical model of health, data concerning morbidity, disability and mortality are appropriate measures to use for evaluation purposes. For those who adopt a more social model of health, a much broader range of measures (including, for example, measures of socioeconomic status or the quality of the environment) will be appropriate. For people who prioritize the educational model, measures of knowledge and attitude change will be paramount.

The golden rule must be to measure the objectives set during the planning process. (For more details on programme objectives, see Chapter 19.) Although this sounds straightforward, in practice it can be difficult, and a surprising number of evaluation studies violate this principle. Different stakeholders might have different objectives and the evaluation needs to take this into account. The objectives set may concern areas where there is a lack of consensus over appropriate measurement. For example, process objectives such as increased multiagency collaboration or increased community involvement are difficult to measure. To collect relevant data would require a special effort because they are not measured routinely. Change in people's attitudes or beliefs is particularly problematic to measure.

The success of a health promotion intervention is not solely about achieving behavioural changes or reductions in disease rates. For example, a needle exchange scheme should not be judged solely by a reduction in the rate of human immunodeficiency virus (HIV) infection among drug users. Other markers of success, such as the take-up rate, are also important. In many cases, expecting a clear change in morbidity from a behaviour change would be unrealistic. Although there is a link between needle-sharing and HIV infection, there are other risk factors, and expecting a preventive outcome from this initiative might be unwise.

A programme may have several different objectives, some of which are easier to measure than others. It then becomes tempting to measure the easiest objectives and extrapolate from these findings. But if the measurements are of different classes of events (e.g. combining behavioural, environmental and attitudinal objectives), it is not legitimate to do this.

Box 20.11

A programme has been launched with the objective of reducing child accidents.
Key stakeholders include community and hospital-based health practitioners, community groups (parents' and neighbourhood groups) and local authority staff, including environmental health officers and health and safety officers.
The following indicators have been suggested as suitable means of evaluating the programme. For each indicator discuss:
- Is it appropriate?
- Is it feasible?
- Who do you think suggested it?

1. Take-up of campaign literature
2. Campaign awareness
3. Sales of child safety equipment
4. Making changes to the home environment to improve safety e.g. installing stair gates
5. Making changes to the local environment, e.g. traffic-calming measures
6. Establishment of local child accident prevention working groups
7. Reduction in the number of accidents to children
8. Reduction in the number of severe accidents to children that require hospitalization.

Who evaluates?

Success means different things to different groups of people, or stakeholders, who each have their own agendas and interests. Different stakeholders have unequal power to impose their evaluation agendas on others. Different groups of people engaged in health promotion interventions will each have invested something but may well be looking for different results. For example, funders of a project may be looking for efficiency or results which can be interpreted as cost-effective. Practitioners may be looking for evidence that their way of working is acceptable to clients and achieves the objectives set. Managers may be looking for evidence of increased productivity, measured by performance indicators. Clients may be looking for opportunities to take control over some health-related aspects of their lives.

It is therefore important to be clear at the outset about whose perspectives are being addressed in any evaluation. A starting point is simply to acknowledge that different vested interests are involved and try to identify them. The ideal is then to go on to represent the views of the different stakeholders by collecting data from each group. This process is called pluralistic evaluation (Smith & Cantley 1985). Using the process of methodological triangulation, which employs a wide range of data sources, an overall picture may be built up. Pluralistic evaluation which takes into account different stakeholders' views is more complete, although the findings may be complex and lack clarity. Pluralistic evaluation is a means of building capacity and empowering clients and service users as well as practitioners.

In practice, pluralistic evaluation may appear too complex and costly, and evaluation is often carried out by external researchers or by practitioners. The former tend to be larger-scale and more ambitious in their remit. There are advantages and drawbacks to each of these options, as Box 20.12 demonstrates.

 Box 20.12

A dental health project has been launched, and needs to be evaluated. There are two choices: either an in-house evaluation conducted by the people involved in running the project, or an external evaluation conducted by outside researchers. These are some of the pros and cons of each option. Can you identify any others?

	Insider evaluation	Outside evaluation
Pros	Knows background to project Cheaper Acceptable to everyone	Unbiased attitude Research expertise Fresh perspective
Cons	Too involved in project No research expertise Biased to prove success	Expensive May appear threatening Unfamiliar with project

How to evaluate: gathering and analysing data

The process of evaluation involves making decisions about what methods to use to gather and analyse relevant data. Each of these stages is next discussed separately.

Gathering data

Practical difficulties arise when trying to obtain data and trying to combine different forms of data to provide an overall picture. Some relevant data are already available and accessible, for example morbidity and mortality data. Other data already exist and may be obtained, for example policy documents or health surveillance data. However, some data will need to be specially collected and, particularly in areas such as attitude change or empowerment, there are no easy or accepted means of doing this.

A wide range of data, both qualitative and quantitative, may be used in evaluation studies. Guiding principles to use when selecting methods of data collection are to use appropriate and feasible tools. Appropriate means gathering data that will help meet the objectives of the evaluation. Feasible means gathering data within budgetary and time constraints. Process evaluation often concentrates on qualitative data whereas outcome evaluation is more likely to use quantitative data. However both forms of data may be applicable in various ways at different times.

The medical model of research dominant within health care settings prioritizes the RCT as the most rigorous form of quantitative methodology. However RCTs may be inappropriate for evaluating health promotion interventions, where the context is an important and acknowledged element. RCTs may also be misleading and unnecessarily expensive (Morgan 2006). The call for evaluation to be a health-promoting process in itself also mitigates against the use of specialist quantitative methodologies such as RCTs. For participation in an evaluation to be empowering, stakeholders need to be able to understand, contribute and oversee the process.

Evaluation seeks to assess process and effect, and it is therefore vital to have baseline data to use for comparison purposes. Unless baseline data are collected, it will be impossible to state that impacts or outcomes are due to the intervention. Planning needs to take account of this and allocate sufficient resources to allow for the collection of pre- and postintervention data.

Analysing the data

There are various ways of analysing data, depending on whether the data are quantitative or qualitative, what kind of intervention or study was carried out, and what resources and expertise are available. There are many excellent textbooks that discuss data analysis in depth (e.g. Bowling 2002) and the reader is referred to these for a more detailed discussion of methods. However data analysis is not just a question of methodological awareness and expertise. Values also have an impact on data analysis processes. The assumption is that, faced with a certain set of findings, everyone would agree on their significance or meaning, but this is not necessarily the case. There may also be dispute about which findings are relevant or significant. Data analysis should be an inclusive and capacity-building exercise for all participants, enabling everyone to have a say about what data are significant and why.

Evaluating complex interventions

Many health promotion interventions are deliberately complex, involving multiple stakeholders and many different programme components. Interventions may also be context-specific, i.e. take account of, and try to use, specific features of the context. Community programmes such as Health Action Zones and Sure Start are examples of complex interventions. The goals may include not just direct effects, but triggering changes that will impact on the context and magnify the effects.

The use of scientific methods of evaluation, such as experimental trials, to evaluate such interventions is therefore inappropriate. Instead of screening out all factors apart from the intervention, evaluation of complex interventions seeks to unpack and examine the trigger effects of the intervention. Pawson & Tilley (1997) describe this process as looking inside the black box to explore what is happening at the inputs–outcomes interface. Outcome and process evaluation need to take place together. Pawson & Tilley's (1997) realist approach to evaluation provides a means of doing this, and may be summarized as:

context + mechanisms → outcomes

Realist evaluation seeks to understand how causal mechanisms work within specific contexts – what works for whom and under what circumstances. Once the whole picture is understood, the results may be appropriately transferred to other situations.

The Theory of Change approach has developed as a response to the challenge of evaluating complex community initiatives (Fulbright-Anderson et al 1998). This approach seeks to make explicit stakeholders' assumptions about cause and effect, and how ministeps build and combine to create long-term outcomes. There are five stages in the Theory of Change approach to evaluation:

1. Identify long-term goals and assumptions behind them.

2. Backwards mapping to reveal the necessary preconditions to achieve goals.

3. Identify the initiative's interventions that will lead to the desired changes.

4. Develop outcome measurement indicators in order to assess the initiative.

5. Write a narrative to explain the logic of the initiative.

A good theory of change is plausible, do-able and testable (Connell & Kubisch 1998).

Box 20.13

You have been asked to evaluate a community initiative aimed at reducing nuisance behaviour and crime (youths hanging around in public areas, noisy and inconsiderate behaviour, muggings and street robberies). How could you use the Theory of Change model to plan your evaluation?

Green & South (2006, p. 84) identify six elements of good practice in the evaluation of community health projects:

1. Building evaluation into the project

2. Maximizing stakeholder involvement

3. Measuring changes in individual and community health

4. Using appropriate evaluation methods

5. Examining processes

6. Learning in practice.

Box 20.14

How would you evaluate the community project described below, using Green & South's six criteria for good practice?

Community health project

A community health project is launched in a deprived inner-city area. The project has two dedicated community health workers and its aims are to increase participation, reduce health inequalities, work collaboratively with existing agencies and achieve sustainable results. The project workers link up with existing groups, e.g. church groups and parents' groups, and set up four new groups focusing on carers, older people, unemployed people and young people. Activities include the establishment of a community garden, setting up a buddying system for vulnerable people in the community and a weekly drop-in support group for carers. The project workers also establish links with local statutory services, e.g. schools, general practices and social services. Two years on, you are invited to contribute to the project's evaluation.

What to do with the evaluation: putting the findings into practice

Dissemination of findings is important in order to publicise good practice and also to flag up interventions that were not as successful as had been anticipated. Knowing what doesn't work is as valuable as knowing what does work, but there is a great emphasis on producing and publicising positive results. As Hawe et al (1994) state:

> Sometimes to avoid 'failure', health promoters may avoid evaluation ... At any one time many of the current initiatives may turn out to be those that fail to produce intended results. There is no shame in this ... Stigma should not be attached to programmes that fail, only to

> those programmes that fail to learn from these experiences or to those programmes that fail to evaluate.

Putting findings into practice can take many forms. The results of evaluation should ideally feed into an ongoing cycle of action and reflection, allowing more knowledgeable and reasoned interventions to take place. Evaluation may also enable stakeholders to progress activities and gain more support to do so. Evaluation helps to establish the cost-effectiveness of health promotion and contributes towards its evidence base.

Cost-effectiveness

Part of the reason for evaluation is to determine whether desired results were achieved in the most economical way and whether allocating resources to health promotion can be justified. There are many different ways of calculating the economic pluses and minuses of health promotion. Cost–benefit analysis is a way of calculating whether, and to what extent, something is worth doing. Cost–benefit analysis relies on pricing both the inputs and the benefits of a health promotion programme. An attempt is then made to calculate the cost of each benefit. This is known as a cost–benefit ratio. Putting a price on health outcomes or benefits is a very difficult exercise. One approach to this problem is to compare the cost–benefit ratio for a health promotion intervention with the cost–benefit ratio for some other health intervention. It is often assumed that prevention is cheaper than cure and that health promotion saves money, but this is not necessarily the case.

Box 20.15

An effective smoking prevention campaign is associated with the following costs. Money is saved by:
- Not having to treat people with smoking-related diseases on the NHS

- Not having to pay sickness benefit and disability pensions to people with smoking-related diseases
- Increased production in industry because fewer employees are off sick.

Money is lost by:
- Retirement pensions paid to people who live longer
- Unemployment benefits to people in tobacco production and retail industry made unemployed due to fall in demand
- Loss of government revenue from tobacco taxation.

Overall, do you think this campaign is cost-effective?

Once a decision has been made to implement an intervention, economic analysis can help to determine the most efficient way of resourcing it. Efficiency refers to the maximum benefit that can be derived from the least cost. Cost-effectiveness is a comparison in monetary terms of different methods used to achieve the same outcomes. 'Cost-effectiveness analysis addresses *technical* efficiency in the sense that it can tell us the best way to do something but not whether or not that something is worth doing' (author's italics; Cohen 2008, p. 337). Opportunity costs refer to what is sacrificed or forgone when resources are allocated to something, e.g. a health promotion project.

Economic appraisal is an important element in evaluation because there are always competing claims for limited resources. Using economics to make health-related decisions might seem a distasteful idea and people may shy away from attempts to put a value on people's health, well-being or life. But the reality is that people, societies and governments are constantly making choices and decisions that are influenced by economic considerations. It is therefore important to make the decision-making process transparent and include economic principles and concepts in evaluation studies.

Using evaluation to build an evidence base for health promotion

Evaluation helps build a basis of research to demonstrate which health promotion interventions succeed in meeting objectives. Evaluation therefore identifies effective health promotion practice which others can adopt. Evidence-based practice is firmly established in medicine and nursing, where RCTs of alternative treatment protocols are used to establish which form of treatment is most effective for most people. In health promotion, creating evidence-based practice is more problematic.

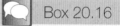 Box 20.16

Why might it be difficult to establish evidence-based health promotion practice?

There are several reasons why proving an evidence base exists for health promotion is problematic. These include knowing when to evaluate, knowing what constitutes success, being able to attribute results to interventions and the inappropriateness of using RCTs.

Knowing when to evaluate is a challenge, and the timing of an evaluation can affect its results. If an evaluation is seeking to determine the outcomes of an intervention, a longer timescale is desirable. However this has problems. Health promotion is a long-term process and contexts and settings are constantly changing, so it can be difficult to be sure that any changes detected are due to the health promotion input, and not to any other factor. Health-related knowledge, attitudes and behaviour are constantly changing, regardless of health promotion programmes. Societies and environments are also changing in response to many different factors. One response to this problem might be to evaluate sooner and use a shorter timescale. However to do so might mean that longer-term sustained outcomes are missed. The best solution is to evaluate over different time periods, but this requires more resources.

Knowing the threshold for success is another challenge, and is illustrated in Example 20.17. A balance needs to be struck between setting the threshold too high, leading to interventions that are unjustly deemed to be ineffective, and setting the threshold too low, leading to a judgement that health promotion is not worth the effort. Striking the correct balance involves knowing what changes are likely to take place in the absence of the intervention, and then setting a realistic goal of what additional change is feasible and represents an efficient use of resources.

Box 20.17

What constitutes evidence of success?

A smoking cessation programme is launched which includes clinics for those wishing to give up smoking. A clinic run by a health promoter attracts 20 clients who attend all six sessions. At a 6-month evaluation, 25% of the participants have stopped smoking.

- Is this a success?

The health promoter may be pleased with these results. People attend clinics often as a last resort, and 6 months is a reasonable time period to assess long-term behaviour change. However, the health promoter's manager may point out that 20% is an average success rate for people trying to quit, regardless of what methods are used. Clinics are time-consuming and 20 people is not a large group. The result, 25% quitters, is five people, four of whom might have quit using other less intensive or expensive methods. So one additional ex-smoker might be the result of the smoking cessation clinic.

The third problem is being able to attribute any changes that occur to the health promotion input. The many different individual, organizational, social,

economic and environmental factors affecting health are in a constant state of flux and it is very difficult to pin any changes down to specific causes. A health promotion intervention may trigger a variety of changes, some immediate, some intermediate, and some longer-term. It is challenging to record and capture changes happening at different times.

The most solid evidence that is used to prove cause and effect is derived from quantitative methodologies such as RCTs. However there are several reasons why the RCT is often inappropriate for health promotion interventions, and this is the fourth problem. Many interventions are complex and multicomponent and are designed to trigger effects and spread into other contexts and groups. So attempts to isolate the intervention are at odds with health promotion principles and practice.

There are also ethical problems with adopting the RCT model of evidence. When and how does the practitioner or agency decide there is sufficient proof to roll out a programme? Is it ethical to deny what is very likely to be an effective intervention in order to obtain more scientific evidence of its efficacy? These methodological and ethical problems mean the RCT is often inappropriate for health promotion interventions.

Although the RCT is often inappropriate, this does not mean that there is no evidence on which to base health promotion work. Meta-analyses or systematic reviews of research studies pool together findings from different studies in effectiveness reviews. Effectiveness reviews are a means of building up a knowledge base which can tell us what are reasonable expectations of success in health promotion. Success in health promotion is complicated because the aim is not just to change knowledge or behaviour, but to change the social determinants of health, and this requires qualitative as well as quantitative evaluation.

There is now an independent national body, the National Institute for Health and Clinical Excellence (NICE), devoted to providing evidence-based guidance on the promotion of good health and the prevention and treatment of ill health. NICE publications include guides on providing environments to encourage physical activity (NICE 2008a) and smoking cessation (NICE 2008b). In conclusion, the evidence base for health promotion is developing and includes a variety of approaches and methodologies. Syntheses of evaluations are being produced, enabling practitioners to start to practise evidence-based health promotion.

Conclusion

Evaluation contributes to the accountability and development of evidence-based health promotion practice, and so is an important aspect of the health promoter's work. This involves evaluating health promotion activity with which you are involved. There are often pressures to adopt unrealistic measures of success, such as reduced mortality rates or demonstrable cost benefits. Most health promoters are engaged in more modest activities which seek to achieve changes in knowledge, behaviour, attitudes, service take-up or the policy process. These are more appropriate outcomes to use for evaluation purposes.

Evaluation is a practical activity which feeds into the theoretical debate about the nature and purpose of health promotion. This debate cannot be confined to professionals, or those who hold managerial or financial power. It must include the public, those who are the targets of health promotion activity. This is why pluralistic evaluation, which enables participants to have a voice in determining effectiveness, is so important.

Evaluation is not a simple activity and it consumes resources which might otherwise be spent on doing health promotion. The decision about whether, when and how to evaluate is therefore important. The question of evaluation should be considered at the outset of any planned health promotion intervention. If it is to be done, it should be done in the best possible way. If this is not feasible, then it is better to admit the impossible, and not attempt to evaluate. Ongoing monitoring may be the best one can do. This is acceptable, but there is a distinction between routine monitoring of activities through the

use of performance indicators and a more thorough-going evaluation. It is important not to confuse the two and to be clear about which it is you are doing.

Box 20.18

Guidelines for good practice in evaluation
Which of the following suggested guidelines for good practice in evaluation do you think should be included in a checklist of criteria to be met if undertaking evaluation?
Are there any other guidelines you would wish to add?
- Evaluate early on before vested interests have had time to solidify.
- Evaluate only if it will make a difference.
- Evaluate only when it is appropriate.
- Evaluate only when you can include the perceptions of different groups, e.g. only when you can do a pluralistic evaluation.
- Publicise the results of evaluation widely in relevant formats.
- Evaluate only when there is a chance of scientific accuracy.
- If you cannot meet these criteria, do not evaluate.

Questions for further discussion

- What factors would influence your decision about whether to evaluate a particular health promotion activity?

- What factors would you wish to consider when evaluating a health promotion intervention?

Summary

This chapter has looked at how evaluation is defined, the different kinds of research methodologies used in evaluation research, and why health promotion needs to be evaluated. Different kinds of evaluation have been identified, including process, impact, outcome and whole-systems evaluation. The process of evaluation, including principles and stages, has been outlined. The importance of demonstrating the cost-effectiveness of health promotion and the role of evaluation in building an evidence base for health promotion have been discussed.

Further reading

Douglas J, Sidell M, Lloyd C et al 2007 Evaluating public health interventions. In: Earle S, Lloyd CE, Sidell M (eds) Theory and research in promoting public health. Sage Open University, London, pp. 327–354. *A succinct chapter that includes a detailed discussion of how the evaluation criteria can be applied to public health and health promotion interventions.*

Green J, South J 2006 Evaluation. Open University Press, Maidenhead. *A very readable account of the theoretical underpinnings of evaluation and the practicalities of doing evaluation. The real-life challenges and complexities of evaluation are discussed in depth.*

Rootman I, Goodstadt M, Hyndman B et al (eds) 2001 Evaluation in health promotion: principles and perspectives. Denmark, WHO. *A very thorough and comprehensive account of the theoretical and methodological issues relating to the evaluation of health promotion interventions.*

National Institute for Health and Clinical Excellence (NICE) produces guidance documents and effectiveness reviews on a variety of topics, including public health and health promotion issues such as obesity and nutrition, exercise and smoking cessation. Their website is www.nice.org.uk.

References

Bowling A 2002 Research methods in health: investigating health and health services, 2nd edn. Open University, Maidenhead.

Cohen D 2008 Health economics. In: Naidoo J, Wills J (eds) Health studies: an introduction, 2nd edn. Palgrave Macmillan, Basingstoke. Chapter 10.

Connell J P, Kubisch A C 1998 Applying a theory of change approach to the evaluation of comprehensive community initiatives: progress, prospects and problems. In: Fulbright-Anderson K, Kubisch A C, Connell J P (eds) New approaches to evaluating community initiatives, vol. 2: theory, measurement and analysis. Aspen Institute, Washington DC.

Douglas J, Sidell M, Lloyd C et al et al 2007 Evaluating public health interventions. In: Earle S, Lloyd C E, Sidell M (eds) Theory and research in promoting public health. Sage, Open University, London. Chapter 11.

Fulbright-Anderson K, Kubisch A C, Connell J P (eds) 1998 New approaches to evaluating community initiatives, vol. 2: theory, measurement and analysis. Aspen Institute, Washington DC.

Green J, South J 2006 Evaluation. Open University Press, Maidenhead.

Hawe P, Degeling D, Hall J 1994 Evaluating health promotion: a health worker's guide. Maclennan and Petty, Sydney.

Morgan A 2006 Evaluation of health promotion. In: Davies M, Macdowall W (eds) Health promotion theory. Open University Press, Maidenhead, pp. 169–187.

Naidoo J, Wills J 2005 Public health and health promotion: developing practice, 2nd edn. Baillière Tindall, London.

National Institute for Health and Clinical Excellence 2008a Promoting and creating built or natural environments that encourage and support physical activity. NICE, London.

National Institute for Health and Clinical Excellence 2008b Smoking cessation services in primary care, pharmacies, local authorities and workplaces, particularly for manual working groups, pregnant women and hard to reach communities. NICE, London.

Nutbeam D 1998 Evaluating health promotion – progress, problems and solutions. Health Promotion International 13: 27–44.

O'Connor-Fleming M L, Parker E 2001 Health promotion principles and practice in the Australian context, 2nd edn. Allen and Unwin, Sydney, Australia.

Parry-Langdon N, Bloor M, Audrey S et al 2003 Process evaluation of health promotion interventions. Policy and Politics 31: 207–216.

Pawson R, Tilley N 1997 Realistic evaluation. Sage, London.

Rootman I, Goodstadt M, Hyndman B (eds) et al. 2001 Evaluation in health promotion: principles and perspectives. WHO, Denmark.

Smith G, Cantley C 1985 Assessing health care: a study in organisational evaluation. Open University Press, Milton Keynes.

Springett J 2001 Appropriate approaches to the evaluation of health promotion. Critical Public Health 11: 139–152.

Thorogood M, Coombes Y 2004 Evaluating health promotion: practice and methods, 2nd edn. Oxford University Press, Oxford.

Advocacy the combined efforts of individuals and groups to gain political, social or organizational support for a specific health programme or goal

Behaviour change the purposeful changes in behaviour and activity that individuals make in order to promote, maintain and protect their health

Capacity building developing sustainable skills, structures, resources and policies to embed and multiply health gains

Collaboration working together towards agreed goals. Collaboration usually refers to different agencies working together to achieve a synergistic effect (intersectoral collaboration)

Communication the use of media, mass media, multimedia and new technologies to raise awareness and convey information and messages about health issues

Community a group of people, often living in the same geographical area, with a shared culture, values and norms. Community members share social networks and derive part of their identity from their community membership. In modern society people may belong to several different communities focused around different aspects of life, e.g. workplace, neighbourhood, religious, leisure interests

Community development action taken to develop community infrastructures and capacity to articulate and meet needs

Determinants of health those factors that have an impact on health status, including personal, social, economic and environmental factors

Disease an objective malfunctioning of some part of the body, detectable through medical testing and monitoring

Disease prevention measures taken to prevent disease or slow its progress, e.g. reducing known risk factors, screening or presymptomatic intervention

Empowerment the process of gaining greater control over the decisions and actions that affect one's health. This involves developing skills and confidence, articulating needs and strategies, and taking action to meet needs

Enablement taking action through partnerships to mobilize resources for health

Equity fairness and the distribution of resources for health on the basis of needs

Evidence-based practice practice based on the best available current, valid and relevant evidence. Evidence is derived from formal research and systematic investigation into the causes of health and ill health and the impact of interventions

Globalization the worldwide connections and networks of people and organizations that span national, geographic and cultural borders and boundaries

Health The World Health Organization (1948) defines health as 'complete physical, mental, spiritual and social well-being and not merely the absence of disease or infirmity'. Health is a resource for living and is a positive concept emphasizing social and personal resources as well as physical capabilities (World Health Organization 1986)

Health behaviour action purposefully taken by individuals in order to promote, protect or maintain their health

Health education the communication of health-related information and the development of the attitudes, skills and confidence necessary to enable people to take action to improve their health

Health impact assessment (HIA) a systematic process designed to assess the impact of an intervention or policy on the health of a defined population

Health literacy the cognitive ability, personal skills and motivation to access, understand and use health information to promote health

Health needs assessment (HNA) an assessment of a population to determine if and how their health can be improved

Health promotion a broader concept than health education, encompassing not just individual action but also social, political and environmental action to change the determinants of health and thereby improve health. Health promotion is the process of enabling people to increase their control over, and improve, their health (World Health Organization 1986)

Health protection social, organizational, fiscal or legal measures taken to prevent disease and protect the health of individuals and communities. May refer to actions to control communicable diseases

Developing healthy public policy policy that is explicitly concerned to promote health and equity and is accountable for its health impact. Healthy public policy is often focused on providing supportive environments that enable people to lead healthy lives

Illness the subjective state of being unwell and unable to function normally. Illness may or may not coexist with disease

Inequalities   variations that are not fair or just. Health inequalities are variations in health status due to socio-economic factors such as income

Life skills   the personal cognitive, social and physical skills that enable people to control and direct their lives

Lifestyles   the pattern of personal behaviours adopted by people. Lifestyles are the result of the interplay of individual, social, economic and environmental living conditions

Mediation   reconciling the conflicting interests of individuals, communities and sectors in a health-promoting manner

Medical model   a model of health based on scientific medicine, encompassing positivistic methodologies and an objective stance

Ottawa Charter   the first seminal World Health Organization conference on health promotion in 1986 produced the Ottawa Charter, which outlined core health-promoting areas for action (developing personal skills, strengthening communities, reorienting services, building healthy public policy and creating supportive environments) and strategies (enablement, mediation and advocacy) that are still widely cited and used today

Outcomes   changes in the health status of individuals, groups or societies that are attributable to planned health promotion interventions, policies or services

Participation   the active involvement of people in interventions, research or evaluation. Participation enables people's views and opinions to be heard, valued and integrated into action, leading to feelings of ownership and commitment

Personal skills   individuals' knowledge, attitudes, skills and feelings of self-efficacy that enable them to take action

Public health   the organized efforts by society to protect and promote the health and well-being of populations and to prevent illness, injury and disability

Quality of life   the subjective assessment individuals make of their position in life, encompassing physical, social, psychological, spiritual, independence and environmental factors. Quality of life is affected by cultural, social and personal expectations. Quality of life overlaps with concepts of health

Risk behaviour   behaviour that is proven to be associated with an increased risk of ill health or disease

Risk factor   social, economic or biological status, behaviours or environments that are proven to be associated with an increased risk of ill health or disease

Settings   places where people conduct their everyday lives and where personal, organizational, social and environmental factors interact to affect health

Social capital   social support, trust and neighbourliness that results from social networking and community participation and contributes to health and well-being

Social justice   a concern with equality and democracy, encompassing measures taken to narrow the gap in income, wealth and power that exists between different groups in society

Social marketing   the use of commercial marketing techniques (e.g. advertising, media coverage) to achieve beneficial health-related behaviour changes

Social model   a model of health based in the social sciences, encompassing interpretivist methodologies, subjective meanings and socioeconomic factors

Stakeholder   any person or organization with a direct interest in an intervention. Stakeholders refers to both the people implementing an intervention and those receiving it

Sustainability   meeting the needs of the present generation in a way that does not compromise the ability of future generations to meet their needs. Sustainable health promotion actions are embedded in services and structures so that their positive effects continue beyond the life of the programme or intervention

Wellness   the optimal state of health of individuals and groups

Further reading

Smith B J, Tang K C, Nutbeam D 2006 WHO health promotion glossary: new terms. Health Promotion International 21: 340–345

The World Health Organization has produced a comprehensive and detailed glossary of health promotion terms that is regularly updated. See Nutbeam D 1998 Health promotion glossary. WHO, Geneva or visit www.who.int/hpr/NPH/docs/hp_glossary_en.pdf

The UK public health website also has a useful glossary: www.publichealthy.com/glossary.aspx#h and http://www.polity.co.uk/healthpromotion/student/glossary/

References

World Health Organization 1948 Constitution. WHO, Geneva

World Health Organization 1986 Ottawa charter for health promotion: an international conference on health promotion, November 17–21. WHO, Copenhagen

Index